KV-198-706

Matthew B. Werd · E. Leslie Knight
Editors

Athletic Footwear and
Orthoses in Sports Medicine

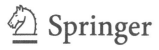 Springer

Editors
Matthew B. Werd
Foot and Ankle Associates
2939 S. Florida Ave.
Lakeland FL 33803
USA
dr.werd@floridafootandankle.com

E. Leslie Knight
ISC Division of Wellness
P.O.Box 8798
Lakeland FL 33806
USA
isc@gate.net

ISBN 978-0-387-76415-3   e-ISBN 978-0-387-76416-0
DOI 10.1007/978-0-387-76416-0
Springer New York Dordrecht Heidelberg London

Library of Congress Control Number: 2010922999

© Springer Science+Business Media, LLC 2010
All rights reserved. This work may not be translated or copied in whole or in part without the written permission of the publisher (Springer Science+Business Media, LLC, 233 Spring Street, New York, NY 10013, USA), except for brief excerpts in connection with reviews or scholarly analysis. Use in connection with any form of information storage and retrieval, electronic adaptation, computer software, or by similar or dissimilar methodology now known or hereafter developed is forbidden.
The use in this publication of trade names, trademarks, service marks, and similar terms, even if they are not identified as such, is not to be taken as an expression of opinion as to whether or not they are subject to proprietary rights.
While the advice and information in this book are believed to be true and accurate at the date of going to press, neither the authors nor the editors nor the publisher can accept any legal responsibility for any errors or omissions that may be made. The publisher makes no warranty, express or implied, with respect to the material contained herein.

Printed on acid-free paper

Springer is part of Springer Science+Business Media (www.springer.com)

Foreword

As the preface to this book tells us, its intent "is to provide a comprehensive resource on athletic footwear and orthoses for the entire sports medicine team, from all backgrounds and training." This goal is achieved. The book covers it all, from the complex science that underlies those underlayments found in the athletic shoes of many athletes, the orthosis, to the aim of, as the authors say at the beginning of Chapter 14, Prescribing Athletic Footwear and Orthoses, "maximizing athletic performance and minimizing injury through the use of an appropriate prescription for athletic footwear and orthoses." To the best of the editors' knowledge, this is the first book of its type. And the editors, Drs. Matthew Werd and Les Knight, have done an outstanding job in assembling a talented and knowledgeable group of authors for their effort.

Speaking as someone who owns a variety of athletic shoes, running, pace walking, cycling, and downhill skiing, and does not take a step in any of them without an orthosis between my foot and the shoe's insole, I was fascinated to discover how much there is to know and learn about this subject. For example, we learn in some detail the history of the development of the modern running shoe, which development goes back to the time of the ancient Greeks. There is a comprehensive review of the history and literature on the development of orthoses, a theoretical and practical science that continues to evolve. A whole chapter is devoted to the design and characteristics of the various types of athletic socks. Separate chapters detail virtually every type of specialty athletic footwear, from the running shoe to the snow sport boot (downhill and cross-country skiing and snowboarding).

This book will indeed be useful for all health professionals who deal with patients who are athletes of one kind or another. All sports other than swimming require a shoe of one kind or another. Many patients and clients who are athletes, or thinking simply of becoming regular exercisers, will have questions about shoes and about orthoses. Many who might benefit from the latter do not know about them or might think that one bought from a drugstore shelf will do the trick when indeed that is not the case. While for the podiatrist this book presents a good deal of technical information in one place, for the non-podiatric health care provider this book provides very helpful information on when and how to make appropriate referrals. Some chapters provide the detail required by the specialist, while others provide more general information useful to all potential readers.

Finally, this book does not have to be read through to be very helpful, and in fact most readers will likely not read it from cover to cover. Therefore, the repetition of essential information that does appear is very useful, for that repetition increases the chances that every reader will get to see it. Whether your patients are looking for basic comfort, improved performance, or injury avoidance/prevention in their footwear, this is the guidebook for you.

Steven Jonas, MD, MPH
Stony Brook, NY

Preface

The intent of this book is to provide a comprehensive resource on athletic footwear and orthoses for the entire sports medicine team from all backgrounds and training, including physicians (MD, DO, DPM, DC), athletic trainers (ATC), physical therapists (PT, DPT), researchers (MA, PhD), massage therapists (LMT), and all other professionals who are involved in sports medicine and the evaluation and treatment of the athlete.

We were approached to author this text as a result of the overwhelming interest stimulated on this topic through numerous lectures and workshops which have been presented at the American College of Sports Medicine regional and national meetings by the American Academy of Podiatric Sports Medicine.

This book should serve to educate professionals to make an informed decision on recommending and prescribing athletic footwear and orthoses, as well as to provide insight to appropriate referral to a specialist.

The approach to this text has been to include as much evidenced-based medicine as available, and contributors have referenced the most current studies and literature. The science and research is available which clearly documents the efficacy of functional foot orthoses in treatment of lower extremity biomechanical pathology. The use of proper athletic footwear and orthoses has been shown to optimize an athlete's performance, as well as to help limit the risk of certain injuries.

Questions such as "What is the best athletic shoe?" and "What is the best orthotic device for this condition?" and "Which athletic shoe or orthosis is most appropriate for that sport?" are frequently posed in a busy sports medicine practice; however, very little written information is available that addresses these important concerns. Although several excellent books are currently available regarding lower extremity biomechanics, *Athletic Footwear and Orthoses in Sports Medicine* offers a unique focus on athletic footwear and orthoses, as well as sport-specific recommendations.

The American Academy of Podiatric Sports Medicine is represented prominently throughout this text and has provided the majority of contributors through its members, fellows, and past-presidents. AAPSM's shoe review committee is comprised of practicing sports medicine podiatric physicians, and it maintains a current unbiased list of recommended athletic shoes based on a number of objective criteria, which is posted on the Academy's website, www.AAPSM.org. We hope that this book will be a valuable and practical resource on athletic footwear and orthoses in sports medicine for the entire sports medicine team.

Matthew B. Werd, DPM, FACSM
Lakeland, FL

E. Leslie Knight, PhD, FACSM
Lakeland, FL

Acknowledgments

Each contributing author has been selected for their recognized expertise and experience as leading educators and practitioners in the area of athletic footwear, orthoses, and lower extremity biomechanics. The time and effort given by each contributor in order to help educate the general sports medicine profession has been tremendous, and each contributor is to be commended. Special thanks also to Steven Jonas, MD, PhD, for his critical review of the manuscript and his comments in the Foreword.

A number of extremely talented individuals who share a passion for sports medicine have provided both inspiration and motivation in pursuing a career in sports medicine. Credit goes to my mentor and residency director at South Miami Hospital, Dr. Keith B. Kashuk, for his influence on my career and for his commitment as an educator, who is always challenging students, residents, and physicians to be their best.

The American Academy of Podiatric Sports Medicine's members, fellows, board members, and past-presidents should be commended for their enthusiasm and continued support of the Academy and its mission. Special thanks to Dr. James Losito, who provided me early guidance and opportunities within the Academy, as well as colleagues including Drs. Edward Fazekas, Marvin Odro, Timothy Dutra, Gerald Cosentino, Rich Bouche, and Douglas Richie, as well as AAPSM's Executive Director, Rita Yates, for being a steadying force and tremendous resource.

The American College of Sports Medicine provides an opportunity to interact and collaborate with sports professionals from diverse fields, all of whom share the same common passion for sports medicine. Several key individuals should be recognized for their guidance, friendship, and inclusion of podiatric sports medicine, including Drs. E. Leslie Knight, William Roberts, Robert Sallis, and Jeffery Ross.

The Prescription Foot Orthosis Laboratory Association (PFOLA) is a non-profit professional worldwide association dedicated to promoting and improving the efficacy of custom, prescription foot orthoses to the medical professions. PFOLA has been instrumental in the dissemination of on-going research on the effectiveness of functional foot orthoses; many of our book contributors are also leaders within PFOLA.

I am also grateful to my colleagues at Florida Southern College and the athletic training program and staff for including me as part of the outstanding sports medicine team, especially Sue Stanley-Green, ATC, Al Green, ATC, and Drs. Mick Lynch and Susan Ott.

I am grateful to my parents, wonderful wife Heather, and my children Madalyn, Matthew, and Melody. Their smiling faces provide inspiration each and every day and provide a constant reminder of the value and importance of balance in life.

A special thanks to the editorial staff at Springer for their persistence and guidance, including Margaret Burns, Portia Bridges, Kathy Cacace, Susan Westendorf, Lydia Shinoj (Project Manager, Integra) and especially Sadie Forrester, who was instrumental in identifying the need for this text and helping to lay the original framework.

Matthew B. Werd, DPM, FACSM
Lakeland, FL

Contents

Contributors

Richard T. Bouché Private Practice, The Sports Medicine Clinic, Seattle, WA, USA

Robert M. Conenello Private Practice, Orangetown Podiatry, Orangeburg, NY, USA

John F. Connors Private Practice, Little Silver, NJ, USA

David M. Davidson Department of Orthopedics, State University of New York, Buffalo; Department of Orthopedics, Kaleida Health System, Buffalo, NY, USA

Tim Dutra Student Health Services, California State University, Hayward, CA, USA

David Granger Private Practice, York, PA, USA

Kirk Herring Private Practice, Inland Northwest Family Foot Care, Spokane Valley, WA, USA

R. Neil Humble Department of Surgery, University of Calgary, Calgary, AB, Canada

Steven Jonas Department of Preventive Medicine, Stony Brook University, Stony Brook, NY, USA

Keith B. Kashuk Department of Orthpaedics and Rehabilitation, University of Miami School of Medicine, South Miami, FL, USA

Christy King Department of Podiatry, California School of Podiatric Medicine, Samuel Merritt University, Oakland, CA, USA

Kevin A. Kirby Department of Applied Biomechanics, California School of Podiatric Medicine, Oakland, CA; Precision Intricast Orthotic Laboratory, Payson, AZ, USA

Chatra Klaisri Department of Podiatry, California School of Podiatric Medicine, Samuel Merritt University, Oakland, CA, USA

E. Leslie Knight ISC Division of Wellness, Lakeland, FL, USA

Paul Langer University of Minnesota Medical School, Minneapolis, MN, USA

David Levine Private Practice, Frederick, MD, USA

James M. Losito School of Podiatric Medicine, Barry University, Miami Shores; Mercy Hospital, Miami, FL, USA

Patrick Nunan Fit Feet/Healthy Athletes/Special Oympics, Inc.; Podiatry Section, Jewish Hospital of Cincinnati, West Chester, OH, USA

Anthony Poggio Private practice, Alameda, CA, USA

Douglas H. Richie, Jr. Private Practice, Alamitos Seal Beach Podiatry, Seal Beach, CA, USA

Jeffrey A. Ross Department of Medicine, Baylor College of Medicine, Houston, TX, USA

Maxime Savard Department of Podiatry, South Miami Hospital, South Miami, FL, USA

Lisa M. Schoene Private Practice, Gurnee Podiatry & Sports Medicine, Park City, IL, USA

Paul R. Scherer Department of Applied Biomechanics, Samuel Merritt College of Podiatrics, San Francisco, CA, USA

Hilary Smith Dr. William M. Scholl College of Podiatric Medicine, Rosalind Franklin University of Medicine and Science, North Chicago, IL, USA

Tanisha Smith Department of Orthopedics, South Miami Hospital, South Miami, FL, USA

Steven I. Subotnick Department of Surgery, Eden Hospital, San Leandro Hospital, San Leandro, CA, USA

Mher Vartivarian Department of Podiatry, California School of Podiatric Medicine, Samuel Merritt University, Oakland, CA, USA

Shawn Walls Department of Surgery, The Jewish Hospital of Cincinnati, Cincinnati, OH, USA

Matthew B. Werd Past President, American Academy of Podiatric Sports Medicine; Chief of Podiatric Surgery, Lakeland Regional Medical Center; Team Podiatrist, Florida Southern College; Private Practice, Foot and Ankle Associates, Lakeland, FL, USA

Josh White SafeStep**, Milford, CT**; Department of Orthopedics, New York College of Podiatric Medicine, New York, NJ; Department of Applied Biomechanics, California School of Podiatric Medicine, Oakland, CA, USA

Bruce Williams Private Practice, Breakthrough Podiatry, Merrillville, IN 46410, USA

Part I
Fundamentals of Athletic Footwear and Orthoses

Chapter 1
Evolution of Athletic Footwear

Steven I. Subotnick, Christy King, Mher Vartivarian, and Chatra Klaisri

History of the Running Shoe

Shoes are vital to man's sole. It is no secret that feet manage the challenges of daily life with the help of shoes. Shoes can stabilize, allow for flexibility or rigidity, cushion, and, in some cases, even injure feet. With the evolution of fast-paced lifestyles, shoes have been scientifically engineered to provide the most comfort and to perform at the highest level for the individual who wears them, but shoes have not always been as systematically constructed.

The earliest footwear ever recorded was discovered by Luther Cressman inside Fort Rock Cave in Oregon and dated to the end of the last ice age, making it almost 10,000 years old [1]. The simple construction incorporated sagebrush bark knotted together, creating an outsole with ridges for traction, a covering for the forefoot, and straps to go around the heel. Although people did not devote much attention to detail when making shoes in the past, even early human beings realized that a basic piece of material covering their feet could afford them the opportunity to explore a larger part of their world.

Ancient History

As the Olympics gained much success in a remarkable empire, the society began to devote more attention to shoes. Most ancient Greek athletes barely wore any clothes let alone running shoes, but these dedicated competitors began to observe that champions from colder climates wore race sandals [2]. Thus, the Greeks gave up the initial notion that their rivals were cheating and realized that this type of foot covering actually increased traction. As the popularity of competitive events in ancient civilizations grew so did the advancement of running sandals.

S.I. Subotnick (✉)
Department of Surgery, Eden Hospital, San Leandro Hospital, 13690 East 14th St, Suite 220, San Leandro, CA 94578-2538, USA

M.B. Werd, E.L. Knight (eds.), *Athletic Footwear and Orthoses in Sports Medicine*, DOI 10.1007/978-0-387-76416-0_1, © Springer Science+Business Media, LLC 2010

The ancient Etruscans attached the sole of the sandal to the upper with metal tacks, while the Romans used tongs to wrap the shoe as close to the foot as possible to maximize traction [2]. The Romans ultimately excelled in shoemaking and created many styles from sandals to boots to moccasins. Personal commitment to athletic sovereignty and to the success of the empire drove the ancient Greeks and Romans to investigate ways to increase human performance through the use of manmade enhancements like shoes.

The Running Shoe Revolution

It wasn't until the 17th and 18th centuries in Britain that careful thought was once again given to sports and the running shoe. The first sports-specific shoe was not developed for running but for cricket [1]. The Spencer cricket shoe, a low-cut, leather construction with three spikes under the forefoot and one under the heel, was developed in 1861, and these spiked shoes became an essential part of competing. Then from 1864 to 1896 the sport of track flourished and runners began to compete with low-cut shoes made of kangaroo leather uppers, leather soles with six mounted spikes on the forefoot, and leather half-sole [1]. Once runners decided that the circular track was too confining, they took a step away from the track, began to run long distance races, and the running shoe took another leap forward.

Initially, marathon runners of the early Modern Olympic Games competed in heavy boots or shoes with leather uppers and soles, allowing for little plasticity. With the increasing popularity of the running events, the Spalding Company addressed the need for running shoes among the public and advertised a high cut, black leather shoe with a reinforced heel and a sole of gum rubber, but the outsole did not last long and further improvements needed to be made [1]. In the 1940s the famous marathon runners, Johnny Kelly and Jock Semple, were having serious problems with the crude manufacturing of their running shoes, so Richings, a retired English shoemaker, created a pair with a seamless toe box, laces on the side of the shoe, a separate heel, a low-cut rear part without a counter, and a repairable outsole [1]. The race of another sort was on as individuals from around the world joined in the shoemaking effort to see who could devise the better shoe.

Reebok Begins the Race

Joseph William Foster opened up a family-owned shoe business called J. W. Foster and Sons Limited in 1895 in Bolton, United Kingdom. This dedicated company made thin leather shoes constructed of rigid leather to be worn by Lord Burghley in the 1924 Olympics [2]. A notable advancement occurred when Foster's company began to stitch a leather strip around the top of the shoe [2]. However, in 1958 the grandsons of Foster, Jeffrey, and Joseph, left their grandfather's business and conceived Reebok. The company's name originated from a Dutch word that refers to a type of antelope or gazelle. In the 1980s Reebok explored the market of women's shoes by designing a flimsy but eye-catching shoe, and the aerobic era added to Reebok's faithful following [2]. The Reebok Freestyle was developed to be worn in or out of the gym. Later in the decade, Reebok created the Pump, consisting of an air bladder in the tongue of the shoe, to hold the ankle in a more fixed position.

The Amazing Dassler Brothers

In Germany Adolf Dassler began making shoes in 1920 and was later joined by his brother, Rudolph. Their popular shoe was worn by successful German athletes and even donned by Jesse Owens in at least one of his races at the 1936 Munich Olympics [1]. Despite their success, a bitter family feud in 1948 divided the brothers, their small community in West Germany, and the thriving shoe company. Adolf Dassler created Adidas while Rudolph formed Puma, and the two companies have been competing in the runner's world ever since. Adidas assumed the trefoil sign that represented Adolf's three sons [1]. He used arch support lacing which is an early form of speed lacing and the classic, three stripes to help support the foot in his shoes [1]. On the other side of town, Puma chose the leaping puma as its logo to convey speed and power.

Tiger Shoes and ASICS Join the Chase

Onitsuka Co. Ltd. started constructing shoes in 1949. At the 1951 Boston Marathon a young, Japanese runner by the name of Shigeki Tanaka won the coveted race and displayed the Tiger shoes as he crossed the finish line. This shoe was designed with the traditional, Japanese shoe, the Geta, in mind and had a separate compartment for the big toe. The shoe with the divided toe box could only be worn by Japanese athletes with a large space between the first and second digits [1]. Eventually, the shoe company known as Tiger became ASICS, which is a Latin acronym for "healthy mind in a healthy body."

New Balance and Intelligent Design

William J. Riley founded the Riley Company, the predecessor to New Balance, and began crafting shoes in the New England area in 1906. In 1961 the new owner of New Balance, Paul Kidd, took the experience he had gleaned from making orthopedic shoes, poured his knowledge into a running shoe, tested it scientifically, and invented the first modern running shoe, the New Balance Trackster [1]. Due to interest by runners, New Balance modified its Trackster by increasing the heel height, adding a continuous outsole, and placing a wedge of rubber under the back part of the heel. As the aerobic revolution began in 1968, New Balance extended its grasp on the sports shoe arena and Americans were encouraged to walk away from the couch and start exercising [1]. In response to the need for dual usage, New Balance introduced the Speed Star that was designed to be worn on and off the track.

The Modest Beginnings of the Nike Shoe Empire

University of Oregon track coach, Bill Bowerman, knew what he wanted in a running shoe, and he even created shoes for his track team members because his understanding of running form and shoe construction presented higher standards than those set by the current market. In 1964 Bowerman joined forces with one of his ex-athletes, Phil Knight, and began a small shoe company called Blue Ribbon Sports that made a line of shoes with the Tiger shoe company in Japan [3]. Bowerman and Knight were extremely busy, so through the extra efforts of Jeff Johnson, a former collegiate runner at Stanford, the Tiger Marathon and Roadrunner became the most popular running shoes on the market in 1967 [1]. The Tiger Marathon had a light rubber outsole with a separate heel and forepart, including a reverse leather upper. In 1967 they continued to modify the running world as they offered all nylon uppers. Johnson created the idea of a continuous midsole by removing the outsole of the Tiger shoe and replacing it with a shower slipper with an outer layer of rubber.

In 1972 Tiger and Blue Ribbon Sports separated over distribution disputes [1]. Fortunately, the American following of Bowerman and Knight's did not falter with the disintegration of this partnership. With the addition of a "swoosh" logo from one of Knight's students at Portland State College and the appropriate naming of Nike for the winged, Greek goddess of victory from Jeff Johnson's dream, this fresh company was able to continue production by establishing a deal with one of Tiger's competitors [1, 3]. Further changes in their shoes occurred as Bowerman and a colleague, Jeff Holister, used urethane and a waffle iron to construct extremely light running shoes [1]. Since its conception, the Nike Company has dominated the shoe world and continues to strive for perfection.

Breakthrough by Brooks

The Brooks Company began in 1914 by making ice skates and cleated shoes. During the running craze in the 1970s, the company flourished in the running shoe market. In 1974 Jerry Tuner called a chemical engineer who introduced the light, shock absorbing material of ethylene vinyl acetate, more commonly known as EVA, to anxious customers [1].

For decades running shoe companies have been dueling to make a better shoe and perhaps a bigger profit, but it wasn't until podiatrists and researches became involved that shoes were able to evolve once more to deliver maximum performance.

Key Contributors in Athletic Shoe Development

The athletic shoe market in America is a huge industry. Early on, shoes were an extremely basic item. With the emergence of competitive sports, shoes became more high-tech and added many more features. Podiatrists became involved in the designing of shoes in the 1970s. They provided ways to reduce injuries and enhance performance of athletes through modifications of shoes [4]. Here we will feature ten people who jump-started the evolution of the modern athletic shoe and their contributions to the field of shoe designing.

As mentioned, *Bill Bowerman* was most noted for as the track coach for the University of Oregon. Initially, he came to Oregon to study and play football. As he saw his first track meet, he decided he wanted to run [1]. After school, Bowerman coached football and basketball for a few years, but starting in 1949, he began a productive 24-year venture of coaching track and field. He coached many Olympians, All-Americans, and other world-class runners [5].

Making shoes for his runners was his main area of contribution. One of Bowerman's focuses was to reduce the weight of the shoe in order to allow the runner to use less energy and to reduce blisters [5]. He would do this by taking a standard last and shaving it down to fit a specific foot type. Through his intelligent coaching and expertise in custom shoe making, runners soon topped the list of the nation's best athletes. See the previous discussion (The Modest Beginnings of the Nike Shoe Empire) of Bowerman and Phil Knight's development of the company that would become Nike.

Now, Bill Bowerman is a member of the National Distance Running Hall of Fame, the USA Track and Field Hall of Fame, the Oregon Sports Hall of Fame and Oregon's Athletic Hall of Fame, but his contributions to shoe making has left the biggest mark in this world today [6].

As mentioned, *Phil Knight* was another prosperous product of Oregon. As a kid, he loved to run. He was part of Bill Bowerman's team at University of Oregon. He was not the best runner on the team, so he was one of the athletes to consistently test the shoes Bowerman designed [3].

After college, Knight enrolled at the Graduate School of Business at Stanford. Knowing that the more expensive German shoes were more comfortable than the cheap Japanese shoes, Knight wrote a paper for a class project on "Can Japanese Sports Shoes Do to German Sports Shoes What Japanese Cameras Did to German Cameras?". He designed a better, less expensive shoe than the Germans [3].

Knight then visited Japan and went to the Onitsuka shoe factory. He was astonished by how good the quality was and how inexpensive the shoes were. Knight made a deal with Onitsuka and began to distribute the Tigers in the United States. He partnered with his former coach, Bill Bowerman, who became the designer of the shoes for their business. Their company then split from Onitsuka in 1972. As Knight was thinking of a new name for the company, Jeff Johnson came up with the name Nike, after the winged goddess of victory. Johnson became the marketer of the business [3].

Phil Knight is now in the Oregon Sports Hall of Fame [7]. A simple graduate school project eventually led him to develop one of the biggest running shoe companies in the world known to produce quality shoes.

Steve Subotnick, DPM, DC, is a podiatrist who has been practicing in northern California since 1971. In addition to sports biomechanics and medicine, he also has a background in naturopathy, homeopathy, chiropractic, and foot and ankle surgery [8]. He is one of the founders and past presidents of the American Academy of Podiatric Sports Medicine and a past Fellow of the American College of Sports Medicine. Dr. Subotnick has written three paperback books and three medical text books on sports medicine.

In 1976, Subotnick gave the Brooks Shoe Company advice on an innovation to their running shoes. Dr. Subotnick strongly believed in the use of sport-specific biomechanics for shoe design, and he suggested the use of a varus wedge because of the functional varus inherent in running [4]. This design raised the inside of the heel compared to the outside by incorporating a 4° angle into the midsole. It is used to bring the subtalar joint into a neutral position during unidirectional running. With this innovation came the Brooks Vantage, which was a top-rated shoe at the time for 5 years. The varus wedge evolved into variable durometer midsoles with reinforced counters to help decrease excessive pronation [1].

Through his expertise in running shoes and sports biomechanics and kinesiology, Subotnick became an Olympic team podiatrist and an NBA team podiatrist for the Golden State Warriors.

Harry Hlavac, DPM, Ed.D, is a podiatrist who recently retired after practicing in California for over 35 years. He is one of the founders and past presidents of the American Academy of Podiatric Sports Medicine. He founded a foot-care company, developed the Hlavac Strap, and wrote a book on sports medicine advice for athletes [9].

In the 1980s, Hlavac worked with Nike on a modification for their shoes, which resulted in the use of the cobra pad in one of its popular shoes, the Equator [4].

Rob Roy McGregor, DPM, is a podiatrist who practiced in Massachusetts for over 50 years. He focused mainly on diabetic feet until he helped with the Boston Marathon. After this marathon, McGregor began to devote his practice mainly to runners [1].

In the 1970s, Dr. McGregor worked with Etonic shoes [4]. He designed a "one-piece heel and arch support." This became known as the Dynamic Heel Cradle. The Dynamic Heel Cradle is a compressible insert in the shoe that has a heel cup all around the rearfoot and gives support to the arch by thickening in the inside arch [1].

McGregor's design was one of the first items to hit the market that was designed by a podiatrist [1]. It would be safe to say he was one of the podiatrists to kick-start the evolution of the running shoe.

Lloyd Smith. DPM, is a podiatrist who has been practicing in Massachusetts for many years. He is a former president of the American Podiatric Medical Association. Smith has been working with runners and shoes for a long time. Dr. Smith, along with Drs. Dianne English and John McGillicuddy, obtained histories and diagnoses on almost a thousand runners. They also looked at whether the number of injuries changed within a decade [1].

Smith eventually worked with New Balance and also obtained a few patents of his own. One patent involved an external counter and cushion assembly for an athletic shoe. This is used to control pronation while still providing comfort through the increased cushioning and wedge in the midsole [10]. Another patent was an internal dynamic rocker element in casual or athletic shoes. This is a rocker element placed at the forefoot end of the midsole to provide comfort [11]. Dr. Smith continues to practice and devotes much of his practice to sports injuries and shoes [12].

Barry Bates, PhD, was the director of biomechanics at the University of Oregon for 25 years. The focus of his research was mainly on lower extremity function of runners [13]. In the mid-1970s, Bates, along with Drs. Stan James and Louis Osternig, gathered and presented data on injuries to runners. They wrote the epic paper on the biomechanics of running. This was the first time this type of data was presented based upon a physical examination of the runner [1].

Bates determined that shoes in extreme temperatures lose their stability. In the 1990s, Bates worked with Asics and invented a shoe comprising a liquid cushioning element [14]. He felt that shoes with this component were less affected by extremely hot temperatures [15]. This was known as the Asics gel.

Dr. Bates is very well known for his concept of running backward. He states that backward running helps with muscle balance and injury prevention among many other things. Bates also says that backward running has rehabilitation benefits. These include rehabilitation from Achilles' tendon injuries and ankle sprains [16].

Peter Cavanaugh, PhD, was an Associate Professor of Biomechanics at The Pennsylvania State University, whose main area of research is in locomotion and footwear studies. Cavanaugh is the author of *The Running Shoe Book* and *Physiology and Biomechanics of Cycling*, which is by far the best book written on the history and development of running shoes [1].

Cavanaugh worked with Puma and produced footwear having an adjustable width, foot form, and cushioning. This is done by varying the material of the midsole [17]. He performed a study showing that running shoes help relieve plantar pressure in diabetics. The basis of Cavanaugh's studies has been that shoes aid in shock absorption and stability. These contribute to motion control which prevents injury [18].

Benno Nigg, PhD, is the director of the human performance lab at the University of Calgary. Prior to Calgary he was in Zurich. He focuses his research on human locomotion, including mobility and longevity, as well as products related to movement, such as shoes and orthoses. Dr. Nigg has over 290 publications and has written/edited ten books [19].

Nigg states that shoes should be an "additional shell of skin around the foot, allowing the foot to do what it does naturally." As a result of a study he conducted on ski boots, he found ski boots are the opposite of running shoes since they "anchor the foot in a block." Running shoes allow for controlled motion, whereas ski boots stabilize the foot and ankle, allowing for only a forward bend at the ankle, while transferring pressure from the ankle and foot to the ski edges [20].

Throughout the hundreds of Nigg's studies and contributions, the one he is most known for is his work with Adidas. Adidas came to his lab and asked to create a soccer shoe for David Beckham. The result of this was the Adidas Predator Pulse. Dr. Gerald Cole describes, "Dr. Nigg is one of the pioneers of footwear biomechanics research" [21].

Howard Dannenberg, DPM, is a podiatrist who practiced in New Hampshire for many years. He made huge contributions to the world of high heels and running shoes. For high-heeled shoes, he developed the Insolia shoe insert to aid in the back pain and sagittal plane dysfunction of these patients [22].

Dannenberg is the inventor of the Kinetic Wedge, which provided comfort to running shoes. He introduced this product to the Brooks Shoe Company [4]. The Kinetic Wedge formed the foundation of the very successful Brooks shoes.

Early Research on Athletic Shoes

In the early 1970s, there was limited research and development being done in running and athletic shoes. Addidas was doing work with Benno Nigg, PhD, on various projects, and his lab also did research and development on ski boots. Phil Knight, in the early days, consulted with Hlavac and Subotnick. Personal experience recalls gluing Coach Bowerman's waffle outsoles, which he actually made in a waffle iron, to the bottom of running shoes using a glue gun, then going for long runs in the Hayward hills, only to have the outsoles fall off. Later Nike was to develop a sophisticated research and development center.

Shortly thereafter, Jerry Turner from Brooks consulted me to help develop an improved running shoe. Peter Cavanagh, PhD, did research for Puma. Various others did research and consulting with different shoe companies. At one time the Rockport had a podiatry advisory board.

The American Academy of Podiatric Sports Medicine (the Academy), under the guidance of Tom Sgarlato, DPM, Robert Barnes, DPM, and Dick Gilbert DPM, was formed in the early 1970s. The Academy, in conjunction with the college, had large, multidisciplinary sport medicine seminars and invited the directors of the major university biomechanics laboratories. Peter Cavanagh, PhD, Benno Nigg, PhD, and Barry Bates, PhD, were among the early participants. These "real scientists" took rather primitive research back to their respective labs and elevated the research to much higher levels.

Early work with other podiatrists such as John Pagliano, DPM, was based on the observation that runners running on a crowned road had supination of one foot with pronation of the other. The pronated foot resulted in a functional valgus at the knee with lateral mal tracking of the patella. Runners on level surfaces had a functional varus due to the narrow base of gait in runners. The pronated foot had one set of lower extremity problems while the supinated foot had others. By controlling foot function, with shoe design, foot orthoses, and training technique, the entire lower extremity from the toes to the low back could be affected.

High-speed motion pictures of runners with various types of shoe and orthotic modifications verified our early observations. Stress plate research and research with electromyography using telemetry were performed to observe the effect that foot function had on muscle fiber recruitment and muscle phasic activity. This early research supported the thought that a myriad of running-related problems could be prevented and treated by attempting to alter foot function. This was the early premises of sports podiatry and the biomechanics PhD's took this premises and proved its validity with sophisticated research that far exceeded early attempts. As an Academy, the first fledging members planted a seed that forever changed the development of athletic shoes and the diagnoses, prevention, and treatment of running injuries. The Academy also became involved in the prevention and treatment of various types of sports injuries ranging from skiing, soccer, football, basketball, hockey, baseball, tennis, to golf and virtually all sports, even bowling.

Sports podiatrists joined the medical teams for high school, college, and professional sports, and a few became members of the Olympic medical team and worked at the various Olympic training centers with the sports physiologists, orthopedists, trainers, and biomechanics researchers.

Now most major universities in the United States, Canada, and Europe have biomechanics departments with multiple research projects on-going; many of which are sponsored by various sports shoe companies. The entire field of sport biomechanics and kinesiology has grown and expanded over just a few decades.

Running Shoe Anatomy: Past and Present

Refer to Chapter 5 for a complete discussion of running shoe anatomy; the following discussion lists shoe anatomy and then compares and contrasts the evolution of current shoe materials.

It is important for both the athlete and the sports medicine practitioners to have a working knowledge of the anatomy and function of a running or athletic shoe. This understanding can both prevent injury and enhance recovery from injury or any shoe-related problem. An example is the athlete with a Haglund's disease, which is a retrocalcaneal exostosis and bursitis, or *pump-bump* aggravated by the counter of the shoe digging into the posterior heel and Achilles insertion. Simply removing the counter of the shoe, or changing shoe models or brands, can convert a very painful and disabling condition to a pain-free past memory in short order. In many cases, it's been the difference for Olympic athletes qualifying in the Olympic trials. It is no secret that's its easier to operate on a shoe and the results are consistently better than operating athletes prematurely.

Basic knowledge of the parts of a running shoe, the anatomy, can be as important as knowledge of functional anatomy when treating an athlete with a shoe-related problem. Being aware of the different options and varieties of material used may help determine the athletic shoe that will best fit not only its purpose but the athlete's feet. The running shoe is composed of two main parts: the upper and the bottom.

The upper covers the foot and the bottom provides a barrier between the foot and the environment, be it a trail, track, court, field, slope; whatever surface the foot contacts.

The Upper

The *vamp* is the portion of the shoe covering the forefoot. The remainder of the upper covering is referred to as inside and outside quarters. Featherline is where the upper meets the sole of the shoe. Traditionally, the vamp is constructed from one piece of material minimizing the number of seams and therefore irritation to the foot.

The *upper* has several intricate details as there are several attachments that need to be placed on it to complete the running shoe. The upper starts as one large piece, usually nylon. Leather, or synthetic leather-like materials, is added as reinforcement in needed areas. The *eyelet* forms the *throat* of the shoe acting as the anchor for lacing. The *tongue* is a padded piece that lies beneath the lacing to provide cushioning to the top of the foot against the pressure of the laces. The reinforcement sewn on the upper at the level of the arch is to help support the eyelet. *Reinforcement* on the outside is known as *saddle*. Reinforcement on the inside of the upper is known as the *arch bandage*.

Foxing is the suede covering at the back of the shoe. The *toe box* is the front of the upper that has leather overlay known as a *wing tip*. A leather tip that does not meet the throat and covers only the rim of the toes is referred to as a *mudguard tip* or *moccasin toe box*. To make the toe box sturdier a stiffener can be placed underneath the wing tip.

The padded vinyl or stretch nylon that covers the upper where there is contact of the foot just below the ankle to the shoe is called the *collar*. The *collar* has a projection that comes up above the heel to help protect the Achilles tendon from irritation. The *heel counter* is at the back of the shoe surrounding the heel of the foot. It has a pocket for a stiffener to help control the rearfoot during motion. Heel counters are firm and inflexible to prevent excessive motion during running. It helps to hold the foot in place [1]. It also can be a significant source of rubbing and irritation to the posterior heel or Achilles insertion.

Upper Materials: Past and Present

The upper is vital for fit and managing moisture, making the choice of materials important in the construction of the running shoe. Leather has several properties that make it resourceful in shoes. It can permanently change its form to fit the foot, store perspiration, transmit water vapor from the foot to the outer air, withstand tension, and resist abrasion. Yet, leather is not often used alone as the upper. Runners and other athletes have no limitations when it comes to weather. Rain or shine athletes will be outdoors working out or competing. Under unfavorable weather conditions such as rain, leather becomes plastic, stretching to a different length and not returning to its original size. Leather also takes longer to dry after exposure to water. It is now used as an accessory to reinforce the upper [1].

More recently, uppers are constructed from synthetic fabric with patches of synthetic leather for durability. Synthetic fabrics tend to cover the area from the laces and down the side of the shoe to the sole. This decreases the weight of the running shoe, making the shoe washable and breathable, so the feet don't become too hot. The synthetic materials are better at wicking and heat transfer. Nylon taffeta is a plain weave that is smooth on both sides. It is more resistant to permanent deformation and dries easily after exposure to water. However, shoes made from it do not allow the foot to breathe well because of its tight weave. Making the holes between the strands bigger with less taffeta threads compromises the integrity, causing it to lose its resistance to abrasion. Therefore, nylon mesh which is knitted instead of woven is more popularly used. Its strength doesn't depend on the tightness of the weave [1]. These newer "high-technology" materials have greatly improved the function, durability, and comfort of athletic shoes, and the same is true of athletic clothing and gear.

The Bottom

The bottom of the athletic shoe is made up of three main components: midsole, wedge, and outsole. The *midsole* lies between the upper and both the outsole and the wedge. Its purpose is for shock absorption, attenuation, and dampening. The cushioning effect is balanced with the stability function. This is an important and often crucial factor. The more cushioning, the less stability while the softer the midsole materials, the less stability. This makes the midsole one of the most important components of the running shoe. All too often a runner will purchase a new shoe based on that "soft, cushy feel" only to develop excessive pronation and associated injuries that are directly related to the shoe selection.

The *heel wedge* lies between the midsole and the outsole at the rear of the shoe. It helps with both heel impact and shock attenuation and provides a heel lift.

The *outsole* is the layer that contacts the ground. While it also contributes some to shock absorption, its main purpose is durability and traction. It is where the "rubber meets the ground." It can be the difference between life and death in activities such as rock climbing. It helps determine the amount of torsion rigidity and flexibility of a shoe. There is an *insole board* on top of the midsole that is found in most shoes.

The *sock liner* covers the insole board. Different materials for wicking and comfort are used to line the inside of the shoe [1].

Materials: Past and Present

The midsole no longer used leather soles because of the poor shock absorption it offered. Natural sheet rubber was included for a little while, but it was heavy and had a minor improvement in absorbing shock. Foam rubber with small bubbles of encapsulated air was lighter and a better shock absorber than sheet rubber. There is a chemical blowing agent that reacts with other chemicals in the mixture under right temperatures to produce gas. The small bubbles of air trapped within the material are known as closed cell foam and appears to be lighter and a better shock absorber than sheet rubber. Closed cell foams absorbed energy because the walls of the air cells deformed to absorb energy, and the small bubbles of air compressed to act as shock absorbers. There was then a movement to use foams from polymers. It reduced the weight and density by a factor of four and improved shock absorption [1].

Today, the most common midsole material now is a type of foam called ethylene vinyl acetate (EVA) [23]. It provides cushioning, increases shock absorption, and decreases shearing. Polyurethane (PU), another form of polymer, resists compression and is more durable than EVA, but is heavier and harder. Some midsoles are made with the combination of both EVA and PU. EVA is placed in the forefoot and PU in the rearfoot. The logic behind this change is that the heel takes on 2–3 times the body weight of a runner; therefore it needs material that is more resistant to compression and can absorb the impact of that force [1]. A dual density midsole is made from materials of two different densities. Multi-density midsoles contain more than two different densities [23]. The purpose of different densities is to accentuate the areas that need more support. Often times, the higher density material is placed on the medial side of the shoe to reduce over-pronation. Mixed materials are also used for the midsole [24]. EVA impregnated with solid rubber can improve the resistance to compression and have a quicker rebound [1]. Different manufacturers are finding ways to come up with more cushioning devices such as gel and air in the midsole to maintain cushioning that lasts longer than EVA, but it may come at more of an expense [25].

Wedges

Wedges are also known as medial post. They are designed by tapering the midsole so the medial side is thicker than the outside border. It was created because feet tend to pronate or roll in beyond the neutral position. The wedge helps reduce over-pronation in running and increases stability on the inner part of the shoe [1]. To properly serve its function, wedges are often made from a material with higher density foam or thermal plastic unit to prevent the medial arch from collapsing. Thermal plastic unit creates stiffness in the midsole and makes the shoe lighter [23].

Outsole

Rubber has been the material of choice for the outsole because it is both soft and durable [1]. There are several different types of rubber that can be used. Tire rubber is durable but heavy. Gum rubber offers a good grip [26]. Despite the various options, the outsole is usually made from blown rubber and carbon rubber [27]. Blown rubber is air-injected rubber, making the outsole lighter and softer to provide cushioning and flexibility. However, it wears quickly making it less durable than carbon rubber [23]. Carbon rubber is both light and the most durable type of rubber. With its distinct properties, blown rubber serves better purpose at the forefoot of the shoe and carbon rubber at the heel. Like the midsole, outsoles can also be made from mixing different materials [26].

Motion control shoes help with both the subtalar joint and the midtarsal joint, while stability shoes control only the subtalar joint. Therefore the shape and design of the outsole is an important factor in determining what kind of control runners need [26]. The straighter the shoe, the more motion control it offers, so it is usually for those with a pes planus foot type [27]. Slightly and semi-curved outsoles have less motion control and are for those with a more "normal" foot type. Curved outsoles are in neutral shoes, allowing for no motion control, so this type of running shoe is generally for sprinters and can give supinators more cushion [26].

Furthermore, outsole designs help runners maximize the use of their shoes [1]. Stud or waffle outsoles are ideal for running on dirt or grass because it improves traction and stability. Ripple soles are better for running on cement or asphalt [25].

Insole and Sockliner

The insole board is stable and flexible. It should serve as a rigid base for the shoe, but flexible enough to allow the foot some movement once in the shoe. It is made of cellulose fibers. Because the insole is exposed to sweat from the feet, better boards include components to inhibit bacterial and fungal growth from the moisture in the shoe [1].

The sockliner is the layer that lies between the foot and the insole board. Its principle functions are to absorb perspiration, energy absorption, and comfort. Because each foot is shaped differently, good sockliners should conform to match the foot shape. EVA foam is conducive to this. Terrycloth lining works well for wicking away perspiration. Sockliners also need to generate enough friction to prevent the foot from sliding inside the shoe. Blisters on the dorsum of the foot can occur from rubbing with the upper because of too much movement. Velour has also been used as a sockliner because it creates friction [1].

Putting It All Together

The construction of the running shoe to attach the upper to the sole has three options: board lasting, slip lasting, or combination lasting. Board lasting is a fiber board that runs from the heel to the forefoot. Shoes with this type of lasting have the most stability. Slip lasting has no board at all. It provides stability and the most comfort. A combination last has a board at the rearfoot for stability and is slip lasted in the forefoot for flexibility and comfort. Removing the insole and exploring the inside of the shoe can determine which kind of last the running shoe has [1, 26].

References

1. Peter C: The Running Shoe Book. Anderson World Inc., Mountain View, CA, 1980.
2. Kippen C: The History of Sports Shoes. 1 March 2007, http://podiatry.curtin.edu.au/sport.html.
3. Krentzman J: The Force Behind the Nike Empire. The Stanford Magazine. 1 March 2007, http://www.stanfordalumni.org/news/magazine/1997/janfeb/articles/knight.html.
4. Pribut SM, Douglas HR: 2002: A Sneaker Odyssey. 4 May 2007, http://www.drpribut.com/sports/sneaker_odyssey.html.
5. Bill B: Wikipedia, The Free Encyclopedia. 9 Jun 2007, 11:40 UTC. Wikimedia Foundation, Inc. 4 May 2007, http://en.wikipedia.org/w/index.php?title=Bill_Bowerman&oldid=13702 1879.
6. Guide to the Bill Bowerman papers: Northwestern Digital Archives. 4 May 2007, http://nwda-db.wsulibs.wsu.edu/ark:/80444/xv98511.
7. Phil K: Wikipedia, The Free Encyclopedia. 7 Jun 2007, 23:55 UTC. Wikimedia Foundation, Inc. 4 May 2007, http://en.wikipedia.org/w/index.php?title=Phil_Knight&oldid=136720572
8. Subotnick SI: Podiatry: Foot and Ankle Surgery. 4 May 2007, http://www.drsubotnick.com/.
9. Harry H: Wikipedia, The Free Encyclopedia. 17 Dec 2006, 14:53 UTC. Wikimedia Foundation, Inc. 4 May 2007, http://en.wikipedia.org/w/index.php?title=Harry_Hlavac&oldid=94893048.
10. Athletic shoe with external counter and cushion assembly: Patent Storm. 4 May 2007. http://www.patentstorm.us/patents/4731939.html.
11. "Shoe with internal dynamic rocker element." Free Patents Online. 4 May 2007, http://www.freepatentsonline.com/4794707.html.
12. Smith L, James S: Newton Center Podiatry. 4 May 2007. http://www.drsmithstewart.com/.
13. Bates B: Biomechanics 4 May 2007, http://darkwing.uoregon.edu/~ems/EMS02/bates.html.
14. Shoe comprising liquid cushioning element. Delphion. 4 May 2007. http://www.delphion.com/details?pn10=US05493792.
15. Summer sports safety. Ladies Home Journal. 4 May 2007, http://www.bhg.com/lhj/story.jhtml?storyid=/templatedata/bhg/story/data/summersafety_07032001.xml&catref=bcat83.
16. Bates B: Backward Running: Benefits 4 May 2007, http://darkwing.uoregon.edu/~btbates/backward/backward1.htm.
17. Article of footwear having adjustable width, footform and cushioning. Free Patents Online. 4 May 2007, http://www.freepatentsonline.com/5729912.html
18. Chapel RJ: Making the shoe fit: good design can help prevent injuries caused by an unusual stride – selecting running shoes. Feb. 1986. Nation's Business. 4 May 2007, http://findarticles.com/p/articles/mi_m1154/is_v74/ai_4116365
19. Kinesiology: University of Calgary. 4 May 2007, http://www.kin.ucalgary.ca/2002/profiles/nigg.asp
20. Blanchard F: Putting the Best Shoe Forward. 4 May 2007, http://www.ucalgary.ca/UofC/events/unicomm/Research/nigg.htm
21. Urquhart D, Mark R: U of C scores soccer assist. On Campus Weekly. 4 May 2007, http://www.ucalgary.ca/oncampus/weekly/may7-04/soccer-shoe.html
22. Inventor of the Week: Lemelson-MIT Program. March 2006. MIT School of Engineering: 4 May 2007, http://web.mit.edu/invent/iow/dananberg.html
23. Deconstructing Shoes: Running Warehouse. 1 March 2007, http://www.runningwarehouse.com/LearningCenter/ShoePhD.html.
24. How to buy a running shoe: CBS Sports Store. 15 March 2007, http://www.cbssportsstore.com/sm-running-shoe-buyers-guide--bg-222919.html.
25. Anatomy of a running shoe: American Running Association. 1 March 2007, http://www.americanrunning.org/displayindustryarticle.cfm?articlenbr=1430.

26. Reeves M: The Athletic Shoe. California School of Podiatric Medicine Biomechanics II Class. Samuel Merritt College. Room TC 9, 4 April 2007.
27. Super D: Anatomy of a running shoe. Roadrunner sports. 3 March 2007, http://www. roadrunnersports.com/rrs/content/content.jsp?contentId=content1106.

Chapter 2
Evolution of Foot Orthoses in Sports

Kevin A. Kirby

Foot orthoses have been used for over 150 years by the medical profession for the treatment of various pathologies of the foot and lower extremity [1]. Starting from their simple origin as a leather, cork, and/or metallic in-shoe arch support, foot orthoses have gradually evolved into a complex assortment of in-shoe devices that may be fabricated from a multitude of synthetic and natural materials to accomplish the intended therapeutic goals for the injured patient. For the clinician that treats both athletic and non-athletic injuries of the foot and lower extremity, foot orthoses are an invaluable therapeutic tool in the treatment of many painful pathologies of the foot and lower extremity, in the prevention of new injuries in the foot and lower extremity, and in the optimization of the biomechanics of the individual during sports and other weightbearing activities. Because of their therapeutic effectiveness in the treatment of a wide range of painful mechanically based pathologies in the human locomotor apparatus, foot orthoses are often considered by many podiatrists, sports physicians, and foot-care specialists to be one of the most important treatment modalities for these conditions.

Definition of Foot Orthoses

To the lay public and many medical professionals, foot orthoses are often described by the slang word *orthotics* to describe the wide variety of in-shoe devices ranging from non-custom arch supports to prescription custom-molded foot orthoses. Because of this potentially confusing problem with terminology, this chapter will use the term *foot orthosis* to describe all types of therapeutic in-shoe medical devices that are intended to treat pathologies of the foot and/or lower extremities.

It is appropriate within the context of laying down proper terminology for foot orthoses that a proper definition also be given. *Dorland's Medical Dictionary* gives

K.A. Kirby (✉)
Department of Applied Biomechanics, California School of Podiatric Medicine,
Oakland, CA, USA

M.B. Werd, E.L. Knight (eds.), *Athletic Footwear and Orthoses in Sports Medicine*,
DOI 10.1007/978-0-387-76416-0_2, © Springer Science+Business Media, LLC 2010

a relatively generic definition of an orthosis as being "an orthopedic appliance or apparatus used to support, align, prevent, or correct deformities or to improve the function of movable parts of the body" [2]. However, it is clear from the prevailing research that will be reviewed in this chapter that foot orthoses have a much more complex function than simply "supporting or aligning the skeleton." Due to the need for a more modern definition of these in-shoe medical devices, especially considering the extensive scientific research that has been performed on foot orthoses within the past few decades, Kirby has proposed the following definition for foot orthoses:

> An in-shoe medical device which is designed to alter the magnitudes and temporal patterns of the reaction forces acting on the plantar aspect of the foot in order to allow more normal foot and lower extremity function and to decrease pathologic loading forces on the structural components of the foot and lower extremity during weightbearing activities [3].

Historical Evolution of Foot Orthoses

Ever since 1845, when an English chiropodist, Durlacher, and other practitioners and boot-makers of his era described the use of built-up in-shoe leather devices, the medical literature has described foot orthoses as being valuable medical devices for the treatment of painful pathologies and deformities within the foot and lower extremity [1, 4]. The early literature describes the efforts of pioneering podiatrists and medical doctors, such as Whitman [5, 6], Roberts [7], Schuster [1], Morton [8], Levy [1], and Helfet [9], to create more effective foot orthoses for treatment of mechanically based foot pathologies.

Even though foot orthoses were being used by select medical practitioners in the first half of the 20th century, it was not until 1958 that the era of modern foot orthosis therapy began. It was at this time, when a California podiatrist, Merton Root, began to fabricate thermoplastic foot orthoses made around feet casted in a subtalar joint (STJ) rotational position (which he coined as the "neutral position" in 1954) that the era of modern prescription foot orthoses was born [10, 11]. The introduction by Root and coworkers of a new lower extremity biomechanical classification system based on the STJ neutral position and of eight "biophysical criteria" of the foot and lower extremity that were required to be present in the foot and lower extremity before it could be considered ideal, or "normal," has served as the biomechanical basis for clinicians involved in foot orthosis therapy for nearly a half-century [12]. Later refinements and modifications to the modern foot orthosis made by Henderson and Campbell [13], Blake [14–16], Kirby [3, 17, 18], and others [19] have added significantly to the potential therapeutic effectiveness and range of pathologies that may be treated with foot orthoses.

Research and Theory on Orthosis Function

The early medical literature on foot orthoses, even though it was probably quite valuable for the clinician of that era, unfortunately consisted of only a few sparse anecdotal accounts from practitioners regarding the therapeutic effectiveness of foot orthoses on their own patients. However, in today's medical environment, which demands more evidence-based research to inform the clinician of the most effective medical therapy to choose for their patients, anecdotal reports of a single clinician's results with foot orthoses are no longer considered to be evidence of high value [20]. Fortunately, due to the numerous computer-based technological advances that have occurred over the past few decades, both clinical specialists and researchers within the international biomechanics community have now combined their efforts to produce a virtual explosion in foot orthosis research [21]. The effective collaboration between clinician and researcher has started to progress the medical specialties toward better scientific validation of the observations that clinicians have been claiming for over a century in the successful treatment of their injured athletes and non-athletes with foot orthoses.

Research on Therapeutic Effectiveness of Orthoses

Numerous research studies have now provided for solid validation of the therapeutic effectiveness of the treatment of injuries within both the athletic and non-athletic population. In the recreational and competitive runner, the success rate at treating various foot and lower extremity injuries has been reported as being between 50 and 90% [22–25]. A complete resolution or significant improvement in symptoms was found in the foot orthosis treatment of injuries in 76% of 500 distance runners [26]. In 180 patients with athletic injuries, 70% of the athletes reported that foot orthoses "definitely helped" their injuries [27]. In addition, 76.5% of patients improved and 2% were asymptomatic after 2–4 weeks of receiving the custom foot orthoses in a study of 102 athletic patients with patellofemoral pain syndrome [28].

Further evidence of the therapeutic effects of foot orthoses comes from the research literature on treatment of non-athletic injuries. In a study of 81 patients treated with foot orthoses, 91% were "satisfied" and 52% "wouldn't leave home without them" [29]. In a study of 520 patients treated with foot orthoses, 83% were satisfied and 95% reported their problem had either partially or completely resolved with their orthoses [30]. The majority of the 275 patients that had worn custom foot orthoses for over a year had between 60 and 100% relief of symptoms, with only 9% reporting no relief of symptoms [31]. In a recent prospective study of 79 women over the age of 65, the group of subjects that received custom foot orthoses and was given guidance on shoe fitting had significant improvements in mental health, bodily pain, and general health compared to their non-orthosis wearing controls so that foot orthosis intervention was determined to be "markedly effective not only in the physical but also in the mental aspect" [32].

In scientific studies that involved the foot orthosis treatment of specific pathologies, very positive results have also been reported. In a prospective study of infantry recruits, those recruits wearing foot orthoses had an 11.3–16.3% reduction in incidence of stress fractures than in the non-orthotic control group [33]. Another prospective study in military recruits found that foot orthoses reduced the incidence of femoral stress fractures in those recruits with pes cavus deformity and reduced the incidence of metatarsal fractures in those recruits with pes planus deformity [34]. In a study of 20 female adolescent subjects with patellofemoral syndrome, foot orthoses were found to significantly improve symptoms versus muscle strengthening alone [35]. In research on 64 subjects with osteoarthritis in the foot and ankle, 100% of the patients wearing orthoses had significantly longer relief of pain than those patients receiving only nonsteroidal anti-inflammatory drugs [36]. A review of the literature regarding the treatment of medial compartment knee osteoarthritis with laterally wedged foot orthoses led researchers to conclude that their "data indicate a strong scientific basis for applying wedged insoles in attempts to reduce osteoarthritic pain of biomechanical origin" [37]. In addition, a 75% reduction in disability rating and a 66% reduction in pain rating occurred in patients with plantar fasciitis when they wore custom foot orthoses [38]. In certain other medical conditions, foot orthoses have also been found to be therapeutic. In subjects with hemophilia A treated over a 6-week period with foot orthoses, there was found to be significant control of ankle bleeds, decreased pain, decreased disability, and increased activity [39]. Significant improvement in pain and a decrease in foot disability occurred in patients with rheumatoid arthritis (RA) when they wore custom foot orthoses [40–42]. In addition, in a recent randomized control trial of 40 children with juvenile idiopathic arthritis, it was found that the children wearing custom foot orthoses had significantly greater improvements in overall pain, speed of ambulation, foot pain, and level of disability when compared to those that received shoe inserts or shoes alone [43]. A review of the research literature, combined with the author's personal experience of treating over 12,000 patients within the past 22 years with custom foot orthoses, makes it very clear that foot orthoses can offer significant therapeutic benefit to both athletic and non-athletic patients.

Theories of Foot Orthosis Function

Even though the therapeutic efficacy of foot orthoses has been well documented within the medical literature for the past quarter century, the biomechanical explanation for the impressive therapeutic effects of foot orthoses has been a matter of speculation for well over a century. In 1888, Whitman made a metal foot brace that worked on the theory that the foot could be pushed into proper position either by force or by pain, by the use of medial and lateral flanges that would rock into inversion once the patient had stepped on it [5]. Morton, in 1935, believed that a "hypermobile first metatarsal segment" was the cause of many foot maladies and that his "compensating insole" with an extension plantar to the first metatarsophalangeal joint would relieve "concentration of stresses on the second metatarsal segment" [8]. Even though early authors claimed excellent clinical results with foot orthoses [9, 44, 45], none offered coherent mechanical theories that described how foot orthoses might accomplish their impressive therapeutic results.

In the late 1950s and early 1960s, Root and his coworkers from the California College of Podiatric Medicine in San Francisco developed a classification system based on an ideal or "normal" structure of the foot and lower extremity that used Root's original concept of the subtalar joint (STJ) neutral position as a reference position of the foot [10–12, 46, 47]. Root and coworkers also integrated their ideas of "normal" structure into an orthosis prescription protocol that had the following goals: (1) to cause the subtalar joint to function in the neutral position, (2) to prevent compensation, or abnormal motions, for foot and lower extremity deformities, and (3) to "lock the midtarsal joint" (Root and Weed, 1984, Personal communication).

New ideas on foot function came in 1987 when Kirby first proposed that abnormal STJ rotational forces (i.e., moments) were responsible for many mechanically based pathologies in the foot and lower extremity and that abnormal STJ axis spatial location was the primary cause of these pathological STJ moments [48]. A foot with a medially deviated STJ axis was suggested to be more likely to suffer from pronation-related symptoms since ground reaction force (GRF) would cause increased magnitudes of external STJ pronation moments (Figs. 2.1 and 2.2). A foot with a laterally deviated STJ axis would tend to suffer from supination-related

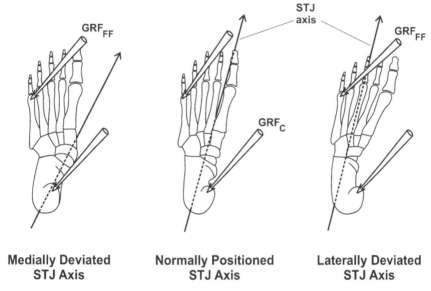

Medially Deviated   **Normally Positioned**   **Laterally Deviated**
STJ Axis   **STJ Axis**   **STJ Axis**

Fig. 2.1 In a foot with a normally positioned subtalar joint (STJ) axis (*center*), the ground reaction force plantar to the calcaneus (GRF$_C$) will cause a STJ supination moment since it acts medial to the STJ axis. Ground reaction force acting plantar to the 5th metatarsal head (GRF$_{FF}$) will cause a STJ pronation moment since it acts lateral to the STJ axis. In a foot with a medially deviated STJ axis (*left*), since the plantar calcaneus now has a decreased STJ supination moment arm when compared to normal, GRF$_C$ will cause a decreased magnitude of STJ supination moment. Since the 5th metatarsal head has an increased STJ pronation moment arm, GRF$_{FF}$ will cause an increased magnitude of STJ pronation moment when compared to normal. However, in a foot with a laterally deviated STJ axis (*right*), since the plantar calcaneus now has an increased STJ supination moment arm, GRF$_C$ will cause an increased magnitude of STJ supination moment and since the 5th metatarsal head has a decreased STJ pronation moment arm, GRF$_{FF}$ will cause a decreased magnitude of STJ pronation moment when compared to normal. Therefore, the net result of the mechanical actions of ground reaction force on a foot with a medial deviated STJ axis is to cause increased magnitude of STJ pronation moment and the net mechanical result of a laterally deviated STJ axis is to cause increased magnitude of STJ supination moment. (From [50] with permission of JAPMA)

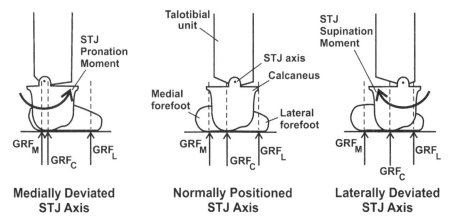

**Medially Deviated   Normally Positioned   Laterally Deviated
STJ Axis   STJ Axis   STJ Axis**

Fig. 2.2 In this model, a posterior view of the right foot and ankle is modeled as consisting of the talus and tibia combined together to form the talotibial unit which articulates with the foot at the subtalar joint (STJ) axis. The external forces acting on the foot include ground reaction force (GRF) plantar to the calcaneus (GRF_C), GRF plantar to the medial forefoot (GRF_M), and GRF plantar to the lateral forefoot (GRF_L). In a foot with a normal STJ axis location (*center*), the more central location of the STJ axis relative to the structures of plantar foot allows GRF_C, GRF_M, and GRF_L to cause a balancing of STJ supination and STJ pronation moments so that more normal foot function occurs. In a foot with a medially deviated STJ axis (*left*), the more medial location of the STJ axis relative to the plantar structures of the foot will cause a relative lateral shift in GRF_C, GRF_M, and GRF_L, increasing the magnitude of STJ pronation moment and causing more pronation-related symptoms during weightbearing activities. In a foot with a laterally deviated STJ axis (*right*), the more lateral location of the STJ axis relative to the plantar structures of the foot will cause a relative medial shift in GRF_C, GRF_M, and GRF_L, increasing the magnitude of STJ supination moment and causing more supination-related symptoms

symptoms since GRF would cause increased magnitudes of external STJ supination moments [48]. Medial and lateral deviations of the STJ axis were also proposed to cause changes in the magnitudes and directions of STJ moments that are produced by contractile activity of the extrinsic muscles of the foot [48, 50] (Fig. 2.3). When STJ axis spatial location was combined with the mechanical concept of rotational equilibrium, a new theory of foot function, the "Subtalar Joint Axis Location and Rotational Equilibrium (SALRE) Theory of Foot Function," emerged to offer a coherent explanation for the biomechanical cause of many mechanically based pathologies of the foot and lower extremity [48–50].

In 1992, Kirby and Green first proposed that foot orthoses functioned by altering the STJ moments that were created by the mechanical actions of ground reaction force (GRF) acting on the plantar foot during weightbearing activities [47]. They hypothesized that foot orthoses were able to exert their ability to "control pronation" by converting GRF acting lateral to the STJ axis into a more medially located orthosis reaction force (ORF) that would be able to generate increased STJ supination moments during weightbearing activities. Using the example of a foot orthosis with a deep inverted heel cup, known as the Blake Inverted Orthosis [14–16, 51], they proposed that the inverted heel cup orthosis produced its impressive clinical

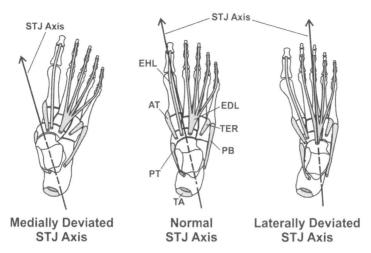

Medially Deviated   **Normal**   **Laterally Deviated**
STJ Axis   **STJ Axis**   **STJ Axis**

Fig. 2.3 In a foot with a normal STJ axis location (*center*), the posterior tibial (PT), anterior tibial (AT), extensor hallucis longus (EHL), and Achilles tendons (TA) will all cause a STJ supination moment when they exert tensile force on their osseous insertion points since they all insert medial to the STJ axis. However, the extensor digitorum longus (EDL), peroneus tertius (TER), peroneus brevis (PB) tendons will all cause a STJ pronation moment when they exert tensile force on their insertion points since they all insert lateral to the STJ axis. However, in a foot with a medially deviated STJ axis (*left*), since the muscle tendons located medial to the STJ axis have a reduced STJ supination moment arm, their contractile activity will cause a decreased magnitude of STJ supination moment when compared to normal. In addition, since the muscle tendons lateral to the STJ axis have an increased STJ pronation moment arm, their contractile activity will cause an increased magnitude of STJ pronation moment. In addition, in a foot with a laterally deviated STJ axis (*right*), since the muscle tendons medial to the STJ axis have an increased STJ supination moment arm, their contractile activity will cause an increased magnitude of STJ supination moment when compared to normal. Since the muscle tendons lateral to the STJ axis have a decreased STJ pronation moment arm, their contractile activity will cause a decreased magnitude of STJ pronation moment. Therefore, the net mechanical effect of medial deviation of the STJ axis on the actions of the extrinsic muscles of the foot is to cause increased magnitudes of STJ pronation moment and the net mechanical effect of lateral deviation of the STJ axis on the actions of the extrinsic muscles of the foot is to cause increased magnitudes of STJ supination moment

results in reducing rearfoot pronation and relieving pronation-related symptoms by increasing the ORF on the medial aspect of the plantar heel so that increased STJ supination moments would result [47]. Kirby later introduced a foot orthosis modification called the *medial heel skive technique* (Fig. 2.4) that also produced an inverted heel cup in the orthosis to increase STJ supination moment and more effectively treat difficult pathologies such as pediatric flatfoot deformity, posterior tibial dysfunction, and sinus tarsi syndrome [17].

Foot and lower extremity pathologies caused by excessive magnitudes of external STJ supination moment, such as chronic peroneal tendinopathy and chronic inversion ankle sprains, were also proposed by Kirby to be caused by the interaction of GRF acting on the foot with an abnormally laterally deviated STJ axis [3, 18, 49, 50]. It was suggested that the abnormal STJ supination moments would be best

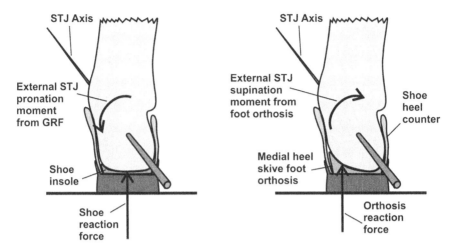

Fig. 2.4 In the illustrations, the posterior aspect of the right foot with a medially deviated subtalar joint (STJ) axis is shown in a shoe without an orthosis (*left*) and also in a shoe with a medial heel skive foot orthosis (*right*). In the shoe with only the insole under the foot (*left*), the medially deviated STJ axis will cause increased STJ pronation moment since the shoe reaction force is more centrally located at the plantar heel. However, when the varus heel cup of a medial heel skive foot orthosis is added to the shoe (*right*), the resultant medial shift in orthosis reaction force will cause a decrease in STJ pronation moment and an increase in STJ supination moment. Therefore, foot orthoses with varus heel cup modifications, such as the medial heel skive, are more effective at treating symptoms caused by excessive foot pronation due to their ability to shift reaction forces more medially on the plantar foot and, thereby, greatly increase the STJ supination moment acting on the foot

treated with an increased valgus construction within the foot orthosis, including a *lateral heel skive technique* [52] within the heel cup of the orthosis. In this fashion, the orthosis would mechanically increase the magnitude of external STJ pronation moments by shifting ORF more laterally on the plantar foot to more effectively treat supination-related symptoms.

In the late 1980s and 1990s, a number of other authors also started focusing on the idea that orthosis treatment should not be determined by the results of measuring "deformities" of the foot and lower extremity, as proposed by Root and coworkers, but rather be determined by the location and nature of the internal loading forces acting on injured structures of the patient. The idea that pathological internal loading forces acting on the foot and lower extremity in sports and other weightbearing activities may be effectively modeled to develop better treatment strategies was pioneered by Benno Nigg and coworkers at the University of Calgary, Canada. Nigg and coworkers realized that since invasive internal measurements could not be made on patients to determine the absolute magnitudes of internal loading forces, reliable estimates of these forces could instead be made with more effective models of the foot and lower extremity [53–55].

However, it was not until 1995, when McPoil and Hunt first coined the term "Tissue Stress Model," that one of the most recent foot orthosis treatment models was given a proper name. McPoil and Hunt suggested that foot orthosis therapy should be directed toward reducing abnormal levels of tissue stress in order to more effectively design mechanical treatment aimed at healing musculoskeletal injuries caused by pathological tissue stress. They felt that by focusing the clinician's attention on the abnormal stresses causing the injury, rather than on measuring "deformities" of the lower extremity, optimal mechanical foot therapy could be better achieved [56].

Following up on the ideas embodied within the Tissue Stress Model, Fuller described, in 1996, how computerized gait evaluation and modeling techniques could be effectively used to guide foot orthosis treatment by aiding in the prediction of abnormal stresses within the foot and lower extremity [57]. Three years later, Fuller described how the location of the center of pressure on the plantar foot, relative to the spatial location of the STJ axis, may help direct orthosis therapy for foot pathologies resulting from abnormal STJ moments [58]. In later published works, Fuller and Kirby further explored the idea of reducing pathological tissue stress with orthoses and how this could be integrated with the SALRE Theory of Foot Function and an analysis of midtarsal joint kinetics (Fig. 2.5) to guide the clinician toward a better understanding of foot orthosis function and toward more effective foot orthosis treatments for their patients with mechanically based foot and lower extremity injuries [3, 59, 60].

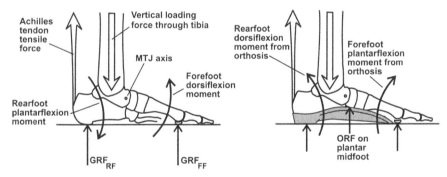

Fig. 2.5 During standing without a foot orthosis (*left*), ground reaction force acting plantar to the rearfoot (GRF$_{RF}$), Achilles tendon tensile force acting on the posterior rearfoot, and vertical loading force from the tibia acting onto the superior talus work together to mechanically cause a rearfoot plantarflexion moment which tends to cause the rearfoot to plantarflex at the ankle. In addition, ground reaction force acting plantar to the forefoot (GRF$_{FF}$) causes a forefoot dorsiflexion moment which tends to cause the forefoot to dorsiflex at the midtarsal joint (MTJ). Both the resultant rearfoot plantarflexion moment and the forefoot dorsiflexion moment tend to cause the longitudinal arch of the foot to flatten. However, when a custom foot orthosis is constructed for the foot that applies a significant orthosis reaction force (ORF) to the plantar aspect of the longitudinal arch (*right*), the resultant increase in ORF at the plantar midfoot combined with the resultant decrease in GRF$_{RF}$ and GRF$_{FF}$ will cause an increase in rearfoot dorsiflexion moment and an increase in forefoot plantarflexion moment. By this mechanical method, foot orthoses help resist longitudinal arch flattening to produce one of the strongest biomechanical and therapeutic effects of orthoses on the foot and lower extremity

Another new theory of foot orthosis function, the "Preferred Movement Pathway Model," was proposed by Nigg and coworkers that was claimed to be a "new paradigm for movement control." Basing their new theory on previous scientific research, Nigg and coworkers proposed that foot orthoses do not function by realigning the skeleton but rather function by producing a change in the "muscle tuning" of the lower extremity via their alteration of the input signals into the plantar foot during athletic activities. It was suggested that if the preferred movement path is counteracted by the orthosis/shoe combination, then muscle activity would be increased, but conversely, if the preferred movement path is allowed by the orthosis/shoe combination, then lower extremity muscle activity would be reduced [61, 62]. Even though their theory has received considerable attention within the international biomechanics community, their theory, and all the other above-mentioned theories, will require much further research to either support or reject their validity. These and other theories of foot function have been described in much greater detail in the excellent review articles by Payne [63] and Lee [11].

Research on Biomechanical Effects of Foot Orthoses

As mentioned earlier, over the last few decades, there has been a surge in the quality and number of foot orthosis biomechanics research studies on both athletes and non-athletes. Much of the improvement in the quality of research studies on foot orthoses is likely due to many new technological advances that are now available within the modern lower extremity biomechanics laboratory. These facilities are able to perform advanced biomechanical analyses in a relatively short period of time on subjects using accelerometers, force plates, pressure mats, pressure insoles, strain gauges, and computerized three-dimensional motion analysis. In addition, advanced computer modeling techniques, such as inverse dynamics analysis and finite element analysis, have allowed researchers to better understand the kinetics of gait and investigate the changes in internal loading forces that occur in feet with different orthosis designs. All of these technological advances have allowed researchers to provide very meaningful insights into how foot orthoses biomechanically produce their significant positive therapeutic effects in the treatment of foot and lower extremity injuries [21].

Since early research on the effects of foot orthoses on running biomechanics showed that there was little to no change in the kinematics of gait function with foot orthoses, many doubted whether foot orthoses had any significant biomechanical effect on the foot and lower extremity of the individual [64–67]. However, as the sophistication of biomechanics research has progressed over the past few decades, important new research has now demonstrated how foot orthoses may change the mechanical function of the foot and lower extremities and help heal injuries in athletes and non-athletes [68–72]. With the newer, more sophisticated research, the multiple alterations that occur in the internal forces and internal moments (i.e., kinetics) of the lower extremities with foot orthoses can now be determined, which has produced considerable research evidence regarding how foot orthoses may produce their biomechanical effects.

Foot Orthoses Alter Foot and Lower Extremity Kinematics and Kinetics

Foot orthoses have now been conclusively shown to alter the motion patterns (i.e., kinematics) of the foot and lower extremities in numerous scientific research studies. Research has now shown a decrease in maximum rearfoot eversion angle [64, 65, 72, 73], a decrease in maximum rearfoot eversion velocity [65, 72], a decrease in maximum ankle dorsiflexion angle [72], a decrease in maximum internal tibial rotation [71, 73–75], and a decrease in knee adduction [71, 73,75].

Foot orthoses have also been shown to conclusively alter the internal forces and internal moments (i.e., kinetics) acting on the segments of the foot and lower extremity during running. Recent research has shown a decrease in maximum internal ankle inversion moment [70–72] (Fig. 2.6), changes in maximum knee external rotation moment [70], and changes in knee abduction moment [71] during running with foot orthoses. In addition, a decrease in impact peak and maximum vertical loading rate was seen in runners treated with foot orthoses [70].

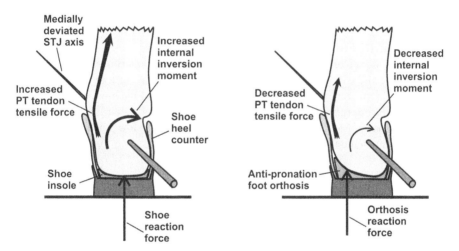

Fig. 2.6 Research has shown that foot orthoses change the kinetics of gait by altering the internal forces acting on the segments of the foot and lower extremity. In the model illustrated above of the posterior aspect of a right foot with a medially deviated STJ axis, when the posterior tibial muscle contracts with increased force to cause increased tensile force on its tendon, an increased internal inversion moment will be measured (*left*). However, when an anti-pronation custom foot orthosis is designed for the foot to shift the orthosis reaction force more medial on the plantar heel and longitudinal arch, the resultant increase in external STJ supination moment from the orthosis (see Fig. 2.4) will cause a decrease in posterior tibial muscle contractile force and a decrease in tendon tensile force which will also result in a decrease in measured internal inversion moment (*right*). It is by this proposed mechanism that foot orthoses may relieve symptoms and heal injuries in the athlete and non-athlete but, in doing so, may also cause little change in measured foot and lower extremity gait kinematics

In addition to the more prevalent research on the biomechanical effects of foot orthoses on running, recent studies have now shown that foot orthoses significantly affect the biomechanics of walking. Decreased rearfoot pronation and decreased rearfoot pronation velocity with varus-wedged orthoses and increased rearfoot pronation with valgus-wedged orthoses were shown in subjects that walked on both varus-wedged and valgus-wedged foot orthoses [76, 77]. In addition, patients with RA that wore foot orthoses for 12 months showed significant reductions in rearfoot eversion and internal tibial rotation [78]. These studies conclusively demonstrate that foot orthoses are able to alter both the motion patterns and internal forces and moments acting within the foot and lower extremity during both running and walking activities. The more recent research on the kinetics and kinematics of foot orthosis function also support the theories mentioned earlier that proposed that foot orthoses work largely by altering the internal forces within the foot and lower extremity by changing the moments acting across the joints of the human locomotor apparatus [3, 18, 47, 50, 53–55, 58–60].

Foot Orthoses Alter Contractile Activity of Lower Extremity Muscles

Research has also shown that foot orthoses significantly affect the contractile activity of muscles during running and other activities. Foot orthoses were found to alter the EMG activity of the biceps femoris and anterior tibial muscles during running [79] and to significantly change the EMG activity of the anterior tibial muscle during walking [80]. Recent research has shown that changes in foot orthosis design may cause significant changes in EMG activity in many of the muscles of the lower extremity during running [81]. A correlation between perceived foot comfort with different types of foot orthoses and the EMG activity of the lower extremity muscles has also been demonstrated [82].

Foot Orthoses Improve Postural Stability

There is experimental evidence that foot orthoses can also improve the postural stability of individuals. Postural sway was reduced when subjects wearing foot orthoses were subjected to inversion–eversion and medial–lateral platform movements which indicated that undesirable motion at the foot and ankle may have been restricted and/or the ability of joint mechanoreceptors to detect motion perturbations may have been enhanced by orthoses [83]. Subjects balancing on one foot were likewise shown to have significant decreases in frontal plane CoP length and velocity with medially posted orthoses, which possibly indicated foot orthoses enhanced their postural control abilities [84]. In another study involving subjects with excessively pronated feet, foot orthoses produced reductions in medial–lateral sway during bipedal standing indicating improved balance [85].

Foot Orthoses Reduce Plantar Forces and Pressures

Research on the ability of foot orthoses to reduce the forces and pressures on injured or painful areas of the plantar foot provides yet another therapeutic mechanical action of foot orthoses (Fig. 2.7). In a prospective study of 151 subjects with cavus foot deformity, those subjects wearing custom foot orthoses after 3 months showed significant decreases in foot pain, increases in quality of life, and showed three times the forefoot plantar pressure reduction when compared to sham insoles [86]. In 42 subjects with metatarsalgia, foot orthoses were found to not only decrease the metatarsal head pain but also significantly decrease the force impulse and peak pressure at the metatarsal heads [87]. Significant reductions in plantar pressures and loading forces were shown in another study that measured the effects of foot orthoses on both normal and RA subjects [88]. In 81 patients with Type II diabetes, maximum peak plantar pressures were reduced by 30% with foot orthoses [89] and in 34 adolescent Type I diabetic patients both peak pressure and pressure–time integral were reduced while wearing foot orthoses [90]. In a study of eight patients with plantar neuropathic ulcerations that had become healed with custom foot orthoses, it was found that their custom foot orthoses significantly reduced peak vertical pressure, reduced the pressure/time integral, and increased the total contact

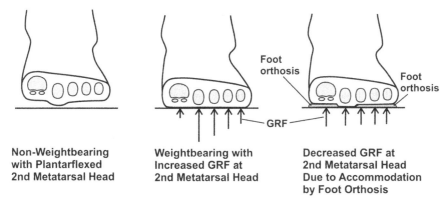

Non-Weightbearing with Plantarflexed 2nd Metatarsal Head   **Weightbearing with Increased GRF at 2nd Metatarsal Head**   **Decreased GRF at 2nd Metatarsal Head Due to Accommodation by Foot Orthosis**

Fig. 2.7 Research has shown that foot orthoses may be designed to reduce the plantar pressures and forces acting on the foot. In the model shown, a frontal plane cross-section of the metatarsal heads in a foot with a plantarflexed second metatarsal is illustrated. When the forefoot is close to contacting with the ground, but still is non-weightbearing, the plantarflexion deformity of the 2nd metatarsal is obvious (*left*). However, once the forefoot becomes weightbearing, the increase in ground reaction force (GRF) that occurs at each of the metatarsal heads will be particularly increased at the 2nd metatarsal head (*middle*) which may cause injuries to the osseous and/or soft tissue structures of the 2nd metatarsal or 2nd metatarsophalangeal joint. To treat the increased compression forces and stresses at the 2nd metatarsal head, a foot orthosis may be designed to increase the GRF plantar to the 1st, 3rd, 4th, and 5th metatarsal heads and decrease the GRF plantar to the 2nd metatarsal head (*right*). This redistribution of GRF on the plantar foot, away from high-pressure areas toward lower pressure areas, is the most likely mechanism behind the ability of foot orthoses to reduce pathologic pressures away from specific areas of the plantar foot surface area versus the no-insole condition [91]. In another study using computer-simulated three-dimensional finite element analysis of a foot exposed to different orthosis constructions, orthosis shape was found to be more important in reducing peak plantar pressures than was orthosis stiffness [92].

Conclusion

Foot orthoses have been used for well over a century by clinicians as a means to reduce pain, improve gait mechanics, and heal injury to the foot, lower extremity, and lower back. There is considerable research evidence that supports the therapeutic efficacy and significant mechanical effects of foot orthoses on standing, walking, and running activities. Theoretical explanations as to how foot orthoses actually produce their therapeutic and mechanical effects have been previously proposed and are being continually refined as exciting new research evidence is brought to light and discussed in academic forums. There is great promise for increased understanding and further development of foot orthoses as a valuable therapeutic tool in the treatment of mechanically based musculoskeletal injuries for the athletic and non-athletic population of today and for future generations.

References

1. Schuster RO: A history of orthopedics in podiatry. J Am Pod Assoc, 64:332, 1974.
2. Dorland's Illustrated Medical Dictionary, 25th ed., W.B. Saunders, Philadelphia, 1974.
3. Kirby KA: Foot and Lower Extremity Biomechanics II: Precision Intricast Newsletters, 1997–2002. Precision Intricast, Inc., Payson, AZ, 2002.
4. Dagnall JC: History of foot supports. British J Chiropody, 32 (1):5–7, 1967.
5. Whitman R: Observations of forty-five cases of flat-foot with particular reference to etiology and treatment. Boston Med Surg J, 118:598, 1888.
6. Whitman R: The importance of positive support in the curative treatment of weak feet and a comparison of the means employed to assure it. Am J Orth Surg, 11:215–230, 1913.
7. Roberts PW: The initial strain in weak foot, its mechanics, and a new method of treatment. N Y Med J, 102(9):441–442, 1915.
8. Morton DJ: The Human Foot: Its Evolution, Physiology and Functional Disorders. Columbia University Press, New York, 1935.
9. Helfet AJ: A new way of treating flat feet in children. Lancet, 1:262–267, 1956.
10. Root ML: How was the Root functional orthotic developed? Podiatry Arts Lab Newsletter, 1981.
11. Lee WE: Podiatric biomechanics: an historical appraisal and discussion of the Root model as a clinical system of approach in the present context of theoretical uncertainty. Clin Pod Med Surg, 18:555–684, 2001.
12. Root ML, Orien WP, Weed JH, RJ Hughes: Biomechanical Examination of the Foot, Volume 1. Clinical Biomechanics Corporation, Los Angeles, 1971.
13. Henderson WH, Campbell JW: U.C.B.L. shoe insert casting and fabrication. Technical Report 53. Biomechanics Laboratory, University of California at San Francisco and Berkeley, 1967.
14. Blake RL, Denton JA: Functional foot orthoses for athletic injuries: A retrospective study. JAPMA, 75:359–362, 1985.
15. Blake RL: Inverted functional orthoses. JAPMA, 76:275–276, 1986.
16. Blake RL, Ferguson H: Foot orthoses for the severe flatfoot in sports. JAPMA, 81:549, 1991.

17. Kirby KA: The medial heel skive technique: improving pronation control in foot orthoses. JAPMA, 82: 177–188, 1992.
18. Kirby KA: Foot and Lower Extremity Biomechanics: A Ten Year Collection of Precision Intricast Newsletters. Precision Intricast, Inc., Payson, AZ, 1997.
19. Valmassy RL (ed.): Clinical Biomechanics of the Lower Extremities. Mosby, St. Louis, 1996.
20. Sackett DL, Rosenberg WMC, Gray JAM et al.: Evidence based medicine: what it is and what it isn't. Br Med J, 312:71–72., 1996.
21. Kirby KA: Emerging concepts in podiatric biomechanics. Podiatry Today, 19(12):36–48, 2006.
22. Eggold JF: Orthotics in the prevention of runner's overuse injuries. Phys Sports Med, 9:181–185, 1981.
23. D'Ambrosia RD: Orthotic devices in running injuries. Clin Sports Med, 4:611–618, 1985.
24. Dugan RC, D'Ambrosia RD: The effect of orthotics on the treatment of selected running injuries. Foot Ankle, 6:313, 1986.
25. Kilmartin TE, Wallace WA: The scientific basis for the use of biomechanical foot orthoses in the treatment of lower limb sports injuries-a review of the literature. Br J Sports Med, 28:180–184, 1994.
26. Gross ML, Davlin LB, Evanski PM: Effectiveness of orthotic shoe inserts in the long distance runner. Am J Sports Med, 19:409–412, 1991.
27. Blake RL, Denton JA: Functional foot orthoses for athletic injuries: A retrospective study. JAPMA, 75:359–362, 1985.
28. Saxena A, Haddad J: The effect of foot orthoses on patellofemoral pain syndrome. JAPMA, 93:264–271, 2003.
29. Donatelli R, Hurlbert C, Conaway D, St. Pierre R: Biomechanical foot orthotics: A retrospective study. J Ortho Sp Phys Ther, 10:205–212, 1988.
30. Moraros J, Hodge W: Orthotic survey: Preliminary results. JAPMA, 83:139–148, 1993.
31. Walter JH, Ng G, Stoitz JJ: A patient satisfaction survey on prescription custom-molded foot orthoses. JAPMA, 94:363–367, 2004
32. Kusomoto A, Suzuki T, Yoshida H, Kwon J: Intervention study to improve quality of life and health problems of community-living elderly women in Japan by shoe fitting and custom-made insoles. Gerontology, 22:110–118, 2007.
33. Finestone A, Giladi M, Elad H et al.: Prevention of stress fractures using custom biomechanical shoe orthoses. Clin Orth Rel Research, 360:182–190, 1999.
34. Simkin A, Leichter I, Giladi M et al.: Combined effect of foot arch structure and an orthotic device on stress fractures. Foot Ankle, 10:25–29, 1989.
35. Eng JJ, Pierrynowski MR: Evaluation of soft foot orthotics in the treatment of patellofemoral pain syndrome. Phys Therapy, 73:62–70, 1993.
36. Thompson JA, Jennings MB, Hodge W: Orthotic therapy in the management of osteoarthritis. JAPMA, 82:136–139, 1992.
37. Marks R, Penton L: Are foot orthotics efficacious for treating painful medial compartment knee osteoarthritis? A review of the literature. Int J Clin Practice, 58:49–57, 2004.
38. Gross MT, Byers JM, Krafft JL et al.: The impact of custom semirigid foot orthotics on pain and disability for individuals with plantar fasciitis. J Ortho Sp Phys Ther, 32:149–157, 2002.
39. Slattery M, Tinley P: The efficacy of functional foot orthoses in the control of pain and ankle joint disintegration in hemophilia. JAPMA, 91:240–244, 2001.
40. Chalmers AC, Busby C, Goyert J et al.: Metatarsalgia and rheumatoid arthritis-a randomized, single blind, sequential trial comparing two types of foot orthoses and supportive shoes. J Rheum, 27:1643–1647, 2000.
41. Woodburn J, Barker S, Helliwell PS: A randomized controlled trial of foot orthoses in rheumatoid arthritis. J Rheum, 29:1377–1383, 2002.
42. Mejjad O, Vittecoq O, Pouplin S et al.: Foot orthotics decrease pain but do not improve gait in rheumatoid arthritis patients. Joint Bone Spine, 71:542–545, 2004.

43. Powell M, Seid M, Szer IA: Efficacy of custom foot orthotics in improving pain and functional status in children with juvenile idiopathic arthritis: A randomized trial. J Rheum, 32:943–950, 2005.

44. Rose GK: Correction of the pronated foot. JBJS, 40B:674–683, 1958.

45. Rose GK: Correction of the pronated foot. JBJS, 44B:642–647, 1962.

46. Sgarlato TE (ed.): A Compendium of Podiatric Biomechanics. California College of Podiatric Medicine, San Francisco, 1971.

47. Kirby KA, Green DR: Evaluation and Nonoperative Management of Pes Valgus, pp. 295–327. in DeValentine S.(ed.), Foot and Ankle Disorders in Children. Churchill-Livingstone, New York, 1992.

48. Kirby KA: Methods for determination of positional variations in the subtalar joint axis. JAPMA, 77:228–234, 1987.

49. Kirby KA: Rotational equilibrium across the subtalar joint axis. JAPMA, 79:1–14, 1989.

50. Kirby KA: Subtalar joint axis location and rotational equilibrium theory of foot function. JAPMA, 91:465–488, 2001.

51. Blake RL, Ferguson H: The inverted orthotic technique: Its role in clinical biomechanics, pp. 465–497. in Valmassy RL(ed.), Clinical Biomechanics of the Lower Extremities, Mosby-Year Book, St. Louis, 1996.

52. Kirby KA: Lateral heel skive orthosis technique. Precision Intricast Newsletter. Precision Intricast, Inc., Payson, AZ, September 2004.

53. Nigg BM: The assessment of loads acting on the locomotor system in running and other sports activities. Seminars in Orthopaedics, 3:(4) 197–206, 1988.

54. Nigg BM, Bobbert M: On the potential of various approaches in load analysis to reduce the frequency of sports injuries. J Biomech 23:3–12, 1990.

55. Morlock M, Nigg BM: Theoretical consideration and practical results on the influence of the representation of the foot for the estimation of internal forces with models. Clin Biomech, 6:3–13, 1991.

56. McPoil TG, Hunt GC: Evaluation and management of foot and ankle disorders: Present problems and future directions. JOSPT, 21:381–388, 1995.

57. Fuller EA: Computerized gait evaluation, pp. 179–205. in Valmassy RL(ed.), Clinical Biomechanics of the Lower Extremities, Mosby-Year Book, St. Louis, 1996.

58. Fuller EA: Center of pressure and its theoretical relationship to foot pathology. JAPMA, 89(6):278–291, 1999.

59. Fuller EA: Reinventing biomechanics. Podiatry Today, 13:(3), December 2000.

60. Fuller EA, Kirby KA: Subtalar joint equilibrium and tissue stress approach to biomechanical therapy of the foot and lower extremity. In Albert S (ed.), Lower Extremity Biomechanics: Theory and Practice, pending publication, 2007.

61. Nigg BM, Nurse MA, Stefanyshyn DJ: Shoe inserts and orthotics for sport and physical activities. Med Sci Sports Exerc, 31(Suppl):S421–S428, 1999.

62. Nigg BM: The role of impact forces and foot pronation: a new paradigm. Clin J Sport Med, 11:2–9, 2001.

63. Payne CB: The past, present, and future of podiatric biomechanics. JAPMA, 88:53–63, 1998.

64. Bates BT, Osternig LR, Mason B, James LS: Foot orthotic devices to modify selected aspects of lower extremity mechanics. Am J Sp Med, 7:328–31, 1979.

65. Smith LS, Clarke TE, Hamill CL, Santopietro F: The effects of soft and semi-rigid orthoses upon rearfoot movement in running. JAPMA, 76:227–232, 1986.

66. Novick A, Kelley DL: Position and movement changes of the foot with orthotic intervention during loading response of gait. J Ortho Sp Phys Ther, 11:301–312, 1990.

67. McCulloch MU, Brunt D, Linden DV: The effect of foot orthotics and gait velocity on lower limb kinematics and temporal events of stance. J Ortho Sp Phys Ther, 17:2–10, 1993.

68. Butler RJ, McClay-Davis IS, Laughton CM, Hughes M. Dual-function foot orthosis: Effect on shock and control of rearfoot motion. Foot Ankle Intl, 24:410–414, 2003.

69. Laughton CA, McClay-Davis IS, Hamill J: Effect of strike pattern and orthotic intervention on tibial shock during running. J Appl Biomech, 19:153–16, 2003.

70. Mundermann A, Nigg BM, Humble RN, Stefanyshyn DJ. Foot orthoses affect lower extremity kinematics and kinetics during running. Clin Biomech, 18:254–262, 2003.
71. Williams DS, McClay-Davis I, Baitch SP: Effect of inverted orthoses on lower extremity mechanics in runners. Med Sci Sports Exerc 35:2060–2068, 2003.
72. MacLean CL, Hamill J: Short and long-term influence of a custom foot orthotic intervention on lower extremity dynamics in injured runners. Annual ISB Meeting, Cleveland, September 2005.
73. Eng JJ, Pierrynowski MR: The effect of soft foot orthotics on three-dimensional lower-limb kinematics during walking and running. Phys Therapy, 74:836–844, 1994.
74. Nawoczenski DA, Cook TM, Saltzman CL: The effect of foot orthotics on three-dimensional kinematics of the leg and rearfoot during running. J Ortho Sp Phys Ther, 21:317–327, 1995.
75. Stackhouse CL, Davis IM, Hamill J: Orthotic intervention in forefoot and rearfoot strike running patterns. Clin Biomech, 19:64–70, 2004.
76. Nester CJ, Hutchins S, Bowker P: Effect of foot orthoses on rearfoot complex kinematics during walking gait. Foot Ankle Intl, 22:133–139, 2001.
77. Nester CJ, Van Der Linden ML, Bowker P: Effect of foot orthoses on the kinematics and kinetics of normal walking gait. Gait Posture, 17:180–187, 2003.
78. Woodburn J, Helliwell PS, Barker S: Changes in 3D joint kinematics support the continuous use of orthoses in the management of painful rearfoot deformity in rheumatoid arthritis. J Rheum, 30:2356–2364, 2003.
79. Nawoczenski DA, Ludewig PM: Electromyographic effects of foot orthotics on selected lower extremity muscles during running. Arch Phys Med Rehab, 80:540–544, 1999.
80. Tomaro J, Burdett RG: The effects of foot orthotics on the EMG activity of selected leg muscles during gait. J Ortho Sp Phys Ther, 18:532–536, 1993.
81. Mundermann A, Wakeling JM, Nigg BM et al.: Foot orthoses affect frequency components of muscle activity in the lower extremity. Gait Posture, 23:295–302, 2006.
82. Mundermann A, Nigg BM, Humble RN, Stefanyshyn DJ: Orthotic comfort is related to kinematics, kinetics, and EMG in recreational runners. Med Sci Sports Exercise, 35:1710–1719, 2003.
83. Guskiewicz KM, Perrin DH: Effects of orthotics on postural sway following inversion ankle sprain. J Orthop Sp Phys Ther, 23:326–331, 1996.
84. Hertel J, Denegar CR, Buckley WE et al.: Effect of rearfoot orthotics on postural control in healthy subjects. J Sport Rehab, 10:36–47, 2001.
85. Rome K, Brown CL: Randomized clinical trial into the impact of rigid foot orthoses on balance parameters in excessively pronated feet. Clin Rehab, 18:624–630, 2004.
86. Burns J, Crosbie J, Ouvrier R, Hunt A: Effective orthotic therapy for the painful cavus foot. JAPMA, 96:205–211, 2006.
87. Postema K, Burm PE, Zande ME, Limbeek J: Primary metatarsalgia: the influence of a custom moulded insole and a rockerbar on plantar pressure. Prosthet Orthot Int, 22:35–44, 1998.
88. Li CY, Imaishi K, Shiba N et al.: Biomechanical evaluation of foot pressure and loading force during gait in rheumatoid arthritic patients with and without foot orthoses. Kurume Med J, 47:211–217, 2000.
89. Lobmann R, Kayser R, Kasten G et al.: Effects of preventative footwear on foot pressure as determined by pedobarography in diabetic patients: a prospective study. Diabet Med, 18:314–319, 2001.
90. Duffin AC, Kidd R, Chan A, Donaghue KC: High plantar pressure and callus in diabetic adolescents. Incidence and treatment. JAPMA, 93:214–220, 2003.
91. Raspovic A, Newcombe L, Lloyd J, Dalton E: Effect of customized insoles on vertical plantar pressures in sites of previous neuropathic ulceration in the diabetic foot. The Foot, 10:133–138, 2000.
92. Cheung JT, Zhang M: A 3-dimensional finite element model of the human foot and ankle for insole design. Arch Phys Med Rehab. 2005;86:353–358.

Chapter 3
Athletic Foot Types and Deformities

Tim Dutra

The feet of athletes of all ages can be categorized as belonging to one of three specific types: rectus, planus, or cavus. Some athletes who are affected with congenital deformities and who suffer from chronic pain, discomfort, or reoccurring injuries can be treated. Examples of treatable deformities are discussed in this chapter. A basic knowledge of these foot types is necessary for athletes, certified athletic trainers, and sports medicine professionals. With this knowledge, sensible and informed decisions can be made in selecting appropriate footwear and orthoses in their sport. This chapter briefly discusses foot motion and mechanics as well as reviews common sports injuries relating to the deformities of the foot that can predispose athletes to these conditions.

Normal Foot Motion and Biomechanics During Gait

A brief review of the gait cycle is necessary to understand the pathomechanics of the common athletic injuries we discuss in this chapter [1–5]. The next chapter reviews clinical methods available to perform gait analysis. The gait cycle consists of four key phases: heel strike, midstance, toe-off, and swing phase.

At heel strike, the heel contacts the ground in a slightly supinated position on the lateral aspect of the heel and pronates (more flexible) until the foot contacts the ground. The heel transitions from a supinated position to a more neutral position, and the pronation of the foot allows for adaptation to the ground as the lower leg rotates internally. During midstance, foot pronation decreases as the foot prepares for toe-off. During the toe-off stage, the foot supinates (more rigid) and the heel rises during propulsion. Lastly, the foot goes through the fourth stage, the swing phase as the foot is preparing for heel strike of the opposite foot. Running includes a double float phase in which neither foot is in contact with the surface.

T. Dutra (✉)
Student Health Services, California State University, Hayward, CA, USA

M.B. Werd, E.L. Knight (eds.), *Athletic Footwear and Orthoses in Sports Medicine*,
DOI 10.1007/978-0-387-76416-0_3, © Springer Science+Business Media, LLC 2010

Foot Types

Rectus foot type is a foot with normal foot structure with an average arch and an average calcaneal inclination angle. Injuries to athletes with this foot type typically do not involve instability or abnormal motion available at the joints. Clinically, pes planus and pes cavus foot types are treated most often.

Pes planus is a flat foot, with a moderate or more loss of the longitudinal arch of the foot. Pes planus can be classified clinically into rigid or flexible. Characteristics of a pronated foot include uneven weight distribution, increased flexibility, increased calcaneal eversion, and associated pathologies. Pathologies include hallux valgus, hammertoes, neuromas, medial knee pain, and hip/lower back problems. There are congenital causes and functional causes. Congenital causes include equines, ligamentous laxity, ankle valgus, and peroneal spastic flatfoot. Functional causes include compensated forefoot varus, transverse plane compensation, and leg length difference.

In rigid pes planus, the range of motion is decreased at the tarsal and subtalar joints. The arch does not rise with toe rising. Possible causes include a tarsal coalition and peroneal spasticity. Flexible pes planus is physiologic or pathologic, depending on ligamentous laxity, motor weakness in the foot muscles, or bone abnormalities. These can be categorized further into three types.

Functional flat foot (calcaneovalgus) is the most common type of flat foot with athletes. It is physiologic with a decreased longitudinal arch associated with heel eversion (calcaneovalgus). It is usually not painful or cause of disability in the athlete. Treatment usually consists of adequate heel counter support and orthotic therapy.

Hypermobile flat foot is associated with ligamentous laxity with tight heel chords. Possible causes include tarsal coalition, vertical talus, or accessory navicular. Treatment focuses on stretching exercises for the Achilles tendon and orthotic therapy.

Pes planus with posterior tibial tendon dysfunction evolves through a series of three stages so it is imperative to recognize and treat this type early and aggressive. In stage 1, the posterior tibial tendon is normal length with the tendon showing degenerative changes. Typically there is mild-to-moderate pain symptoms along the posterior tibial tendon. Classically, the pain is localized a few centimeters distal to the tip of the medial malleolus, coursing along to the plantar attachment to the navicular bone. A single heel rise may reveal mild-to-moderate weakness of the tendon. Treatment is conservative with modifying the activity and using orthotic therapy. In stage 2, the posterior tibial tendon elongates, with the rearfoot becoming more mobile. Pain can be along the length of the tendon. The forefoot becomes abducted on the rearfoot, so if viewed from behind "too many toes" are observed. A single heel raise can show significant weakness. Treatment usually requires surgical consideration following an MRI evaluation. In stage 3, there is posterior tibial tendon rupture. The rearfoot becomes rigid and a fixed rigid flatfoot develops. This deformity is a dramatic presentation. A surgical arthrodesis can be required due to the severe pain with this progression.

Pes cavus is a high arched foot with an elevation of the longitudinal arch, which is present with and without weight bearing. The toes can be contracted in the more severe cases. Characteristics include decreased pronation, rigid foot, weight unevenly distributed, and a tendency for later ankle instability leading to frequent inversion ankle sprains. There is limited range of motion and poor shock absorption. In the athlete the cavus foot is usually a static idiopathic presentation. Neuromuscular causes are progressive in nature. Pes cavus can be congenital or functional in nature. Congenital causes include plantar flexed first ray, peroneal spasm/weakness, and metatarsus adductus. Functional causes include leg length difference, uncompensated rearfoot varus, partially compensated rearfoot varus, or compensated rigid forefoot valgus. Treatment consists of shoes with cushioning, orthotics for support, and stretching exercises of the plantar fascia and Achilles tendon.

Functional Foot Disorders

Functional foot disorders can be in the frontal, sagittal, or transverse planes. The frontal plane involves the varus or valgus of the rearfoot or forefoot. These can be uncompensated, partially compensated, or compensated. The sagittal plane involves equines, and the transverse plane involves femoral or tibial torsion.

Examples of Foot Deformities in Athletes

- Rearfoot varus: a frontal plane deformity where the calcaneus is inverted when the foot is maintained in a subtalar joint neutral position.
- Rearfoot valgus: a frontal plane deformity where the calcaneus is everted when the foot is maintained in a subtalar joint neutral position.
- Metatarsus adductus: a transverse plane deformity where the forefoot is adducted when compared to the position of the rearfoot. This is also called a c-shaped foot.
- Plantarflexed first ray: a sagittal plane deformity where the first metatarsal is plantarflexed in comparison to the other metatarsals when the foot is in its neutral position.
- Ankle equinus: a sagittal plane deformity where there is less than 10° of available dorsiflexion at the ankle joint when the subtalar joint is in its neutral position and the midtarsal joint is fully locked.
- Forefoot valgus: a frontal plane deformity where the forefoot is everted in reference to the rearfoot when the foot is maintained in a subtalar joint neutral position.
- Forefoot varus: a frontal plane deformity where the forefoot is inverted in reference to the rearfoot when the foot is maintained in a subtalar neutral position.

Lower Extremity Pathology

Most common lower extremity pathologies are a result of abnormal foot function. This section reviews which foot types are responsible for causing these pathologic conditions. Evidence-based orthotic treatment recommendations for many of the following conditions are included in Chapter 11.

Calcaneal Apophysitis

Calcaneal apophysitis is a painful condition that affects the growth plate of the calcaneus in young athletes in the 8–15 year age group. Pain is experienced with running and jumping activities in a variety of sports such as basketball, baseball, and soccer. Pain can be reproduced with the squeeze test, applying medial and lateral calcaneal compression to the heel. This condition is related to tight posterior muscle group and plantar fascia. Foot types which can be associated with this condition include forefoot varus (compensated or partially compensated), forefoot supinatus, flexible forefoot valgus, or a compensated equinus or transverse plane deformity. With regard to athletic shoes, a negative heel and poor heel counter can contribute to the problem, as well as poor cushioning of the shoe (Fig. 3.1).

Kohler's Disease

Kohler's disease is osteochondritis affecting the navicular bone in young children ages 3–9 years old. Symptoms affect the dorsal medial aspect of the navicular

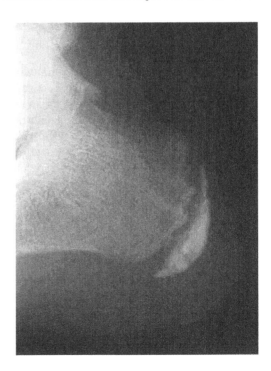

Fig. 3.1 Lateral x-ray view of young athlete with calcaneal apophysitis

area, often causing an antalgic gait with increased lateral column weight bearing to decrease pain.

Freiberg's Disease

Freiberg's disease is osteochondrosis of the lesser metatarsal heads. There is a loss of blood supply to the metatarsal heads, generally affecting the second metatarsal head. Most commonly it occurs in the 13–15 age group. Pain and swelling are localized and motion is guarded.

Heel Spur Syndrome or Plantar Fasciitis

Plantar fasciitis is a common condition with pain at the medial plantar aspect of the calcaneus with pain classically in the morning or following periods of rest. Pain can be present during activity. This pain may be associated with inflammation at the origin of the plantar fascia on the calcaneus or as a periosteal reaction to heel spur formation. Both pes cavus and pes planus can lead to this condition. With pes planus the plantar fascia is chronically stretched during foot flattening with excessive calcaneal eversion. Conversely, with a high arch the plantar fascia that is taut and contracted can also lead to this condition. Most causes of heel spur syndrome are mechanical. X-rays can demonstrate the progression of minimal periosteal involvement which can eventually lead to plantar spur formation (Fig. 3.2).

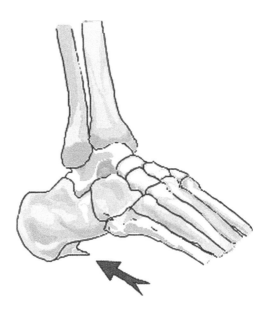

Fig. 3.2 Plantar calcaneal heel spur at origin of plantar fascia

Sesamoiditis

Sesamoiditis causes pain and inflammation plantar to the first metatarsal head from excessive pressure to the area during activity. Pain symptoms are present with joint motion and with muscle testing. Predisposing conditions include plantarflexed first metatarsal, enlarged sesamoids, trauma to the area, and inadequate shoes. X-ray evaluation can be difficult due to bipartite sesamoids. A bone scan may be necessary in some cases. Orthoses can help this condition by controlling pronation and accommodating the sesamoid area with forefoot extensions such as a reverse Morton's extension which supports metatarsals 2–5 and effectively off loads the area (Fig. 3.3).

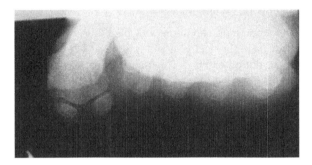

Fig. 3.3 Plantar axial view of the sesamoids demonstrates abnormal tibial sesamoid with fracture. It is important to differentiate between bipartite and fracture of the sesamoid. Sometimes a bone scan is needed to confirm diagnosis

Stress Fracture

Stress fracture is usually caused from repetitive trauma to the area. Faulty foot mechanics can cause and aggravate this painful condition. Pain is usually local with mild edema and erythema and made worse with activity. Commonly the neck or shaft of a lesser metatarsal or a sesamoid is involved. Orthoses can be very helpful in controlling the faulty foot mechanics. Adequate shock absorption is needed with shoe gear and orthotics (Fig. 3.4).

Ankle Sprains

Ankle sprains, especially inversion type, are very common in athletics. The injury involves the ligamentous structures of the ankle, most commonly the lateral collateral ligaments due to inversion stress to the ankle in an unstable position. Frequent ankle sprains or lateral ankle instability can be associated with ligamentous laxity or supinated foot types primarily with the heel inverted, especially with a forefoot valgus deformity or a rearfoot varus (uncompensated or partially compensated)

Fig. 3.4 Stress fracture of the
shaft of the third metatarsal

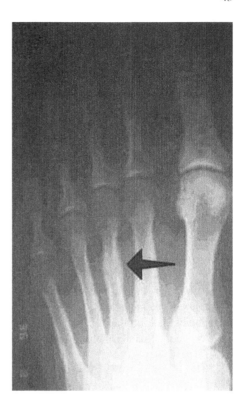

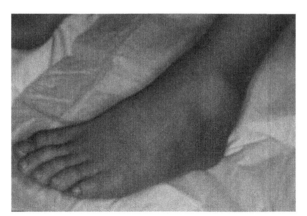

Fig. 3.5 Clinical presentation of acute inversion ankle sprain with erythema and edema of the
lateral aspect of the ankle

deformity. Orthoses addressing the lateral column instability can help with a forefoot posting. Mid-to-high top athletic shoes can provide additional ankle support for
the athlete during activity (Fig. 3.5).

Patellofemoral Dysfunction

With patellofemoral dysfunction patients have chronic symptoms of pain around the patella with activity. Contributing factors include weak vastus medialis, anatomical variation of the patella and knee joint, and abnormal pronation which increases transverse plane torsion at the knee joint. This condition can be controlled with functional orthotics by reducing subtalar joint pronation and internal rotation of the tibia, allowing the patella to track primarily in the sagittal plane.

Interdigital Neuroma

Interdigital neuroma presents with pain located in the interspace, most commonly the third interspace. This pain typically radiates to the adjacent digits. The symptoms increase with activity. Neuromas are aggravated by tight shoes and associated with abnormal subtalar and midtarsal joint pronation which causes an increase in the transverse plane motion at the metatarsals. Orthoses attempt to control the excessive transverse plane motion of the forefoot during midstance and propulsion during gait, specifically between the medial and lateral columns. The medial column is made up of the first three metatarsals articulating with the cuneiforms. The lateral column is made up of the fourth and fifth metatarsals articulating with the cuboid. A metatarsal raise or "met cookie" is helpful in relieving the pain, as well as switching to a wider shoe.

Achilles Tendonitis

The most common area of involvement of the Achilles tendon is the areas proximal to the insertion of the calcaneus. It may be caused by tightness of the Achilles tendon or strenuous activity. A pronated foot type can cause increased frontal plane torquing of the tendon, much like wringing a wash rag. The Achilles pad in the heel of the shoe must not irritate the tendon (Fig. 3.6).

Posterior Tibial Tendonitis

Posterior tibial tendonitis presents with pain behind the medial malleolus or at the insertion of the tendon into the navicular bone. It is usually seen with a pronated foot type that pulls the tendon at the insertion at the navicular bone. Commonly it is associated with an accessory navicular tuberosity (os tibiale externum). A spontaneous rupture or chronic dysfunction can lead to a markedly pronated foot ("too many toes" sign). Orthoses are often necessary to treat this condition and control the pronatory forces.

Hallux Abducto Valgus

Hallux abducto valgus involves a prominence of the medial or dorsomedial aspect of the first metatarsal head. There is an associated increased adduction of the first

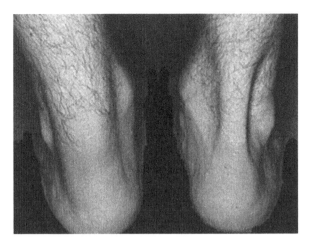

Fig. 3.6   Achilles tendonitis of the *left foot* with severe inflammation as compared with the *right foot*

metatarsal. Commonly there is hypermobility of the first ray with a forefoot adductus type of the foot. There are four basic stages of hallux abducto valgus deformity. In stage 1, there is lateral displacement of the proximal phalanx relative to the first metatarsal head. In stage 2, there is hallux abductus with the hallux abducted against the second toe. In stage 3, there is a development of metatarsus primus adductus leading to an increased angle between the first and second metatarsals. Stage 4 is the end stage with a dislocation of the first metatarsal phalangeal joint with loss of joint congruity. Orthoses are most useful in the treatment of the earlier stages because they can control the abnormal intrinsic and extrinsic muscle function.

Hammer Toe Deformity

Hammer toe deformity involves a contraction of a digit with varus rotation of the toe. Possible causes can be abnormal pronation of the subtalar joint, plantarflexion of the metatarsal, reduced lumbrical muscle function, a forefoot valgus, or hallux abducto valgus deformity.

Tailor's Bunion

Tailor's bunion is a deformity involving a painful enlargement or prominence of the fifth metatarsal head. Causes include increased subtalar joint pronation, dorsiflexion or plantarflexion of the fifth ray, or an uncompensated varus deformity. The fifth ray becomes subluxed. Abnormal pronation alone does not cause this deformity. Often orthoses will not help this condition if abnormal pronation is not the causing this deformity in the athlete.

Treatment

Treatment considerations for athletes with these common conditions involve proper athletic shoes for their sport and often functional orthoses as well. Remember, the orthosis is only as good as the athletic shoe that you put it in. Athletic shoes and orthoses need to be continually monitored for wear and support of the athlete. Depending on the sport, size of the athlete, and the intensity of the sport, the athletic shoe may need to be replaced several times during a season. Shoes that the athlete trains in must also allow for proper support and control for the athlete. Deformities such as hallux abducto valgus, hammer toes, and tailor's bunions must be specially addressed in fitting the athlete for shoe comfort and design. The orthosis must fit well in the shoe and sit properly in the foot bed. Some sports require a low-profile type of orthotic device, as well as less bulky forefoot extensions or cushioning. Often times a rearfoot post will not be fit in the shoe and thus the unposted orthosis will fit in the shoe better. Ultrathin flexible graphite can work well for many of these sports as it is low-profile orthosis.

References

1. Gordon GM, Contompasisi JP: Sports Medicine. Clinics in Podiatric Medicine and Surgery, W. B. Saunders Company, Philadelphia, PA, October 1986.
2. Jones LJ: Shoes, Orthoses, and Related Biomechanics. Clinics in Podiatric Medicine and Surgery, W.B. Saunders Company, Philadelphia, PA, April 1994.
3. MacAuley D, Best TM: Evidence-based Sports Medicine, BMJ Books, London, 2002.
4. Torg JS: Ankle and Foot Problems in the Athlete. Clinics in Sports Medicine, W.B. Saunders Company, Philadelphia, PA, March 1982.
5. Valmassy RL: Clinical Biomechanics of the Lower Extremities, Mosby, St. Louis, 1996.

Chapter 4
Clinical Gait Evaluation of the Athlete

Bruce Williams

How an athlete walks and runs is a key element to the functional capacity of their chosen sport. Being able to fully evaluate these motions can give practitioners a tremendous amount of information in aiding athletic patients. Running and walking mechanics were first recorded using filming techniques in the 1800s [1]. Over the last 40 years, gait analysis techniques have evolved from 2D to full 3D kinematic studies. Ground reaction forces have evolved from force plate analysis to include in-shoe pressure systems. The combination of 3-dimensional (3D) kinematic data and ground reaction forces has led to the potential for specific joint force calculations through kinetics, and now joint coupling techniques to understand how one joint potentially affects another [2, 3].

Many of the techniques used above are available in comprehensive gait analysis laboratories in hospitals and major universities. The literature has many examples of high-tech sports evaluations from ankle sprain rehabilitation to golf swing analysis to the improvement of running form for patellar knee problems [4–6] (Fig. 4.1).

From a clinical perspective, the research gait lab is not usually economically feasible, nor is it timely to evaluate athletes to the levels of a comprehensive gait analysis laboratory. However, there are effective technologies available that can be utilized in-office or in-clinic that are affordable and much less time consuming.

Literature backs the use of in-shoe pressure evaluation as well as 2D video analysis [7–9]. Pressure mapping technologies in small affordable mats are available that can give immediate feedback mimicking stabilometry at a fraction of the cost [10]. In-office cycling setups can incorporate video, power metering, and in-shoe evaluations to see how positioning can improve overall function [11, 12]. Relevant technologies are available for use in the clinic setting which will benefit athletes at every level.

Many evaluation processes started with simple tests or visual analyses of patient function. Visual, or observational, gait analysis is a staple of most sports clinician's evaluations. Because it is extremely subjective, observational gait analysis has been

B. Williams (✉)
Private Practice, Breakthrough Podiatry, Merrillville, IN, 46410, USA

M.B. Werd, E.L. Knight (eds.), *Athletic Footwear and Orthoses in Sports Medicine*,
DOI 10.1007/978-0-387-76416-0_4, © Springer Science+Business Media, LLC 2010

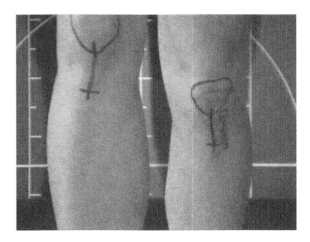

Fig. 4.1 2D kinematic evaluation of patellar tracking

shown to be unreliable as the eye cannot detect certain locomotor events that occur in less than 1/12 of a second [13, 14]. The use of the Romberg test to determine stability of a patient after ankle sprain is common as well [15]. Unfortunately, many of these tests are extremely subjective and decisions made from the performance of the test may be arbitrary. This is often why technology has been introduced into sports and clinical testing. Clinicians want to make sure tests are repeatable and provide information that mimics study equivalent data as often as possible. Technology can help document quantitatively a progression of healing from an injury. A brief overview of the available affordable technologies on the market will be presented.

Technology

What techniques are involved in the clinical environment for in-office gait evaluation of the athlete? Evaluations can be broken down into (1) digital video analysis, where you can choose 2-dimensional (2D) vs. 3-dimensional (3D) analysis; (2) pressure analysis, where options range from force plates to pressure mats to in-shoe analysis. These modalities can be utilized singularly, or for the best possible outcomes, in conjunction.

Digital Video Analysis: 3D Analysis

3D analysis is usually much too expensive and time consuming for the clinical practice. Most labs utilizing this capability are found at major teaching hospitals and universities. The information derived from the utilization of this technology drives clinical research in athletics and gait analysis, but day-to-day multipatient utilization is often beyond a smaller practice business paradigm.

Digital Video Analysis: 2D Analysis

2D video analysis is probably the most inexpensive way to start with gait analysis. A simple video camera can be used to start and provides much more information than just utilizing the naked eye. 2D video analysis also allows for slow motion playback for frame-by-frame analysis. Most 2D systems now offer single or multiple synchronized and non-synchronized camera views. This means that you can watch an athlete from right and left, posterior and/or anterior views, and also overhead. These views can be studied in conjunction, or singularly, which gives great insight into how an athlete moves when they walk, run, or perform their sport from almost any perspective.

Most 2D video analysis software can provide the calculation of joint angles (Fig. 4.2). In joints that function primarily in the Sagittal plane, the knee and hip for example, the angles are very close to what will be calculated from 3D video systems. Foot and camera placement can obviously effect these angle calculations, but generalized determinations can still be calculated and recorded [3].

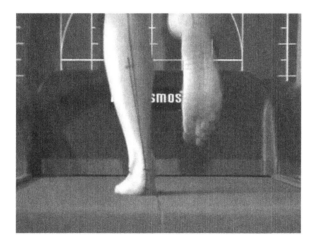

Fig. 4.2 Calcaneal position tracking utilizing 2D kinematics

Pressure Analysis

Pressure analysis consists of utilizing pressure mapping or force plate technology to understand how a patient's foot functions in certain situations of gait or during athletic performance. The devices available for pressure mapping range from the relatively inexpensive, pressure mats, to in-shoe pressure devices and finally the most expensive, force plates.

If true 3D gait analysis is needed to calculate kinetic data to understand the forces at work at differing joints within the lower extremity, then a force plate with 3D kinematic video is necessary. Force plates are expensive and stationary. They will give little to no feedback regarding foot orthosis usage or modification because they can't be used within a shoe. In some studies, force plates have been integrated into treadmills [16]. This has allowed some labs to work closely with runners to affect changes in certain lower extremity pain syndromes just from small technique and positioning modifications to a running gait [5]. Force plates also provide shear force data, which no other pressure evaluation tool can.

Mat scans, or stationary pressure mapping "squares," are very reasonable in cost compared to force plates, and again provide no in-shoe use potential. They offer the potential of acquiring some very useful data for comparing barefoot static stance pressure images of one or both feet, and barefoot single-step functional images right and left separately. Some systems now incorporate a gait walkway that can be 20–40 feet long and allows acquisition of multiple functional barefoot data.

In-shoe pressure analysis serves several functions. The cost of in-shoe pressure analysis is more toward the cost of a mat scan than to that of a force plate (Fig. 4.3). Utilizing in-shoe pressure analysis, calculations can be made by multi-step force vs. time curves that can help quickly identify stoppages in foot motion that can then be addressed through orthosis modification. This is effective for before and after comparisons of orthosis function and works well in a step-wise approach for clinical orthosis outcomes [7, 17, 18].

Most in-shoe modules now come with the option of having a mobile or non-tethered unit, which is advantageous in sports medicine. Recordings with a mobile unit can be done outside of a lab, on a playing field, or wherever a recording is desired. This allows the potential to record an athlete during active running or while performing their sport and can be or great benefit.

Finally, there is opportunity to synchronize 2D or 3D video capture with the pressure analysis systems. This really shows what is going on with each step of the athlete's function and can help to quickly analyze their function as needed.

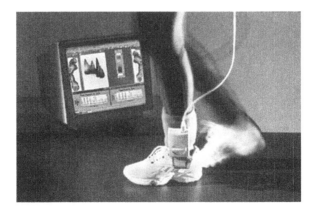

Fig. 4.3 In-shoe pressure analysis module

Methodology

Some form of methodology needs to be described that can uniformly be used for evaluation of video and pressure mapping data gathered in a clinical format.

Video Analysis Methodology

From a strictly 2D perspective when capturing and analyzing video of an athlete's gait and/or sport function, one needs to know exactly what to focus on. Since this textbook deals primarily with shoe and foot orthosis function, a system that works well in private practice will be discussed. Clinical video data capture of walking and running will usually be done utilizing an in-office walkway or a treadmill. The advantage of the walkway is that it will not greatly affect the patient's self-selected speed of walking or running. A disadvantage is that due to space allowances, most walkways abut a wall, which usually only allows a sagittal plane capture from one side, right or left, at a time. Cameras can be set up at either end of the walkway to capture anterior frontal and posterior frontal plane views as well. To capture a full-length sagittal view, some sort of movable tracking system would have to be put in place. Otherwise, the sagittal plane view captured on a walkway will really only have a 3–4 foot wide area that will have the camera as close to 90° as possible to the foot strike.

If a treadmill is used instead, then one can capture a much truer, sagittal plane image from both right and left sides of the athlete while also utilizing anterior, frontal, and posterior frontal views. In some labs, an overhead view is utilized above the treadmill. This can offer some very different information regarding rotation of the trunk on the hips and lower extremities. Treadmills are not without their downsides though as they make it difficult for patients to self-select running and walking speeds and they can alter a patients normal gait pattern until they become used to the treadmill experience [19].

Data capture can be recorded utilizing both barefoot and shod walking and/or running gait. There are many things that can be identified utilizing a barefoot walking gait as well as running gait. The timing of joint motion is one of the first things that can be identified. For example, functional hallux limitus is identified as available full range of motion of the first metatarsophalangeal joint non-weight-bearing, but in weight-bearing the joint will not have its full range of extension motion until weight transfer has been made to the contralateral foot [17]. This is easily identified in barefoot recordings. Ankle joint motion can be estimated using angle calculation, though as stated previously, should not be relied on for accuracy or repeatability. A sign of midtarsal joint compensation is a crease along the lateral aspect of the midfoot from the lateral talo-navicular aspect toward the calcaneal cuboid joint. At times, visualization of heel lift can be witnessed while the forefoot is still completely on the ground and no MPJ extension has occurred. This can indicate severe flatfoot or pathological midfoot and subtalar joint compensations. Early heel lift with the foot in a plantarflexed position is often associated with unilateral ankle joint equinus or a short limb [20].

Concentrate on knee extension/flexion positions as the foot moves into mid-stance and into active propulsion of the stance phase. Many compensations for limb length discrepancies and for ankle joint equinus can be identified with early knee flexion or hyperextension [20].

Finally, hip range of motion can be analyzed from both sagittal and frontal plane views on video. Decreased hip range of motion is often associated with a shortened stride, potentially from the long-sided limb function. Pelvic compensations in the frontal plane can sometimes be identified if marked properly and may be associated with limb length compensations or hip and thigh instabilities [20].

In-Shoe Pressure Methodology

In-shoe pressure analysis systems measure vertical forces. High and low pressures or "hotspots" are seen with pressure mapping devices, but they can offer so much more [21] (Fig. 4.4). For example, the ability to appreciate the changes in the center of pressure as it moves from the heel to the toes, or if it has a more medial, mid-line, or lateral progression on the foot, can be very predictive of function [22–24]. An in-shoe pressure system allows synchronization or visualization of both feet

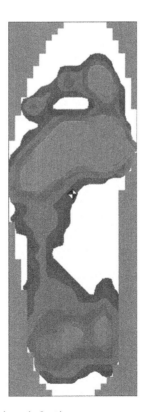

Fig. 4.4 In-shoe pressure analysis static foot image

functioning side by side, statically, or in function from step to step. This appears as if the patient were "bunny hopping" through gait.

Instead of trying to make observations from one right footstep, and then one left footstep, just watch progress from side by side. This allows comparison of many different parameters such as the center of pressure, CoP, icon and trajectory, accelerations of each foot, early loss of pressure or prolongation of pressures, and abnormally high or low areas of pressure in certain areas of the feet.

For instance, when evaluating for a short limb, there may be an early loss of heel pressure on one limb coupled with a much faster acceleration of the CoP icon on that same foot. Evaluation of the CoP trajectory and an increase or decrease in medial arch pressures may help to identify an overly pronated or supinated foot function and/or avoidance of a joint that may be functionally or structurally blocked in gait. High metatarsal pressures could indicate hotspots of metatarsalgia or neuroma, and a lack of sub first mpj pressures with or without high hallux pressures, often indicates a functional hallux limitus. The recordings offer visual information for comparison of asymmetrical functional pathology [7].

The ability to assess and compare force vs. time curves is another important component in evaluating in-shoe pressures. When an athlete is walking, vertical forces are highest under the heel and forefoot, respectively. As the body or center of gravity moves over these parts, this will be reflected as peaks in force vs. time curves. With in-shoe pressure analysis systems, a typical force/time curve would appear as a double hump.

With abnormal gait patterns, you will often identify flat areas in the force vs. time curves. These can be termed either a stoppage of force (not likely) or a stoppage of movement (more likely); you can identify problem areas specifically in the heel, forefoot area, or entire foot itself just by analyzing the specific phase of gait in which a flattening of the curve may take place. Ankle joint range of motion, functional hallux limitus, and midtarsal joint collapse are causes of flattening of the curves suggesting a lack of motion during a prolonged force. With a properly functioning orthosis and/or orthosis modification, symmetric and non-flattened progression throughout the gait cycle may be observed. Comparing and contrasting these curves right to left and from test to test allows tracking of improvements, or detriments in any modifications to custom foot orthoses.

Conclusion

Gait analysis of an athlete's walking and/or running gait can be effectively utilized in a clinical setting. Being able to objectively record and compare digital video and in-shoe pressures allows documentation of a very strong predictive pattern as to what is an athlete's initial functional capacity. Using the previously mentioned methodology allows for a repeatable clinical process for lower extremity evaluation from a digital video and in-shoe pressure standpoint. Tracking potential changes, positive or negative, when attempting technique improvements and/or modifications to shoe gear or custom foot orthoses also allows for objective data that can greatly aid in the improvement of athletic function.

References

1. Cavanagh PR: "The Mechanics of Distance Running: A Historical Perspective," p. 1, in Cavanagh PR (ed.), Biomechanics of Distance Running, Human Kinetics, Champaign, IL, 1990.
2. McClay I: The evolution of the study of the mechanics of running: relationship to injury. JAPMA, 90(3), March 2000.
3. Curran SA, Dananberg, HJ: Future of gait analysis: A podiatric medical perspective, JAPMA, 95(2), March/April 2005.
4. Nesbit SM, Serrano M: Work and power analysis of the golf swing, J Sport Sci Med, 4:520–533, 2005.
5. Davis IS: Gait retraining in runners. Orthop Pract, 17(2),2005.
6. Wikstrom EA, Tillman MD, Chmielewski TL et al.: Dynamic Postural Stability Deficits in Subjects with Self-Reported Ankle Instability. Med Sci Sport Exerc, 39, 2007.
7. Williams BE, Yakel JD: Clinical uses of in-shoe pressure analysis in Podiatric Sports Medicine, JAPMA, 97(1): January/February 2007.
8. Stell JF, Buckley JG: Controlling excessive pronation: a comparison of casted and non-casted orthoses. The Foot, 8: 210, 1998.
9. Genova JM, Gross MT: Effect of foot orthotics on calcaneal eversion during standing and treadmill walking for subjects with abnormal pronation. J Orthop Sports Phys Ther, 30: 664, 2000.[Medline].
10. Richie DH: Effects of foot orthoses on patients with chronic ankle instability. JAPMA, 97(1): January/February 2007.
11. Herring KM: Pertinent pearls on treating overuse injuries in endurance athletes. Podiatry Today, April 2007.
12. Sanner WH, O'Halloran WD: The biomechanics, etiology, and treatment of cycling injuries. JAPMA, 90(7): July/August 2000.
13. Oatis CA: Goals of Gait Assessment, P. 328 in Craik RL, Oats CA (ed.), Gait Analysis, CV Mosby, St Louis, 1995.
14. Gage JR, Ounpuu S: Gait analysis in clinical practice. Semin Ortho 4:72, 1989.
15. Tropp H, Odenick P, Gillquist J: Stabilometry recordings in functional and mechanical instability of the ankle joint. Int J Sports Med 6: 180, 1985.
16. Dingwell JB, Davis, BL: A rehabilitation treadmill with software for providing real-time gait analysis and visual feedback; Transactions of the ASME. J Biomech Eng, 118(2):253–255, 1996.
17. Dananberg HJ: Gait style as an etiology to chronic postural pain: part I. Functional hallux limitus. JAPMA, 83:433, 1993.
18. Dananberg HJ, Guliano M: Chronic low-back pain and its response to custom-made foot orthoses. JAPMA, 89:109, 1999.
19. Sajko SS, Pierrynowski MR: Influence of treadmill design on rearfoot pronation during gait at different speeds. JAPMA, 95(5): September/October 2005.
20. Walsh M, Connolly P, Jenkison A, O'Brien T: Leg length discrepancy – an experimental study of compensatory changes in three dimensions using gait analysis. Gait Posture 12:156–161, 2000.
21. Sarnow M, Veves A, Giurini J, Rosenblum B, Habershaw G: In-shoe foot pressure measurements in diabetic patients with at-risk feet and in healthy subjects. Diabetes Care: 17, 9, 1994.
22. Fuller A: Center of pressure and its theoretical relationship to foot pathology. JAPMA, 89: 278, 1999.
23. Jong Paik N, Sik Im M: The path of center of pressure of the foot during walking. J Korean Acad Rehab Med, 21: 762, 1997.
24. Scherer PR, Sobiesk GA: The center of pressure index in the evaluation of foot orthoses in shoes. Clin Podiatr Med Surg, 11: 355, 199.

Chapter 5
Athletic Shoe Evaluation

David Levine

Athletic footwear has been in existence since the 1800s when track competitors used spikes on their leather shoes. The leather fit poorly and the shoes would get stretched out easily making them useless very quickly. Late in the 1800s the Keds Company was born with the innovation of using rubber soles. Emphasis in the early 1900s was on basketball footwear. The main manufacturers in the athletic shoe market at that time were Adis and Rudolph Dassler – ultimately to become Adidas. They were making athletic footwear by hand for basketball and even some tennis players. The market for athletic shoes changed in the early 1970s when Frank Shorter won the Olympic gold medal in the marathon. By then Nike was building a presence based on their innovations in the running shoe market. This happened to coincide with America's running boom. The demand for running shoes took off and so did Nike. As fitness became a major emphasis in this country, other forms of exercise such as aerobics started gaining popularity. Reebok capitalized on this and aimed its marketing and footwear to this niche.

Competition in the athletic shoe market has intensified over the last 30 years. Athletic footwear is no longer just for athletes. Having the right look and the right shoe is very important to the younger age groups. In addition, the shoe companies have attempted to market as many segments of the population as possible in order to sell more sport-specific shoes. With all of this emphasis on the athletic shoe, the question often asked is whether athletic shoes are actually good for your feet. The answer is not a simple yes or no. In order to provide the best answer to that question, an understanding of the shoe itself, its anatomy, and how it functions will lead to answering that question.

Anatomy of an Athletic Shoe

Review of shoe anatomy, key features, and function will be presented (see Chapter 1 for comparison of historical shoe anatomy designs). All of the parts of a shoe

D. Levine (✉)
Private Practice, Frederick, MD, USA

M.B. Werd, E.L. Knight (eds.), *Athletic Footwear and Orthoses in Sports Medicine*, DOI 10.1007/978-0-387-76416-0_5, © Springer Science+Business Media, LLC 2010

have names, and knowing these names will help to discuss footwear intelligently and consistently. Understanding shoe anatomy and thus shoe function is analogous to learning human anatomy, one needs to understand anatomy before learning physiology.

Last

The last of the shoe ultimately determines how the shoe will fit a particular foot type. Currently, lasts are made of plastic, but in previous times they were made of wood. The last will determine the width toe box, depth of the toe region, toe spring, and heel height. Mass-produced shoes are made from lasts that are typical of common foot structure, whereas custom shoes are made from individual lasts specific for that person and the type of shoe that is desired.

Toe Box

This is the width of the toe region. Some shoes come to a point and some are more squared in their shape. Depending upon the toe shape of the individual will determine what should fit the best. Toe box can also include the depth or height of the toe region. If toes are contracted or overlap each other then as deep a toe box as possible is needed.

Vamp

This is the part of the shoe where the laces are located. Depending upon the angle of the foot in the region of the instep will determine the shape or style vamp that should work the best. For instance if someone has a high instep then increased room is needed in this region.

Balmoral Versus Blucher

Bal is a front-laced shoe in which the quarters meet and the vamp is stitched at the front of the throat. Bal is short for "Balmoral," the Scottish castle where this style was first introduced. Blucher is a style where the quarters flap opens at the vamp, giving extra room at the throat and instep in fitting. Most athletic shoes are made with a modified bal style.

Outer Sole

This is the bottom of the shoe that interfaces with the ground. There are a variety of different materials that are now utilized for outer soles depending upon the activity for which the shoe is designed. Some are more durable than others. In the early

1970s the waffle sole became very popular when its inventor, Bill Bowerman, was experimenting with soling material and a waffle iron.

Midsole

This is the location found between the outer sole and the upper of the shoe. Development of different density midsole materials has affected the design of many athletic shoes. In addition, athletic shoe manufacturers have experimented in this region of the shoe with ways to try and control the biomechanics of the foot.

Upper

This is the part of the shoe that encloses the foot. The upper is what encloses around the foot, decides the shoe style as well as breathability.

Heel Counter

This is within the upper of the shoe and supports the heel around its medial and lateral sides. Some shoes have a substantial heel counter in order to provide motion control and some leave this out completely. Whether a shoe has a heel counter depends also upon the particular activity for which the shoe was designed.

Function of Athletic Shoes

Initially athletic shoes were made with only function in mind, but that was at a time when there was very little information available concerning the biomechanical aspects of the human foot. Basketball, tennis, and football each had shoes specific for their sport in the early 1900s. In the 1950s that changed when sneakers became a fashionable item for the younger generation. The running boom changed that again as function became important again. As important as function is to athletic shoes, fashion is never far behind though. Selling shoes has always been the priority of the footwear industry. In order to sell shoes, appealing design is necessary. Often the fashion characteristics of a shoe outweigh the function in the mind of consumers.

With the popularity of running in the 1970s, sports-specific shoes took off. The difference between the shoes for specific sports is not only how the shoe is made but how the shoes function too. For instance, a running shoe certainly needs to be constructed differently than one for wrestling. This allowed the shoe companies to offer a variety of shoes for different niche markets and expand the population to which they sell.

The starting point in discussing function is how the shoe fits. No matter how well the shoe is constructed, it will not function properly if it does not fit well.

There are some key factors to consider when considering the fit. Certainly measuring the foot and getting the length from heel to toe is important. This serves as a starting point when trying to find the right size shoe. Since shoe sizing is not standardized, sizing between manufacturers is not consistent. Generally, the difference between sizes is consistent with 1/2 sizes equal to 1/3″.

Once the overall length of the foot has been determined, the next measurement to consider is the arch length. This is the measurement from the heel to the ball of the foot. This is also known as the arch length. Arch length and foot length are not necessarily equal. A person can have a long arch and short toes or the opposite situation. Of the two measurements the arch length is actually the more important one. This measurement will determine how the foot fits inside of a shoe which in turn will determine how the shoe will function on the foot.

The ultimate goal is for the foot and the shoe to function together. For this to occur, the shoe needs to flex at the proper location. If the arch length is considered first, then this aspect of shoe fitting will be successful. If only the toe length is considered, then the foot might be placed either too far forward or too far back inside of the shoe. This would then prevent the shoe from flexing in the proper location.

The next consideration is the width of the foot which is measured at the ball region. There are different measurements that footwear manufacturers use for measuring width. There is the letter designation S, N, M, W, and WW as well as the traditional A, B, C, D, E, EE, EEE. Whichever width designation is used, each successive width expands the width of the shoe by one increment.

Although width needs to be considered when fitting the shoe, the volume of the foot needs to be considered as well. Feet that measure the same size can occupy different volumes inside of a shoe. The "thickness" of the foot from top to bottom or how much room the foot occupies inside of a shoe is an important factor in determining fit.

Once the measurements have been obtained, then the last of the shoe needs should be considered. The last that the shoe is made upon determines the shape of the shoe. Since feet come in many different shapes, there are a variety of shoes from which to pick. One shoe cannot be right for everyone. There are feet with a wide forefoot and those with a narrow heel. Lasts will exhibit certain characteristics that will be most suitable for specific foot structures. People often complain about having wide feet, but it is the narrow foot that is hardest to fit.

With hard to fit feet, customizing the fit is often necessary. For some, finding a shoe that fits can be a difficult proposition. Even after obtaining all of the measurements required and picking the shoe that appears to fit the best, the result still may not be as desired. That is when it is necessary to understand the art of shoe fitting so that simple changes can be made that will make the shoe work as well as it can.

These modifications include extra padding in the forefoot in order to snug up the front of the shoe and prevent heel slippage. Addition of tongue pads to enhance fit and alternative lacing patterns to either avoid problem areas on the foot or serve as a way to make the shoe stay on the foot better can also be very successful. Detailed lacing techniques are presented in Chapter 8. Fitting shoes is the first step to having a shoe function properly. The next step is to understand, in more detail, how a shoe functions and how it can either help an individual function better or even prevent injury.

Clinical Assessment of Athletic Shoes

Work is currently being done through the Shoe Review Committee of the American Academy of Podiatric Sports Medicine in order to quantify important characteristics of shoes to allow comparisons between shoes from different manufacturers.

For the purposes of this chapter, running shoes will be the focus. Running is the activity that is in common with most athletic activities and is also the activity which places high demands upon the foot. The standards assessed with running shoes are the ones that are adapted by other sports and then modified depending upon the sport and the specific demands that particular activity places upon the foot.

It is completely inadequate to recommend one shoe for everyone. That is the importance of coming up with standards by which to compare running shoes and the basis from which recommendations can be made for individual athletes.

Fit

The established standards start with the fit, but only in a broad sense. Fit is difficult to quantify because there is much subjectivity involved in how a person perceives the right fit. One person may prefer a tight fit, while another may prefer a looser fitting shoe. Therefore, in a broad sense, fit is quantified, but only by characteristics in the construction of the shoe and what the particular company offers in options. Some companies make one standard width for each size, but there are companies now offering additional widths. This is seen as a bonus as far as achieving the best fit possible. This way the shoe has a better chance of fitting the foot instead of getting the foot to fit the shoe. In the better quality shoes, not only is it just an additional width that is offered but it is how the shoes are constructed. In many shoes the same bottom is utilized for the different widths. In shoes with higher quality, each width is made on a different last meaning that the bottom will proportionally fit the upper. Therefore, a wider shoe is truly a wider shoe including the sole. For wide feet this is important because this will keep the foot from hanging over the sides of a sole that is too narrow.

Insoles

Removable insoles have become universal among running shoe manufacturers, which make replacing them very easy. Most of the insoles that come with shoes are only adequate at best, as they do not offer much in the way of additional cushioning and certainly don't offer much additional support. In fact, most serious runners are better off replacing the inserts that come with the shoes. This is also an area that can be utilized to help obtain better fit. Padding the insoles with additional cushioning can help absorb extra room inside a shoe that would be otherwise considered loose. Even modification of the insoles to relieve areas of pressure can be performed as well. If the individual wears custom orthotic devices, having the ability to remove the insole is very helpful. There is very little difference between shoe manufacturers regarding insoles. Refer to Chapter 9 for more insight on pre-fabricated insoles.

Forefoot Flexibility

This portion of the shoe is very important to assess. This will determine how well the foot and the shoe will function together. There is a very simple test in order to determine this characteristic. Bend the shoe while holding the heel and forefoot. The flex point of the shoe should match the flex point of the foot. The shoe, just like the foot, should bend at the ball of the foot. For optimal shoe and foot function, it is necessary for the foot and the shoe to work together. If the shoe bends anywhere but at the ball of the foot, this is not mechanically advantageous for the foot to function optimally. In shoes where the flex point is not in the proper location, the foot is forcing the shoe to bend thereby altering the function of the shoe and the foot.

Midfoot Sagittal Stability

This characteristic is similar to forefoot flexibility. Bending the shoe between your hands is the test to determine the sagittal stability. If the shoe bends in the middle instead of the ball of the foot, the shoe is considered to be poorly constructed and one that should not be recommended. There is a range within these characteristics though. It is not always absolute as to whether a shoe flexes or not. If there is a slight flex, that would be important to note versus one that is very flexible and a completely wrong location. The goal of all of these functional shoe characteristics is to provide the most optimal environment in which the foot will function. Characteristics that impair this goal are important to note and one should avoid recommending. Athletic shoes which improperly flex through the arch will increase the strain through structures such as the plantar fascia, peroneal tendons, and midfoot.

Midfoot Frontal Stability

This characteristic is similar to the previous two. However, instead of whether the shoe flexes up and down (in the sagittal plane), this characteristic assesses whether there is any torsional component to the flexibility within the shoe (frontal plane). If a particular foot is very flexible in the frontal plane meaning that there is a lot of inversion and eversion occurring, frontal stability of the shoe is important. If the shoe has poor frontal stability, then the shoe will not offer the stability required by the foot and injury risk may be increased.

Lateral Midsole Heel Cushion

Close inspection of the heel of the shoe is important. There are a few characteristics in this region to focus upon that will directly impact foot function. This is the location of the shoe that contacts the ground. Stability and cushioning in this portion of the shoe are critical in preventing injury and promoting proper function. Many shoes are constructed with the idea of trying to control motion within the foot at heel strike. Strategies involved in this area include midsole materials having multiple densities as well as different materials that respond to shock absorption better than others. When people try shoes on, one of the leading subjective perceptions people assess is cushioning. However, if the shoe is too soft this can present problems and actually contribute to injury in the foot or even the knee. Soft materials compress rapidly and accentuate excessive motion within the foot. A supinated heel strike, for instance, will become even more supinated if the shoe compresses too much or too quickly in this region. Therefore, softer is not necessarily better. It is important that the material chosen for the lateral midsole heel cushion is not too soft and not too compressible. Materials have been developed that are now being utilized that have shock absorption, but do not compress too rapidly. One can also note whether other strategies such as special shock absorption materials are employed in addition to the midsole material present.

Medial Midsole Heel Density

This is the opposite side of the shoe. Some shoes exhibit same density material both medially and laterally; for certain feet this may be adequate. But for those individuals that either need extra shock absorption or land in a highly supinated position, differing densities are often necessary. Just as with the lateral midsole heel cushion, the medial midsole heel density is important to note as far as compressibility as well. Certain materials will compress faster than others. This can be noted after a person has worn a shoe for a while. If the material wrinkles that means that it is unable to rebound from the repeated compression that occurs with each step. When assessing this portion of the shoe, one will note whether it is of uniform density between medial and lateral, a medium density, or high density which is a strategy utilized to limit excessive pronation during mid-stance.

Heel Counter

This is the portion of the shoe that wraps around the heel from medial to lateral within the upper of the shoe. Some shoes incorporate a firm material or even plastic in order to help contain the heel and eliminate extra motion. There are also shoes that do not pay any special attention to this portion. In these shoes, the upper is soft and flexible. If the foot has a tendency to either invert at heel strike or pronate excessively during mid-stance, the heel counter will do very little to eliminate the extra motion from occurring.

Outsole Surface Area

Looking at the shape of the bottom of the shoe will determine this particular characteristic. A shoe that has a sole as wide as the upper can be advantageous for extra support. If the sole tapers at the midfoot or even follows the contour of the arch, this can be a negative characteristic as far as providing support. The more surface area in contact with the ground the more support the shoe offers the foot.

Conclusion

Based on the shoe assessment characteristics, a point system was created in order to score shoes (see Table 14.3 in Chapter 14). The score that a shoe receives can be used to compare shoes from different manufacturers. It can also be used as a way to determine shoes that display certain important characteristics such as stability or motion control. If a shoe scores high in all categories, it is a stable shoe with maximum motion control. Not everyone needs this type of shoe though. Therefore, the point system can help decide where to start for the right shoe.

The shoe industry is a competitive one; styles and features of shoes constantly change because consumers desire new products. As a result, what sometimes seems like a great shoe or great feature of a shoe may disappear as fast as it came. Understanding the parts of a shoe and how to assess the function of shoes will help the sports medicine specialist keep abreast of the continually changing offerings that the shoe companies produce.

Chapter 6
Athletic Shoe Fit and Modifications

Josh White

Whether treating professional athletes or weekend warriors, it is critical to select the right shoes and get the correct fit. Some foot-care professionals fit patients themselves, while others refer patients out to stores that decide what is best. Either way, patients' needs are best served by the sports medicine specialist assessing the functional biomechanics of the lower extremity, identifying structural requirements, and creating a plan for the therapeutic objectives to be accomplished. Sports medicine professionals can best help their patients fit appropriate athletic shoes and achieve most favorable outcomes by addressing the four basics of "size, shape, stability, and style."

Shoe Fitting

Size

Size is the first thing one usually considers in fitting shoes. Unfortunately, selecting the right shoe size can be difficult, and as previously stated, there are no manufacturer standards for how a particular length and width must measure. Variability in size exists between brands, among styles of a particular brand and even within a particular style if manufactured by different factories.

Despite this inconsistency, any fit must start with some form of measuring. It is best that patients try shoes that are made in three or four widths per half size and at a store that stocks the various choices. Unfortunately, most manufacturers still make shoes in only one width and most stores carry limited inventory. This results in patients with wide feet frequently wearing shoes longer than they need to get the width they desire.

J. White (✉)
Department of Orthopedics, New York College of Podiatric Medicine, New York, NJ, USA;
Department of Applied Biomechanics, California School of Podiatric Medicine, Oakland, CA, USA

M.B. Werd, E.L. Knight (eds.), *Athletic Footwear and Orthoses in Sports Medicine*,
DOI 10.1007/978-0-387-76416-0_6, © Springer Science+Business Media, LLC 2010

When correctly fit, there should be approximately 1/2″–5/8″ space between the end of the longest toe and the end of the shoe. The shoe should be wide enough such that the foot does not bulge out on the lateral side but not so wide that excess material can be pinched on top. Sometimes, when athletes have been accustomed to wearing shoes that fit too short, the right size will feel too large. The bottom line is that if shoes fit without slipping in the heel, then the bigger the size, the better.

Shape

It sounds simple enough, yet it is often overlooked how important it is to match the shape of the shoe to the shape of the foot. Feet come in an infinite variety of shapes yet shoes are mass produced using a limited number of forms called *lasts*. Lasts are designed to accommodate common foot shape characteristics. Such factors include the breadth of the forefoot, arch morphology, instep height, toe depth, and heel width. Even if sized correctly, picking the wrong shoe shape will result in suboptimal fit.

Most feet demonstrate a medium height arch, mild amount of curvature in the transverse plane, and a broad forefoot. Such feet are best fit in shoes made on what is sometimes referred to as a Universal or SL1 shaped lasts.

A segment of the athletic population has feet that curve medially in the transverse plane. Such feet are best fit on what is sometimes referred to as a *curved* shape lasts. These shoes are lightest in weight and offer a snug, glove-like fit.

Feet that have low-to-flat arches require ample breadth in the midsection of the shoe. These feet are best accommodated with shoes made from what is sometimes referred to as *linear* shape lasts.

Stability

Athletic shoe and orthoses manufacturers have seized on the concept of stability in their marketing and promise everything from limitation of excessive foot motion to allowing feet to move as nature intended. They have developed a slew of design features to provide an appropriate combination of cushioning and control of foot motion. To determine a shoe's stability, squeeze the sides of the heel counter, the rear part of the shoe. Stable shoes resist compression. Additionally, hold the shoe by the heel and at the toes and give it a twist. Torsionally stable shoes resist twisting; flexible shoes twist easily.

The foot's longitudinal arch is important as it helps absorb impact forces during the first half of the stance phase of gait from heel strike to the middle part of midstance. Later in the stride, the arch is supposed to rise, helping the foot to push off and the body to move forward with an efficient, smooth gait. When the arch lowers following heel strike and rises again during the propulsive phase of gait, there is said to be biomechanically efficient gait and the foot itself is referred to as *neutral*.

During walking and running, athletes with neutral-type feet contact on the lateral side of the heel, the foot rolls in toward the medial side, then resupinate through propulsion. Old shoes generally reveal wear on the lateral side of the heel and then even wear across the ball, sometimes continuing to beneath the distal medial aspect.

Neutral are recommended for *neutral* feet as such should be cushioned and flexible enough to allow the foot to progress naturally through the gait cycle without unnecessary correction. They lack extra pronation control devices, which could cause injury to biomechanically efficient runners but should provide good torsional stability.

The majority of athletes demonstrate mild-to-moderate overpronation. Immediately after heel contact, such feet roll in further medially. The shock absorption benefits of pronation are outweighed by the strain created by excessive range of motion. *Stability shoes* are recommended for athletes who are mild-to-moderate overpronators and who have low-to-normal arches. These athletes tend to need a shoe with a combination of good support and midsole cushioning.

Athletic shoe manufacturers incorporate a broad assortment of features designed to support the medial aspect of the heel and prevent compression beneath the plantar medial aspect and thus limit rearfoot pronation. Sometimes, in an attempt to save weight, the mid-part of the midsole is cut out. Torsional stability is restored with plastic reinforcing, sometimes referred to as a *stability web.*

Some runners demonstrate severe overpronation. After the lateral heel makes initial ground contact, the foot rolls in excessively to the point where the natural shock absorption benefits of pronation are diminished and the foot and ankle strain to stabilize joint motion. Such feet make it difficult to walk and run efficiently; they frequently tire easily and are subject to such conditions as heel spurs, bunions, and knee pain. *Motion control shoes* are recommended for athletes with low arches who are moderate-to-severe overpronators who need maximum rearfoot control and extra support on the medial side of their shoes. Supportive features include aggressive stabilization at the medial heel to reign in and convert the inward rolling of the foot and a wider base to provide stable support. This type shoe is also best for larger athletes who need support and durability.

Athletes with rigid or normal to high arch feet that demonstrate minimum pronation are generally well suited for running fast but possess limited shock absorption These runners are usually midfoot or forefoot strikers and are more susceptible to impact injuries such as shin splints, stress fractures, and Achilles tendonitis. These feet demonstrate minimum pronation and generally lack much ankle joint dorsiflexion. Such feet are best accommodated in neutral-cushioned shoes as they feature maximum midsole cushioning and minimum medial support.

Style

There was a time when sneakers with canvas uppers and gum rubber soles were adequate for most any athletic activity. Nowadays, shoes are manufactured for very specific activities and surfaces using a slew of high-tech componentry. A challenge for athletic shoes manufacturers stems from the fact that about 90% of the time, shoes are not worn for the activity for which they are designed. It is important that foot-care providers be able to differentiate the substance from the sizzle of shoe style.

Running shoes are lightest in weight and offer the greatest cushioning. They are designed for linear activity and should never be worn for any sort of court activity. It is okay to wear running shoes for walking but not vice versa.

Athletic walking shoes are similar to running shoes but often have a higher proportion of leather in the upper, giving them greater durability and slightly heavier weight. Athletic walking shoes are also generally not as boldly designed, making them often more appropriate for everyday wear.

Tennis, basketball, and other court sports entail quick changes in direction. Court shoes must integrate superior medial and lateral forefoot support. Tennis also entails a lot of dragging the forefoot and so these shoes often feature extra thickness in the big toe area.

Cross-training shoes come in two different versions, some that are lighter weight and most similar to running shoes and others that are similar to court shoes. Lightweight cross trainers are okay for running up to 2 or 3 miles and fine for working out on exercise machines. For basketball, tennis, and other court activities, the heavier weight cross trainer, generally made from leather is better.

Hiking requires support, protection from the environment, and durability. Such shoes offer heavier, more durable soles, and generally come up higher on the foot to provide greater ankle support. It's desirable that they feature a water proof lining and sealed seams.

The bottom line of shoe fitting is ensuring that they feel good. It's best to take shoes for a test run. While there always is some break-in to be anticipated, the correctly fit shoe will generally feel good right away. Occasionally, when a person has been wearing shoes that fit way too small for a long time, the correct size will feel excessively loose. The athlete must be encouraged to give the correct fit a try if there are no objective signs of looseness like slipping in the heel. Fairly soon, the athlete will appreciate that it is normal to be able to wiggle the toes in properly fit shoes and that feet should not ache by the end of the day.

Athletic Shoe Modifications

There are biomechanical conditions that require more than can be addressed with a combination of shoes and orthoses. One leg may be shorter than the other, there may be significant plantar pressure or no shoe may fit just right.

Limb length discrepancy may be the result of a congenital problem or accident. While limb length is measured in several different ways, anterior superior iliac spine to the ground, ASIS to the medial malleolus, via a level and via x-ray, the best way to determine the appropriate amount of *lift* to add utilizes none of these methods. People compensate for a LLD in different ways. The best way of determining how much lift to add is subjective, determined through trial an error by adding varying amounts of lift beneath the heel and forefoot. The right amount of lift will create a feeling of balance such that the athlete does not feel as though he/she is being pushed right, left, front, or back.

Generally, it is desirable to add as much lift as is possible to the inside of one's shoe. The amount that can be comfortably added depends on the shoe style. Tassel loafer may only allow 1/4″ beneath the heel, while high top athletic shoes may allow the addition of as much as a full inch. If additional lift is required beyond that which fits inside the shoe, it needs to be added outside as an external shoe modification.

The first way to relieve pressure beneath a planar prominence is via an orthotic forefoot accommodation. Additional pressure can be relieved by *carving out the midsole*, from the inside of the shoe, specifically beneath the plantar prominence. The specific areas can be determined by marking the area of the foot with some lipstick and carefully placing the foot, without a sock, into the shoe, all the while taking care not to smudge the marking before it gets to the proper place in the shoe.

Rocker bottoms offer an effective way to both relieve submetatarsal pressure and provide sagittal plane motion where such motion in the ankle, subtalar, midtarsal, or metatarsolphalangeal joints may be limited. Rocker bottom soles are created by adding increased thickness to the shoe midsole beneath the heel, beneath the ball, and then tapering it to the toes. A typical thickness is 1/2″. The rocker bottom allows the shoe to roll forward, maintaining a normal pattern of gait, without requiring sagittal plan dorsiflexion of the foot. It can limit motion when such motion is painful and compensate for a lack of motion with joint motion is restricted. In the absence of a LLD, whatever thickness of rocker bottom that is added to one shoe needs to be added to the other.

Shoe Stretching

Stretching is effective when a foot is irregularly shaped causing shoes to fit correctly in all but a specific area. The ball and ring stretcher is effective for spot stretching over a bunion or dorsally over hammertoes. The two-way type stretcher is better for creating width across the entire forefoot.

Conclusion

These simple guidelines will help sports medicine practitioners address most common shoe fitting issues and frequently seen foot pathology. In this way, injuries will be prevented, patients will heal faster, and they will better be able to participate in athletic activities.

Chapter 7
Athletic Socks

Douglas H. Richie

Socks are an essential component of footwear for the athlete. Previously considered a commodity item, athletic socks are now designed to provide significant functional and protective benefits for the active person. This chapter provides an overview of the key factors in the recommendation of proper socks (hosiery) for the athlete.

Historical Background

The concept of *sport-specific socks* emerged during the 1970s from the invention of the roll top sock, by James Throneburg, owner of THOR LO, Inc., sock company (Rockwell, NC) [1]. Early patented designs from THOR LO placed extra padding in strategic locations of a sock to provide protection during running, tennis, skiing, and cycling. Over the next 30 years, numerous manufacturers have emerged, offering myriad designs for virtually every sport in which shoes are worn. In some cases, the use of a sport-specific sock is valid, while many models and designs have questionable unique functions.

Considerable research has also been conducted on specialized sports hosiery to determine physiologic benefits. This research has suggested that athletic socks can provide significant reduction of plantar pressures [2–5], reduced impact shock [6], reduced incidence of friction blisters [7, 8], and reduced symptoms of venous insufficiency [9, 10]. These medical benefits, validated by scientific study, gave rise to a new category of socks known as *therapeutic hosiery,* designed for patients with diabetes and arthritis.

Basic Sock Design and Construction

Depending on the height of the upper or *foot* portion of the hosiery, an athletic sock has a specific description and sports application (Fig. 7.1). An *over-the-calf* design

D.H. Richie (✉)
Private Practice, Alamitos Seal Beach Podiatry, 550 Pacific Coast Hwy, Suite 209, Seal Beach, CA 90815, USA

M.B. Werd, E.L. Knight (eds.), *Athletic Footwear and Orthoses in Sports Medicine*,
DOI 10.1007/978-0-387-76416-0_7, © Springer Science+Business Media, LLC 2010

Fig. 7.1 Example of sock designs. (**a**) Over-the-calf. (**b**) Crew. (**c**) Mini-crew. (**d**) Roll top. (Courtesy of THOR LO, Inc., Statesville, NC)

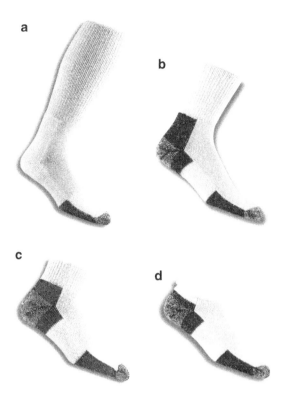

is used for skiing, baseball, soccer, and more recently for endurance running. A *crew length* sock is a standard athletic sock with universal applications. The upper of the crew sock ends just below the calf muscle. The *mini-crew* design ends just above the malleoli of the ankle and is a popular for running and tennis. The *roll top* sock ends at the topline of the shoe and is popular in golf.

The construction of an athletic sock can vary significantly among manufacturers. Depending on the type of knitting machine, a sock can have very dense *terry loop* pads or can have a flat knit design. The gauge of the knitting needle will determine the density of fabric within the sock. In general, more expensive socks use more fabric and tightly woven knit patterns in their construction to provide maximum protection for the foot.

The anatomy of an athletic sock provides further insight into design variations for the athlete. The *leg* or upper portion of the sock can vary in terms of overall compression and elasticity. This portion of the sock can have specialized padding or panels which are sport specific, such as shin pad for alpine skiing. Some manufacturers use specialized fibers in the leg portion of the sock to provide a wicking gradient to pull moisture out of the shoe.

The heel of the sock can be absent, as found in a *tube* sock, or can have a standard heel *gore,* which provides a pocket for the heel bone. A Y-Gore provides the best fit and conformity for the heel. Tube socks do not provide adequate fit requirements for vigorous sport activity.

The foot of the sock can have a cushioned sole portion and cushioned instep portion, or some variation thereof. The arch section may have additional elastic for support. The toe area of the sock has a seam that may be almost imperceptible in finer quality hosiery. The so-called seamless socks are preferred for medical application but this feature may have benefit in reducing pressure over the toes in the active athlete.

A recent trend has been the offering of sport socks shaped specifically for the right and left feet. These socks have a tapered toe area to more closely match the parabolic shape of the forefoot. This may have an advantage in preventing bunching of excessive fabric in the lateral aspect of the toes.

Fiber Composition

One of the primary differentiating features of athletic socks, compared to dress/casual hosiery, is the utilization of high-tech fibers and yarns. Today, the ordinary white cotton sweat sock has been replaced with sport-specific socks composed of synthetic fibers designed to provide better comfort and protection for the feet of the active athlete. Research has shown that synthetic fibers can keep the feet drier, cushion the foot better, and provide better performance than traditional cotton fibers.

Moisture Management

With regard to moisture management on the surface of the foot, the terms hydrophobic (repel moisture) and hydrophilic (retain moisture) are utilized in describing sock fiber performance. In general, cotton fibers and most wool fibers are considered hydrophilic, while synthetic fibers are hydrophobic. The response of socks to exposure to moisture is important from both a comfort and a clinical standpoint.

Moisture can accumulate in the shoe of the athlete from three different sources: the foot itself, the legs and trunk of the athlete, and the outside environment. The foot contains eccrine sweat glands which are innervated by cholinergic fibers activated by the sympathetic nervous system. The palms and soles are unique in having the highest density of eccrine sweat glands in the body: 2000 glands per square centimeter, compared to a density of only 100 glands per square centimeter in the rest of the body [11].

The production of moisture from the sweat glands of the feet during vigorous physical activity is estimated to be as much as 200 cc per hour [12]. The production of moisture from the remainder of the body during exercise can exceed 1 l per hour [12]. The sum total of moisture potentially collecting in the shoe of the athlete during exercise will quickly exceed the absorptive capacity of any sock. Therefore, in order to keep moisture content at a minimal level on the surface of the foot during exercise, a sock must "move" moisture away to the shoe upper for evaporation. This process is known as wicking [13].

Cotton fibers are hydrophilic and absorb three times the moisture as synthetic acrylic fibers which are commonly used in athletic hosiery [14]. Once wet, cotton socks retain moisture and have a ten-fold greater drying time compared to synthetic fiber socks [15]. In sedentary activity, cotton socks may be preferable to acrylic socks, given the low moisture output of the feet, and the better absorptive capacity of these hydrophilic fibers.

However, during vigorous activity, the absorptive capacity of any sock will be exceeded, and only a wicking gradient will allow movement of moisture from the foot surface to the shoe for evaporation to the outside environment. Hydrophilic fibers such as cotton have a 2.4 times greater resistance to moisture transport [15]. This may be related to absorption of fluid and swelling within the fibers themselves. When wet, acrylic fibers swell 5% while wool fibers swell 35% and cotton fibers swell 45% [16]. Swelling of fibers is related also to a loss of shape and conformability to the foot. Cotton socks tend to bunch and elongate when wet, while synthetic fiber socks are more likely to retain shape, cushion, and resiliency, in these conditions.

Fibers Used for Athletic Socks

The common fibers used in the manufacture of specialized athletic hosiery are listed in Table 7.1. The majority of fibers used in the construction of athletic hosiery are from synthetic sources. This is because synthetic fibers have been engineered to have physical properties which are desirable for athletic performance: water resistance, wicking, thermal insulation, wind resistance, anti-microbial resistance, reduced weight, cushion and resiliency, and reduced coefficient of friction. Other important features of athletic socks include durability, maintenance of shape when wet, machine washable, quick drying, and odor resistance. Although cotton fiber socks do not fulfill these functions, other natural fibers may perform just as well as some synthetic fibers.

Wool, being a natural fiber, is hydrophilic but may not have all of the undesirable features of cotton fibers when used for high-performance sock construction. Specialized wool yarns known as Merino wool have been developed that have many of the characteristics of synthetic fibers. Compared with traditional wool, Merino wool has a much finer core diameter of each fiber, giving a softer feel and more air space for moisture movement. Merino wool has fewer tendencies for skin itch, which is common with regular wool socks and apparel. The finer fiber and natural air spaces created by Merino wool have lead manufacturers to claim that this fiber is superior to any synthetic fiber for insulation and wicking.

The most popular synthetic fibers utilized in athletic hosiery are acrylic and polyester. Both acrylic and polyester fibers are hydrophobic and have superior wicking properties and reduced drying time than cotton. COOLMAX fibers (INVISTA, Wichita, KS) have a four-channel geometric configuration to enhance surface area and moisture movement. As a result, studies have shown that COOLMAX and other polyester fibers have a 15% faster drying time compared to acrylic fibers. Both acrylic and polyester remain soft with multiple machine washings, resist wrinkles and stains, and retain their shape with moisture exposure. One shortcoming of

Table 7.1 Fibers used in sock construction

	Brand names	Manufacturer
Merino wool		
Acrylic	Duraspun	Solutia, Inc.
	Cresloft	Sterling Fibers, Inc.
	Microsupreme	Sterling Fibers, Inc.
Polyester		
	COOLMAX	INVISTA, Wichita Kansas
	ComFortrel XP	Wellman, Inc.
	Sensura	Wellman, Inc.
	Spunnaire	Wellman, Inc.
Polypropylene		
	Innova	American Fibers and Yarns
Insulating		
	Thermolite	INVISTA
	Holofiber	Wellman, Inc.
	Outlast	Outlast Technologies, Inc.
	X-static	Noble Technologies
Anti-microbial		
	X-static	Noble Technologies
	MicroSafe	Celanase, Texbac
	BioFresh	Sterling Fibers, Inc

For further information, refer to the following sites:
http://www.fabriclink.com/search/fiber-search.cfm;
http://www.fabriclink.com/Presentations/index.cfm?ID=68 (X-static link);
http://www.fabriclink.com/Presentations/index.cfm?ID=13 (Innova);
http://www.fabriclink.com/Presentations/index.cfm?ID=27 (Comfortrel);
http://www.invista.com/page_product_coolmax_en.shtml (COOLMAX);
http://www.invista.com/page_product_thermolite_en.shtml (Thermolite) replaces
Thermax;
http://www.foxsox.com/SockTechnology/Index.aspx#FiberTech (Fox River).

acrylic is poor insulation. On hot surfaces in summer months, acrylic fiber socks can conduct heat and be undesirable. Hollow core polyester or COOLMAX socks may be preferred in these conditions.

Insulating fibers have been developed for cold climate sporting conditions. Thermolite (INVISTA, Wichita, KS) and Hollofil (Advansa, Hoofddorp, the Netherlands) are examples of hollow core fibers designed to trap air and provide an insulating layer for trapping heat against the skin of the foot. Wool fibers have this same air-trapping framework that has made wool a fiber of choice for cold climates for decades. Newer fibers such as Outlast (Outlast Technologies, Inc., Boulder, CO) have a chemical property to store and release heat, depending on the skin tempera-ture. Silver-impregnated X-static fibers (Noble Biomaterials, Desenzano, Italy) have a natural heat retaining capacity. X-static claims that 95% of body heat is reflected back to the skin by the silver fibers within the sock.

X-static is also one of the newer types of sock fibers that have anti-microbial properties. Other fibers marketed with anti-microbial claims include MicroSafe (Texbac, Germany), Innova (American Fibers and Yarns, Chapel Hill, NC), and

BioFresh (Sterling Fibers, Inc., Pace, FL). The benefits of anti-microbial fibers for sock construction are debatable. Odor reduction is one obvious benefit, but the medical benefits to the consumer are yet to be proven. Socks have not been demonstrated to reduce bacterial or fungal growth on the skin of the feet. These microbes can be eliminated by simple machine washing and heated drying of the sock product. Therefore, the benefits of so-called anti-microbial socks may be one of perception rather than proven by clinical research.

Clinical Benefits of Athletic Socks

Being the closest layer of protection against the foot, hosiery has the potential to protect the skin and the deeper tissues from injury. While most clinicians intuitively examine the role of shoes and orthoses as a cause and preventive mechanism for injury, few look at the role of hosiery in this important area of sports medicine.

In walking and running, the primary stresses on the feet are impact, plantar pressure, friction, and shear [17]. Impact forces result from gravity and inertia as the body propels forward. Plantar pressures are the result of impact, bone deformity, and biomechanical issues. Friction and shear occur when the foot strikes the ground tangential to the supportive surface. Friction and shear also occur when the foot pushes off in propulsion. Frictional forces oppose movement of the skin against the supportive surface [18].

When external movement exceeds the frictional force at the skin interface, shear occurs where layers of skin begin to move upon each other. Initially, shear forces cause exfoliation of the stratum corneum on the skin surface [19]. In the palms of the hands and in the soles of the feet, the integument has a thick stratum corneum and stratum granulosum held tightly to the deeper layers. When high frictional forces secure the surface of the skin to the supportive surface, continued shearing forces can cause a movement interface between the stratum granulosum and the stratum spinosum causing a cleft to develop, resulting in a friction blister [20].

Over the past 15 years research has shown that specialized hosiery can significantly reduce impact shock and plantar pressures on the foot. In addition, there is indirect evidence that specialized hosiery systems can mitigate shearing forces which result in friction blisters.

Impact and Pressure Reduction

Howarth and Rome studied the effects of various athletics socks on shock attenuation during barefoot treadmill walking [6]. Both a padded acrylic and a wool cushion sock significantly decreased impact shock. A cotton sock and double-layer flat knit cotton sock did not significantly reduce impact shock.

Veves et al. conducted several studies of plantar pressure dissipation during barefoot walking on an optimal pedobarograph of specialized padded (THOR LO) hosiery. These densely padded socks showed a 30% reduction of peak plantar pressures during walking in diabetic patients with peripheral neuropathy. Less padded, sport socks also demonstrated significant pressure reduction of 15% which was maintained after 6 months of continuous use [3].

Donaghue et al. also studied padded (THOR LO) hosiery using in-shoe pressure measurements on diabetic patients [4]. Padded hosiery demonstrated a significant 10.7% reduction of peak plantar pressure inside the shoe when padded hosiery was compared to conventional socks. More recently, Garrow et al. utilized in-shoe pressure testing of specialized double-layer acrylic hosiery in diabetic patients [5]. A 10.2% reduction of peak forefoot pressure was measured compared to conventional socks.

Friction Blisters

Studies of friction blisters and hosiery utilized subjects more representative of athletic patients rather than diabetic subjects with neuropathy. Friction blisters are considered the most common skin injury in sport [21]. Because the sequela of these blisters can result in infection and disability, the subject of blister prevention has been of keen interest particularly in the United States Military.

Herring and Richie conducted a prospective, randomized cross-over study of 35 long distance runners wearing padded socks composed of either acrylic fibers or cotton fibers [7]. The runners wearing acrylic socks experienced half as many blisters as those wearing cotton socks. The subjects wearing acrylic fiber socks perceived that their feet were dryer compared to wearing cotton socks. Previous studies had shown that moisture content on the skin surface increased frictional force and tendency to form blisters.

Herring and Richie conducted a similar study comparing acrylic fiber socks to cotton socks, but utilized a less padded thinner sock compared to their original study [8]. The superiority of either fiber to reduce blisters could not be demonstrated with non-cushioned socks, leading the researchers to conclude that both construction and fiber composition were important in a sock's ability to prevent friction blisters.

Knapik et al. studied 357 U.S. Marine recruits during 12 weeks of basic training to determine the rates of blister formation in the feet while wearing one of three types of sock systems [22]. The use of a polyester (COOLMAX) liner combined with a heavily padded wool/polypropylene-blended outer sock resulted in the lowest incidence of blisters compared to the single-layer standard wool sock (40% incidence vs. 69%). Adding a COOLMAX liner to the standard wool sock reduced sick call visits (24.9% standard vs. 9.4% standard with liner).

Other studies of marching soldiers in the U.S. military have confirmed the superiority of synthetic fiber socks, particularly when used as a liner inside of a more heavily padded sock [23, 24]. Double-layer synthetic sock systems have been shown to be more effective than single-layer synthetic fiber socks in the prevention of blisters [25–27].

Studies of socks and friction blisters on the feet suggest that the establishment of a movement interface either within the sock itself or between the layers of a sock system will prevent skin injury. Furthermore, reducing the friction force on the skin surface itself may be dependent upon the fiber composition of the sock, where synthetic fibers appear to work best [28].

Potential Clinical Benefits

Research on newer padded or double-layer socks systems have revealed significant benefits which have direct relevance to the active athlete. Certain socks appear to be able to reduce moisture content on the feet during activity which has direct benefit from both a comfort and a skin injury standpoint. Reduced moisture content of the skin of the feet during vigorous activity will minimize the chance of friction blisters. Damaging skin shear will also be minimized when thicker padded socks are worn, or when a two layer synthetic sock system is worn. Other skin injuries such as calluses, corns, and toenail trauma may also be minimized by the wearing of proper socks.

While shoes and foot orthoses are commonly regarded as the major protection of the feet of the athlete, hosiery has been demonstrated to provide additional protection from impact and pressure which are attributed to be a cause of many foot injuries during running and jumping. Reduction of impact and plantar pressure on the feet can be expected to minimize the risk of common foot injuries such as capsulitis, bursitis, heel bruise, and stress fractures.

There has been recent attention to the potential clinical benefit of compression in the upper of a sock worn by the athlete. In particular, some over-the-calf sport socks have enough elastic compression to aid in venous return of blood flow from the feet and lower legs. Brown and Brown were the first to show the benefits of Thor Lo basketball socks in improving objective and subjective measures in patients with venous insufficiency [9]. Ali et al. showed that over-the-calf sport socks with specially designed uppers for graduated compression would reduce the symptoms of delayed muscle soreness in men after a 10 km road run [10]. Graduated compression over-the-calf socks are now used in professional hockey and in endurance events such as the marathon and triathlon.

Conclusion and Recommendations

When recommending socks for an athlete, it should be recognized that specialized athletic hosiery may change the fitting requirements of the shoe. Heavily padded sports-specific socks may require the addition of a full shoe size to allow proper room for the foot. Therefore, the selection of athletic socks should occur during the measurement and fitting process when athletic shoes are being purchased. The feet should be measured when the athlete is wearing the specialized socks intended to be worn during the sport.

Narrow feet may benefit from specially designed socks for the right and left feet. Such socks may prevent bunching of excessive fabric over the lateral toes. Conformed fit is difficult when socks are offered in sizes covering a broad range (greater than three shoe sizes). Premium sport socks are usually offered in narrow size ranges which more accurately fit the foot. It should be recognized that sock sizes are not the same as shoe sizes: manufacturers may list the sock size, the shoe size, or both.

Certain socks may be recommended depending upon the clinical history or needs of the athlete. In the case of chronic blisters, a double-layer or padded hosiery system is recommended. If there is no significant concern about skin injury, the selection of fiber may be more important than construction style. Acrylic fiber socks are the most versatile of all athletic socks and make a good general sock recommendation. Depending on anticipated exposure to temperature extremes, hollow fiber or wool socks may be indicated.

Finally, the athletic hosiery marketplace is filled with products with consumer benefit claims which have not been substantiated. Many times, promises of blister protection, anti-microbial protection, and insulation have not been proven with adequate scientific study. Furthermore, the true value of a "sport-specific" sock may only be in the packaging rather than in a specific unique construction designed for the activity.

Based on the best available scientific evidence, the following conclusions and recommendations regarding athletic socks can be made:

- Cotton fibers are not recommended for construction and use in athletic socks because of poor performance when exposed to moisture.
- Synthetic fibers are superior to cotton in providing better wicking of moisture from the skin surface of the foot, faster drying time, better maintenance of shape when wet, better durability with multiple machine washing cycles.
- Wool fiber socks, particularly specialized Merino wool, have many positive characteristics of synthetic fibers. Wool fiber socks are superior in cold environments and appear to have adequate wicking capacity to keep the feet drying than cotton fibers.
- Padded hosiery products are preferred to thin, un-padded socks because padding can protect the skin surface from friction and shear. Padded socks also can significantly reduce plantar pressures and impact shock which may reduce the risk of musculoskeletal trauma to the feet.
- The use of a synthetic fiber liner sock, establishing a double-layer sock system, has been demonstrated to reduce the incidence of blisters compared to single-layer sock systems.
- Over-the-calf socks with elastic compression may have clinical and performance benefits for some athletes.

References

1. Richie D: Sock controversy. Phys Sports Med 20(5):55, 1992.
2. Flot S, Hill V, Yamada W, et al.: The effect of padded hosiery in reducing forefoot plantar pressures. Lower Extremity, 2:201–205, 1995.
3. Veves A, Masson EA, Fernando DJS, et al.: Use of experimental padded hosiery to reduce abnormal foot pressures in diabetic neuropathy. Diabetes Care, 12:653–655, 1989.

 4. Donaghue VM, Sarnow MR, Guirini JM, et al.: Longitudinal in-shoe foot pressure relief achieved by specially designed footwear in high risk diabetic patients. Diabetes Res Clin Pract, 31:109–114, 1996.
 5. Garrow AP, van Schie CHM, Boulton AJM: Efficacy of multilayered hosiery in reducing in-shoe plantar pressure in high risk patients with diabetes. Diabetes Care, 28: 2001–2006, 2005.
 6. Howarth SJ, Rome K: A short-term study of shock-attenuation in different sock types. Foot, 6: 5–9, 1996.
 7. Herring KH, Richie DH: Friction blisters and sock fiber composition: a double blind study. J Am Podiatr Med Assoc, 80:63–71, 1990.
 8. Herring KH, Richie DH: Comparison of cotton and acrylic socks using a generic cushion sole design for runners. J Am Podiatr Med Assoc,83:515–522, 1993.
 9. Brown JR, Brown AM: Nonprescription, padded, lightweight support socks in the treatment of mild to moderate lower extremity venous insufficiency. JAOA, 95:173–181, 1995.
10. Ali A, Caine MP, Snow BG: Graduated compression stockings: physiological and perceptual responses during and after exercise. J Sports Sci, 25: 413–419, 2007.
11. Kuno Y: Human Perspiration, pp. 1–65. C.C. Thomas, Springfield, IL, 1956.
12. Grice, K: Sweat glands and abnormalities of their function, pp. 5–68. in Marks R, Sammon PD (eds.), Dermatology. Vol 6. Appleton-Century-Crofts, New York, NY, 1977.
13. Farnworth B: A numerical model of the combined diffusion of heat and water vapor through clothing. Tex Res J, 56:653–665, 1986.
14. Product Knowledge Center for High Performance Fibers, Apparel and Gear. The Acrylic council, Inc., 1285 Avenue of the Americas, 35th Floor, New York, NY, 10019.
15. Euler RD: Creating "comfort" socks for the U.S. consumer. Knitting Times, 54:47, 1985.
16. Harris M: Handbook of Textile fibers, pp. 173–189. Harris Research Laboratory, Inc, Washington, DC, 1954.
17. Spence WR, Shields MN: Prevention of blisters, callosities, and ulcers by absorption of shearing forces. J Am Podiatry Assoc, 58:428–434, 1968.
18. Davis BL: Foot ulceration: hypothesis concerning shear and vertical forces acting on adjacent regions of skin. Med Hypotheses,40:44–47, 1993.
19. Naylor PE: Experimental friction blisters. Br J Dermatol,67:327–335, 1955.
20. Sulzberger MD, Cortese TA, Fishman L, et al.: Studies on blisters produced by friction. I. Results of linear rubbing and twisting techniques. J Invest Dermatol, 47:456–463, 1966.
21. Levine N: Dermatologic aspects of sports medicine. J Am Acad Dermatol, 3:415–423, 1980.
22. Knapik JJ, Hamlet MP, Thompson KJ: Influence of boot-sock systems on frequency and severity of foot blisters. Mil Med161(10):594–598, 1996.
23. Robertson TW, Christopherson MS: Improved sock system customer test. Fort Hunter, US Army Test and Experimentation Command Center, Ligget, CA, 1994.
24. Gackstetter G, Shrifter J: Injury reduction sock study. Epidemiology Division, Lackland Air Force Base, San Antonio, TX, 1994.
25. Allan JR: A study of foot blisters. Research memorandum 1, pp. 64–68. Army Operational Research Establishment, Farnborough, United Kingdom, 1964.
26. Allan JR, MacMillan AL: The effects of heat on unacclimatized paratroops. Exercise Tiger Brew II. Research memorandum 16, pp. 62–75. Army Operational Research Establishment, Farnborough, United Kingdom, 1963.
27. Jagoda A, Madden H, Hinson C: A friction blister prevention study in a population of marines. Mil Med, 146:42–55, 1981.
28. Sanders JE, Greve JM, Mitchell SB, et al.: Material properties of commonly used interface materials and their static coefficients of friction with skin and socks. J Rehabil Res Dev,35:161–176, 1998.

Chapter 8
Athletic Shoe Lacing in Sports Medicine

Matthew B. Werd

Optimal athletic shoe fit and function depends on a number of factors, including foot type, biomechanical foot function, the type of sport, socks, as well as shoe lacing. Athletic shoelaces and lacing patterns are often overlooked, but can enhance better shoe fit and function as well as help minimize painful conditions of the foot.

General shoe lacing tips include loosening the laces before slipping the foot into the shoe, which maintains the integrity of the eyelets and heel counter; tightening the laces from distal (toe end) to proximal (ankle end); and tightening gradually at each set of eyelets. A shoe with more eyelets enables a more custom fit with a variety of lacing patterns.

Athletic Shoelace Materials

Elastic (bungee-like cord) lacing material may be preferred by athletes who want a softer and looser feel and may be beneficial for runners with injuries. The extra flexibility expands and contracts with the foot and may aid healing and reduce pain and discomfort. Shoes with elastic laces may be easy to slip on and off, but they may not provide as much stability and support.

Nonelastic (cotton, braided, or nylon) shoelace material is recommended for athletes with healthy feet who prefer a snug and secure "feel" to their athletic shoes. A combination of outer nylon with inner elastic makes a "finger-trap" system, providing both strength and flexibility.

Velcro straps are sometimes used in place of shoelaces and may be useful for medical patients who may have a difficult time lacing shoes; however, Velcro straps will not provide as much athletic foot support as tie-lacing.

M.B. Werd (✉)
American Academy of Podiatric Sports Medicine; Lakeland Regional Medical Center; Foot and Ankle Associates, Lakeland, FL, USA

M.B. Werd, E.L. Knight (eds.), *Athletic Footwear and Orthoses in Sports Medicine*,   79
DOI 10.1007/978-0-387-76416-0_8, © Springer Science+Business Media, LLC 2010

Athletic Shoelace Shapes

Shapes of athletic shoelaces can also vary, which may affect the ease of tying and tightness of the knot. Different shapes of laces include traditional flat, thick round "cord-like," oval, and even ribbed for additional knot strength.

Athletic Shoelace Lacing Techniques

Difficult to fit feet and conditions such as narrow heels, high or low arches, or narrow or wide feet can be accommodated by changing the way the shoe is laced. Proper lacing can deliver a secure, comfortable, and supportive fit. Often, a small change to the athletic shoe lacing can make a big difference in comfort and performance.

Figures 8.1, 8.2, 8.3, 8.4, 8.5, 8.6, 8.7, and 8.8 demonstrate a variety of useful lacing techniques, which include the purpose of the technique, as well as a list of foot types and/or conditions that may benefit most by each pattern. Notice that, for demonstration purposes, one-half of the shoelace shown in all figures has been colored black and the other half remains white.

Standard Crisscross Lacing Pattern

As shown in Fig. 8.1, the laces begin at the distal eyelets and are crisscrossed proximally through each eyelet of the shoe. This is the traditional lacing technique used most commonly in new shoes that come directly "out-of-the-box." The foot types and conditions for this lacing pattern include the normal-arched foot and pathology-free foot.

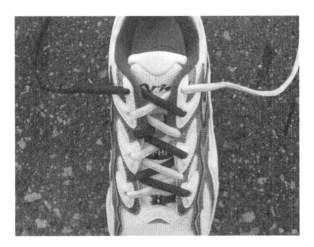

Fig. 8.1 Standard crisscross lacing pattern

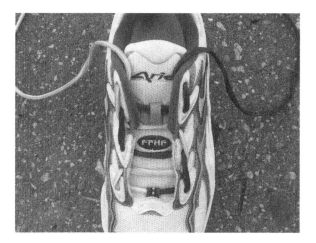

Fig. 8.2 Non-crossing, parallel lacing pattern

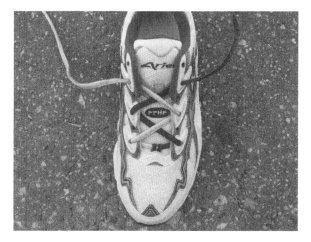

Fig. 8.3 Outside-eyelet, crisscross lacing pattern

Non-crossing, Parallel Lacing Pattern

In Fig. 8.2, beginning at the distal eyelets, each lace is continued proximally after skipping one eyelet and is then crossed. Repeat until all eyelets are laced and tied. Notice that with this lacing pattern, the laces do not crisscross each other. This technique lessens the pressure on the top portion of the arch of the foot, while still securing the foot to the shoe. The foot types and conditions for this lacing pattern are the high-arched foot and shoes that feel too tight on the top of the foot.

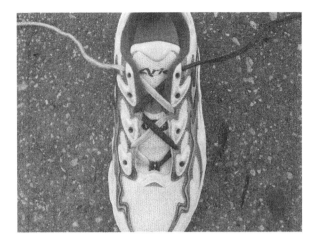

Fig. 8.4 Inside-eyelet, crisscross lacing pattern

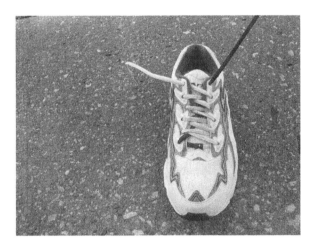

Fig. 8.5 Distal–medial eyelet lacing technique

Outside-Eyelet, Crisscross Lacing Pattern

Figure 8.3 shows the outside-eyelet, crisscross lacing pattern. Shoes with eyelets that zigzag up the placket will work best for this technique. The standard crisscross pattern is modified by using only the outside/widest eyelets of the shoe. Tighten from the outer eyelets, pulling the body of the shoe toward the center. This technique will help to pull up on and support the arch by tightening the shoe to the foot. The foot types and conditions for this lacing pattern include low (flat) arch, posterior tibial tendon dysfunction, and narrow foot.

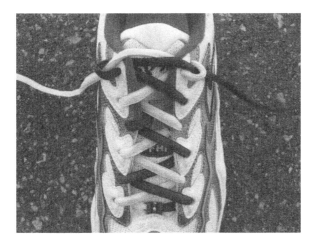

Fig. 8.6 Heel lock lacing modification

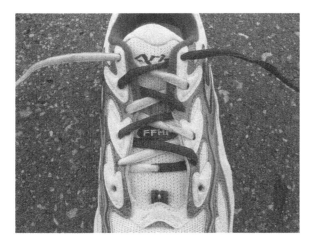

Fig. 8.7 Open distal eyelet lacing technique

Inside-Eyelet, Crisscross Lacing Pattern

Figure 8.4 shows the inside-eyelet, crisscross lacing pattern. Shoes with eyelets that zigzag up the placket will work best for this technique. The standard crisscross pattern is modified by using only the inside/narrowest eyelets of the shoe. Tighten from the inner eyelets, pulling less of the body of the shoe toward the center. This technique helps to alleviate pressure on the top of the arch by loosening the shoe to the foot. The foot types and conditions for this lacing pattern include high arch, dorsal foot ganglion or cyst, dorsal foot exostosis, and nerve impingement syndromes (medial dorsal cutaneus nerve or intermediate dorsal cutaneus nerve).

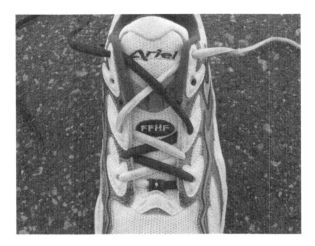

Fig. 8.8 Open eyelet lacing technique

Distal–Medial Eyelet Lacing Technique

Figure 8.5 shows the left shoe. The black half of the shoelace is threaded through the most distal–medial eyelet (closest to the big toe). Next, it is crossed all the way up through the most proximal–lateral (highest, opposite-side) eyelet to the outside. Leave just enough slack at the top to tie a bow. Take the remaining portion of the lace – the white half of the shoelace shown above – straight across toward the outside of the shoe and then diagonally up toward the inside of the shoe. Repeat until all of the eyelets are laced. The purpose of this method is to pull the upper material off of the big toe and decrease the pressure on the great toe and joint. In the above picture, when the black shoelace is tugged and tightened, the distal–medial eyelet (the part of the shoe directly over the big toe) will be pulled away from the great toe and toe-nail, thereby relieving shoe pressure at this area. Foot conditions helped most with this lacing pattern black toenail/subungual hematoma of the great toe, subungual exostosis of the great toe, hallux extensus, hallux valgus/bunion deformity, hallux limitus/rigidus, and turf toe.

Heel Lock Lacing Modification

Lace as normal until one eyelet remains proximally on each side (Fig. 8.6). Draw the lace straight up on the outside of the shoe and bring it through the last eyelet, creating a loop, and repeat on the other side. Cross each lace over the tongue, thread it through the opposite loop, and tie. The loops help to cinch in the material around the ankle, which *locks* the shoe to the heel and prevents the heel from slipping without making the rest of the shoe any tighter.

This technique creates a more secure fit around the ankle without tightening the entire shoe. It should be noted that this technique effectively "locks" the heel into the shoe. This common technique provides a much more stable fit and can easily be combined or added with other lacing patterns. The foot conditions helped most with this lacing modification include narrow heels, heel slippage, heel bullae/blisters, and athletes who wear orthoses and have problems with the orthosis moving inside the shoe.

Open Distal Eyelet Lacing Technique

Skip the most distal set of eyelets (closest toward the toes). Begin lacing at the next set of proximal eyelets (or begin at the second proximal set of eyelets if needed) and continue to lace proximally as usual (Fig. 8.7). An alternative technique is to remove the laces and measure them. Buy two sets (four laces) half of the measured length. On both shoes, use one lace for the bottom three eyelets and a second lace for the upper eyelets. The end result will be two bows on each shoe, allowing the bottom laces to be tied looser (or tied tighter, for a narrow forefoot) to accommodate a wider forefoot. This technique allows more flexibility of the shoe and it loosens the upper of the shoe at the metatarsal–phalangeal joints. The foot types and conditions for this lacing pattern include extra-wide forefoot (or extra narrow forefoot, as noted previously), hallux valgus (bunion), tailor's bunion, Morton's neuroma, hammer toe syndrome, "cramped toes," toenail pathology, Achilles tendon pathology, and posterior heel pathology.

Open Eyelet Lacing Technique

Draw with a marker or place a lipstick smear on the painful area, or "hot spot" on the dorsum of the foot. Insert the bare foot into the shoe, press the tongue of the shoe against the dorsum of the foot, then remove the shoe. The mark on the underside of the tongue will give an indication as to which set(s) of eyelets to skip. Lace the shoe until reaching the eyelet before the spot and take the lace back under and pull it up through the next eyelet on the same side (Fig. 8.8). Next, take the lace across and continue to lace, then repeat this on the other side. There will be an empty spot on the tongue where no laces cross it, which should eliminate the pressure point. Eliminate pressure from a "hot spot" on the top of the foot by lacing around it and not directly over it. Pressure from tight shoes and/or laces is alleviated at the site of impingement. The foot types and conditions for this lacing pattern include high arch, hot spot in which the shoe rubs on one spot on the top of the foot, extensor tenosynovitis, dorsal foot ganglion or cyst, dorsal foot exostosis, and nerve impingement syndromes (medial dorsal cutaneus nerve or intermediate dorsal cutaneus nerve).

Athletic Shoelace Technology

Shoe lacing technologies may be helpful to certain athletes. Many unforeseen problems can occur during a sporting event, including athletic shoes that come untied. Untied shoelaces can be both a frustrating and a dangerous problem and has prompted the development of advanced lacing systems and lacing materials.

Shoelace-locking systems can keep shoelaces tied and can also affect the ability to quickly slip a shoe on or off the foot. Quick shoe application and secure shoelace locking can be important in sports such as triathlon and adventure races, in which a quick transition time (T2) from the bike to the run can be critical. Several common shoelace systems and materials geared to assist improved shoe-fitting through lacing are presented.

Athletic Shoelace Specialized Systems

Athletic shoelaces becoming untied during training or competition can be dangerous as well as harmful to performance. In the past, athletes who have had problems with shoelaces untimely becoming untied during training or competition found it helpful to cinch the shoelaces in a double or triple knot; however, these tend to loosen and need to be re-tied. Another technique used to prevent athletic shoes from becoming untied includes wrapping athletic tape around the outside of the shoes and laces.

Newer patented lace-locking systems such as Lock Laces (www.locklaces.com), Speedlaces (www.speedlaces.com), Xtenex (www.xtenex.com), Tyless (www.tyless.com), Squeezums (www.squeezums.com) and Yankz! (www.yankz.com) use specialty shoelace-locking designs and materials to help prevent loosening and to improve performance and comfort. Once these lacing systems are fit to the shoe, they need minimal readjusting, and they eliminate floppy, loopy laces. However, one potential concern with these lacing systems remains slippage at the lace–lock interface.

Lock laces are a patented elastic lacing system that feature specially designed elastic laces combined with a spring-activated locking device. The lace uses curved tips to allow the lace to pass more easily through the eyelet configurations in athletic shoes. The laces are made with water-resistant banded, multi-strands of elastic/bungee. The lock is a slideable spring-activated device made from a strong, durable, and lightweight plastic which hold the laces in place. The tension springs are made from a metal alloy, resistant to rust and corrosion. Lock laces use a traditional lacing scheme with specialized laces and a locking mechanism in place of a traditional knot.

Speedlaces replace ordinary laces and provide added support and stability, instant tension adjustment, and eliminate the need to re-tie laces again. Speedlaces is a totally secure, closed-loop system in which lace tension is always equal throughout the shoe. Less friction is created at the lace–eyelet interface by using a patented fitting that uses the shoe's existing eyelets. Stretch laces (iBungee) as well as non-stretch laces (Race Runners) are available from Speedlaces.

Xtenex laces incorporate a novel knotted-lace design which does not require any lace tying or extra hardware; these laces were worn by the Olympic gold and silver medalists in the 2008 Olympic Triathlon competition. Tyless and Squeezums incorporate a plastic mechanism which allows quick cinching of the laces without the need to tie a knot.

Yankz! Sure Lace System is another athletic lacing system that uses an elastic shoelace-locking device that tightens the shoe with one pull of the cord.

Athletic Shoelace Lengths

The length of shoelaces can vary for different shoe types. Table 8.1 is intended to be a guideline only for standard shoes. If replacing laces, measure the old laces as a reference.

Table 8.1 Recommended shoelace lengths based on pairs of eyelets

Hole pairs	Shoelace length
3 or 4	27 inches
5 or 6	36 Inches
6 or 7	40 Inches
7	45 Inches
8	54 Inches
9	63 Inches
10 to 11	72 Inches

Summary

Athletic shoelaces and lacing patterns are often overlooked, but can enhance better shoe fit as well as help minimize painful conditions of the foot. Difficult to fit feet and certain foot conditions can be accommodated by simply changing the way the shoe is laced. Proper lacing can deliver a secure, comfortable, and supportive fit, and often, a small change to the athletic shoelacing can make a big difference in comfort and athletic performance. Newer athletic shoelace specialized systems may help reduce loose shoelace-related injury as well as improve performance.

Chapter 9
Prefabricated Insoles and Modifications in Sports Medicine

David M. Davidson

Over-the-counter, ready-made, or prefabricated insoles are marketed widely for relief of foot pain. Shoe stores, sporting goods stores, grocery stores, drug stores have shelves filled with such inserts in all different shapes and sizes. One is able to type "shoe insert" or "over-the-counter foot insert" into a search engine and find more than one million choices. It is not uncommon for the average athlete to self-treat a foot problem using these products prior to seeking professional advice. It is also common for the medical professional to suggest prefabricated insoles before referring them to a podiatric physician or other specialist for care. There are instances when these insoles resolve, or at least improve, the patient's main complaint; however, there are also times when the nonprescription device does more harm than good. Unfortunately, some professionals and nonprofessionals (shoe stores, internet sites, etc.) market over-the-counter insoles as true, corrective orthoses.

Definitions

The American College of Foot and Ankle Orthopedic Medicine in their practice guidelines published definitions that are now widely accepted. An *orthosis* is a device utilized to assist, resist, facilitate, stabilize, or improve range of motion and functional capacity. A *foot orthosis* is defined as a custom or stock orthosis utilized to treat the foot. A *custom foot orthosis* is a device derived from a three-dimensional representation of the patient's foot. *Prescription custom foot orthosis* is created specifically to address the pathomechanical features of a foot condition that may be structural or functional in nature [1].

The dictionary definition of *orthosis* is a device "serving to protect or to restore or improve function..."[2]. A second, accepted definition is "an orthopedic appliance

D.M. Davidson (✉)
Department of Orthopedics, State University of New York, Buffalo, NY, USA; Department of Orthopedics, Kaleida Health System, Buffalo, NY, USA

M.B. Werd, E.L. Knight (eds.), *Athletic Footwear and Orthoses in Sports Medicine*, DOI 10.1007/978-0-387-76416-0_9, © Springer Science+Business Media, LLC 2010

designed to straighten or support a body part" [3]. Kevin Kirby, DPM has eloquently defined *foot orthoses* at the start of Chapter 2. Therefore, it is important for the professional to define terms using specific language to inform the patient exactly what he or she is receiving as treatment for their condition.

In order for a shoe insert to be classified as a true orthosis (i.e., prescription custom foot orthosis), the insert needs to be made from a mold of the foot while the subtalar joint is in the neutral position (neither pronated nor supinated). Once the cast is made, the laboratory constructs a device that, while being worn in the shoe, maintains the subtalar and midtarsal joints in the corrected position during active gait, thereby creating a more biomechanically efficient gait. It should be obvious that a store-bought shoe insert, or an insert taken off the shelf chosen strictly by size of the individual's shoe, does not conform to this description. It has been the experience of this author that retail stores, shoe stores, and some doctor's offices call these store-bought insoles *orthotics* when, in fact, they are not. Common sense should make it clear that simply placing the foot in a foam block and choosing a device based on the configuration of that impression will not satisfy the above definitions. Certainly, pulling a stock shoe insert off the shelf also does not satisfy this designation. Unfortunately, there is no regulation that prevents retail stores from advertising these inserts as orthoses and charging custom orthotic prices for them.

Benefits of Insoles

Dr. Richard Schuster, one of the fathers of lower extremity biomechanics, once said that there is a certain segment of the population that would have fewer symptoms if they were to take a sock and roll it up and place it under the arch in their shoe (Richard Schuster, DPM, 1980, Personal communication). These individuals are usually people with rigid, high-arched feet, which does not allow for shock absorption. This is the reason that many people report feeling better with a simple, store-bought insole (Fig. 9.1).

In practice, prefabricated insoles do have significant value in certain circumstances. For example, many people have a limb length discrepancy, either structural or functional. The body at times compensates for this inequality, but there are times when symptoms develop because of this difference. A leg length difference of 1/2 in. or greater often leads to low back pain, hip pain and, many times, creates pronation of the longer leg creating foot and ankle issues such as posterior tibial tendonitis and plantar fasciitis. Adding a heel lift onto an over-the-counter shoe insert to compensate for the limb length discrepancy will certainly be helpful.

The athlete with an atrophic fat pad and complains of pain under the metatarsal heads and/or under the heel may benefit from a prefabricated insole with additional cushioning [4]. Several years ago, it was believed that injection of collagen would benefit such a patient, using it to replace the natural fat cushion lost in the aging process. This procedure proved both costly and ineffectual as it was often displaced and/or lost after a few weeks of weightbearing. One of the best methods of resolving this complaint is simply cushioning the foot with a full length, soft or semi-rigid,

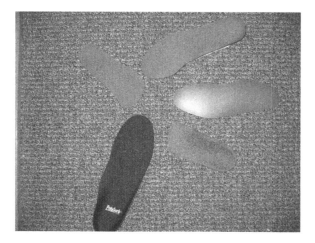

Fig. 9.1 Store-bought insole

over-the-counter device. In addition, athletes who play on unyielding surfaces such as asphalt or concrete may also benefit from such cushioning, especially when they wear thin-soled athletic shoes.

Many forms of arthritis are also characterized by degenerative changes that lead to dorsal subluxation of the toes and plantar prominence of the metatarsal heads. Prefabricated insoles are often beneficial in treatment of these individuals. In addition, modifications can be placed on top of or underneath the insert (Fig. 9.2) to further disperse weight from one particular area.

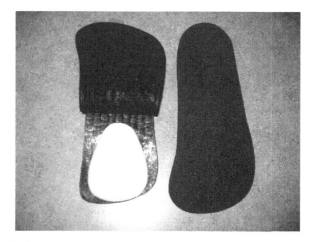

Fig. 9.2 Modifications can be placed on top of or underneath an insert. (From [4], with permission of the American Podiatric Medical Association)

Diabetic athletes may also benefit from a prefabricated insole. Foot problems commonly seen in diabetic patients include vascular impairment, neuropathy, atrophy of the soft tissues, and deformity. The importance of addressing insensitivity, paresthesias, decreased vibratory sense, and motor weakness cannot be stressed enough. Motor neuropathy is commonly believed to lead to weakness in the intrinsic muscles of the foot, upsetting the balance between flexors and extensors of the toes [5]. Atrophy of the small muscles responsible for metatarsophalangeal plantar flexion is thought to lead to the development of hammer toes, claw toes, and prominent metatarsal heads. These deformities are common sites of abnormally high pressure, and repetitive pressure at these sites could result in the buildup of calluses and/or ulceration.

These patients will benefit from prefabricated insoles for the same reason as stated earlier. The insoles can also be easily modified with dispersion using a U-shaped pad or metatarsal pad (Fig. 9.3). These are very helpful in off-loading an area that may be predisposed to ulceration. Diabetic athletes need to be monitored closely and the off-loading material may need to be increased in thickness or placed in other positions if one sees that there is still pressure in a sensitive area.

The same type of off loading a prefabricated insole may be of benefit in athletes who present with forefoot pain due to other pathology such as neuroma or nerve compression, lesser metatarsophalangeal capsulitis, and/or metatarsalgia.

In athletes, whether professional, college, high school, or recreational, prefabricated insoles often have a place in treatment. It is well documented that the forces on the foot are at least three times normal when comparing a running gait to a walking gait [6]. These forces may increase when running downhill or on uneven surfaces, predisposing an athlete to an overuse injury. If an individual's biomechanical examination reveals only a minimal discrepancy, then symptoms may not occur

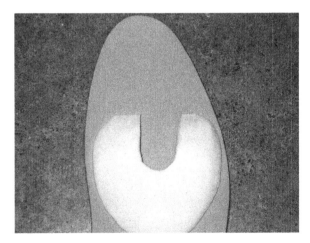

Fig. 9.3 Insoles can also be easily modified with dispersion using a U-shaped pad or metatarsal pad. (From [5]. Copyright © 2007 American Diabetes Association. Reprinted with permission from The American Diabetes Association)

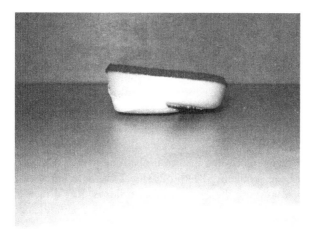

Fig. 9.4 A prefabricated insole may be used as a trial, either alone or with a modification such as a varus wedge

in a walking gait, but may become obvious during running. A prefabricated insole may be used as a trial, either alone or with a modification such as a varus wedge (Fig. 9.4), and may be sufficient to eliminate the athlete's symptoms.

Many times the human body will compensate for imbalances, whether they are structural or biomechanical. Care must be taken not to change an individual's biomechanics solely because an abnormality is documented on examination. It is important to address an athlete's flexibility deficiencies before addressing any biomechanical issues noted on examination. Any shoe insert, whether custom made or not, will not work, for example, if the athlete has a gastrocnemius/soleus equinus as there will be premature heel lift off and will have no effect on the motions of the subtalar or midtarsal joint. When treating with an elite athlete, it is especially dangerous to change the biomechanics unless other attempts at treatment have failed. A professional football running back with early posterior tibial tendonitis, for example, has reached this highest level of achievement with certain biomechanics. Why would one consider changing that with such an individual? One would think this person could be treated without modifying his gait.

It is important for an individual to have an understanding of exactly what he/she receives when a shoe insert is purchased. As stated previously, people use different terms to describe each product. Many people use the word *orthotics* to describe what professionals call a prefabricated insole. The Internet, shoe stores, and even some professionals dispense off-the-shelf inserts and will tell the customer they are receiving a device that will solve all their ills. Wearing such a device, especially in young children, may do more harm than good. It is widely known, for example, that during gait, there is internal rotation of the knee.

Adding an over-the-counter insert in the shoe will change that rotation and may even create rotation in the other direction creating acute symptoms such as lateral knee pain, hip pain, and/or low back pain. In addition, placing a device into a shoe not only fills the arch, which at times is good, it may supinate the foot too much causing an excessive amount of stress laterally and may, in fact, create a stress reaction (or stress fracture) in the fourth or fifth metatarsal. It should be noted that most prefabricated insole are made of a soft or semi-rigid material. Overweight athletes will, therefore, compress the insole to such an extent that it will limit its effectiveness.

Summary

There is a use for prefabricated insoles in the treatment of foot, ankle, lower leg, knee, and low back problems. The professional needs to know when it would be more appropriate to prescribe a custom foot orthosis. It is critical that the athlete makes an educated decision when he or she purchases a prefabricated insole.

References

1. ACFAOM Practice Guidelines, 2005.
2. Dorland's Medical Dictionary. W. B. Saunders, Philadelphia, 2007.
3. Stedmen's Medical Dictionary. Lippincott Williams & Wilkins, Philadelphia, 2004.
4. Özdemir H, Söyüncü Y, Özgörgen M, et al.: Effects of changes in heel fat pad thickness and elasticity on heel pain. J Am Podiatric Med Assoc, 94(1):47–52, 2004.
5. Van Schie CHM, Vermigli C, Carrington AL, Boulton A: Muscle Weakness and Foot Deformities in Diabetes. Diabetes Care, 27:1668–1673, 2004.
6. Nicholas JA, Hershman EB: The Lower Extremity and Spine In Sports Medicine, 396. The C.V. Mosby Company, St. Louis, Vol. 1, Chapter 11,, 1986.

Chapter 10
Orthodigital Devices in Sports Medicine

Matthew B. Werd

Athletes who wear tight-fitting, limited volume shoe gear (soccer/football/baseball/cycling cleats, ballet/dance/aerobic shoes, skating/skiing boots, etc.), and also have digital deformities may benefit from an orthodigital device. An orthodigital device is a custom-made orthopedic appliance used to treat conditions of the digits that has been used successfully for decades [1–3]. These devices can be extremely useful for difficult-to-treat digital conditions in the athlete, which may not respond to traditional care using proper shoe gear and orthoses alone. Orthodigital devices can be used to relieve pressure, immobilize, and reposition the digits (Table 10.1). These devices can be used in place of athletic taping and padding for conditions which may require prolonged splinting.

An orthodigital device is made from a moldable silicone compound that allows the quick fabrication of interdigital wedges, separators, dorsal toe protectors, and orthodigital splints. These devices can be mixed, shaped, and set in less than 5 min, and they are washable, nontoxic, and nonirritating to skin. The material is smooth, soft, and easily kneadable, which – after adding the catalyst hardening paste/curing agent – achieves a putty-like consistency. After 4–5 min, the device hardens into its permanent form and can then be applied to the athlete's foot, and simple modifications can be made by cutting or grinding.

Table 10.1 Indications for orthodigital device in the athlete

Digital deformities requiring immobilization or protection
Heloma durum (hard corns)
Heloma molle (soft corns interdigitally)
Fractures of the digits
Hammer toes
Tight-fitting shoes with limited internal volume (such as soccer/football/baseball/cycling cleats, ballet/dance/aerobic shoes, skating/skiing boots, etc.)

M.B. Werd (✉)
Foot and Ankle Associates, 2939 South Florida Avenue Lakeland, FL, USA

M.B. Werd, E.L. Knight (eds.), *Athletic Footwear and Orthoses in Sports Medicine*, 95
DOI 10.1007/978-0-387-76416-0_10, © Springer Science+Business Media, LLC 2010

Orthodigital devices provide a customizable fit and allow portability (they can be made in an office-setting, in the athletic training room, or even on the sideline). Orthodigital devices provide superior durability versus athletic taping, and they are reusable, washable, and can be removed and re-applied.

Guidelines for Fabrication of an Orthodigital Device

Step-by-Step Process for Fabricating an Orthodigital Device

Step 1: The materials needed are shown in Fig. 10.1 Obtain the approximate volume of material (Figs. 10.2, 10.3, 10.4, 10.5, and 10.6). Prior to adding the hardening agent, estimate the amount of material needed by making a pre-mold of the digits to be splinted.

Step 2: Mix the correct amount of hardening agent with the material. Check the package instructions for the proper ratio of hardening agent to be added to the selected volume. The usual ratio is 1 cm of curing agent per 1 TSP of compound.

Step 3: Mold the mixture to the digits into the correct position. Apply Saran wrap or a plastic bag to the foot to protect the orthodigital device, and then place the athlete's foot into the appropriate athletic cleat/shoe/boot. Allow weight-bearing while the orthodigital device is hardening.

Step 4: Confirm the fit and function of the orthodigital device with the athlete. If the position or hardness of the orthodigital device is not satisfactory, then repeat the process again until correct.

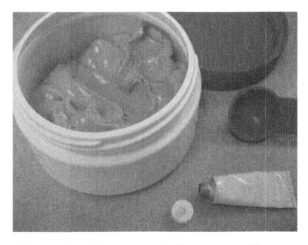

Fig. 10.1 Materials needed to fabricate an orthodigital device: silicon compound, hardening/curing agent, scoop measuring device (1 TSP)

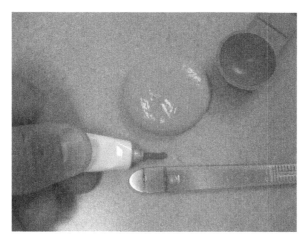

Fig. 10.2 Combine silicon compound with 1 cm of curing agent per one scoop (1 TSP) of compound. For a softer device, add slightly less curing agent. For a more firm device, add slightly more curing agent

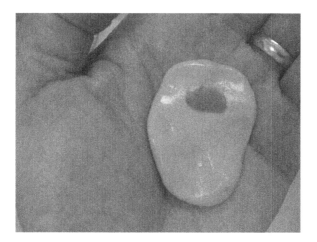

Fig. 10.3 Mix the compound and curing agent

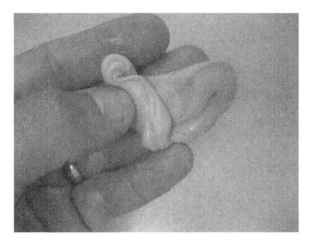

Fig. 10.4 Continued mixing of the compound and curing agent in hand for approximately 20 s

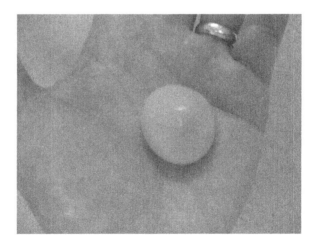

Fig. 10.5 Roll the mixture into a ball

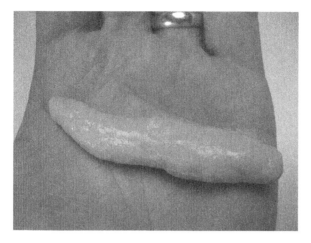

Fig. 10.6 Finally, roll the mixture into an elongated roll before shaping to the athlete's digits, which will help avoid seams in the final shape of the device

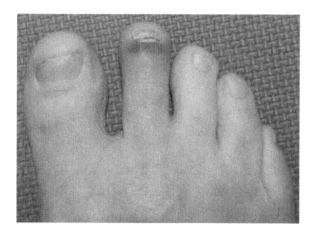

Fig. 10.7 Clinical example of orthodigital device used to support and immobilize a fractured second digit in a competitive triathlete

A clinical example of a common clinical application of an orthodigital device used for an athlete is shown in Figs. 10.7, 10.8, and 10.9.

Fig. 10.8 Orthodigital device shown after molding process

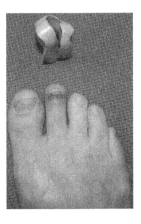

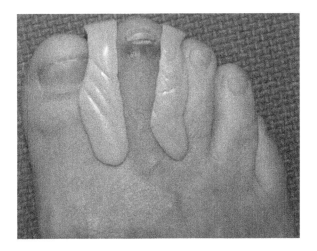

Fig. 10.9 Orthodigital device in place to support the fractured second digit

Summary

Orthodigital devices are custom-made orthopedic appliances which are used to treat multiple conditions of the digits in the athlete. These devices can be extremely useful for difficult-to-treat conditions which may not be amenable to traditional care using taping, padding, shoe gear, and orthoses. Orthodigital devices can be used in place of athletic taping for conditions which may require prolonged splinting. Orthodigital devices provide one more option to the sports medicine practitioner in treating troublesome athletic injuries to the digits.

References

1. Budin HA: Principles and Practice of Orthodigita. Strathore Press, New York, 1941.
2. McGlamry ED, Kitting RW: Postoperative urethane molds. J Am Podiatry Assoc, 58(4): 169, 1968.
3. Whitney KA: Orthodigital Evaluation and Therapeutic Management of Digital Deformity. Churchill Livingstone, New York, 1994.

Chapter 11
Evidence-Based Orthotic Therapy

Paul R. Scherer

The origins of orthotic therapy in sports medicine began in the early 1970s when authors Jim Fixx, M.D. (*The Complete Book of Running*) [1], and Harry F. Halvac, D.P.M. (*The Foot Book: Advice for Athletes*) [2], provided both the public and the medical community anecdotal information about the mechanical origins of foot pathology in athletes and the possible value of custom functional foot orthoses. Most of the American medical community was overwhelmed by the injuries sustained during the latest fitness craze, jogging, and wanted medical solutions to the large numbers of complaints arising from runners.

Primary care physicians, podiatrists, and orthopedic surgeons who had rarely seen stress fractures, ruptured Achilles tendons, and plantar fasciitis were overrun by patients who addicted themselves to recreational jogging and started competing in fun runs or even marathons. The medical literature and continuing education environment provided little help to the medical community, and valid information on either prevention or treatment of the resulting injuries and pathology did not exist. A few texts, written for sports trainers, suggested taping and strapping as a broad solution to many injuries, but this therapy had wildly diverse techniques, methods, and obviously extremely unreliable outcomes.

Somehow, the podiatric medical profession was able to intellectually connect the mechanical origins of many of the sports- and exercise-related injuries to the mechanical benefits of orthoses. With the recommendations of the previously mentioned texts they began an informal national experiment of orthotic therapy on their patients. This adventure and the resulting positive anecdotal evidence created an interest that created sports medicine professional associations, orthotic laboratories, special foot products related to sports, and a huge number of continuing educational opportunities for medical professionals to learn about prescribing and constructing orthoses.

P.R. Scherer (✉)
Department of Applied Biomechanics, Samuel Merritt College of Podiatrics, 825 Vanness Ave., # 204, San Francisco, CA 94109, USA

M.B. Werd, E.L. Knight (eds.), *Athletic Footwear and Orthoses in Sports Medicine*,   103
DOI 10.1007/978-0-387-76416-0_11, © Springer Science+Business Media, LLC 2010

This era was followed by publications, existing and new, supported by professional organizations, dedicated to sports medicine and including some original but not necessarily scientific information related to the effectiveness of functional and soft orthoses. Since the emerging sport shoe industry viewed the origins of pathology, at the time, to impact forces, the original investigation focused on impact reducing orthotic devices rather than functional devices [3, 4].

Slowly the professions and sports medicine community recognized that there will be a continued interest in regular physical activity; that injuries are a common problem in physical activity of healthy individuals; that most pathology is the result of overuse, training errors, and poor foot wear; and finally that many of these problems can be ameliorated or even prevented by custom functional orthoses, especially in the runner with excessively pronated feet [5]. These realizations, in turn, lead to the investigation, with orthotic therapy of individual mechanically induced pathologies and eventually to pathology-specific orthoses for the control, treatment, or prevention of the symptoms related to these pathologies.

Evidence for Orthotic Therapy

This chapter investigates the evidence in the literature of the effectiveness of orthotic therapy in certain pathologies. It is well understood that the pathologies discussed are limited in the context of the total knowledge of the subject. Also, it is understood that the evidence is limited to the available state-of-the-art technology, evolving sport shoe construction and the variety of both sport surfaces and the individual's unique foot and ankle mechanics. There will be more evidence in the near future.

The first significant evidence on the effectiveness of foot orthoses on specific sports medicine pathology was a retrospective cross-sectional survey published in the *American Journal of Sports Medicine* in 1991 [6]. The study, done at a moment in time when there were an estimated 30 million recreational runners in the United States, estimated that 60% of sports participants would experience an injury [7, 8].

Five hundred questionnaires were distributed to runners who were using custom orthoses for the symptomatic relief of lower extremity complaints including plantar fasciitis, patellofemoral disorders, and a variety of tendinitis. Seventy-five and one half percent of the respondents reported complete resolution or great improvement of their symptoms. Ninety percent of the respondents demonstrated a significant satisfaction with orthotic therapy because they continued to use their orthoses even after resolution of their symptoms.

Since publication of this survey there has been much more specific evidence on the effect of custom functional orthoses on specific pathologies. The remainder of this chapter investigates the evidence on plantar fasciitis, functional hallux limitus, patellofemoral and medial knee pain syndrome, and tarsal tunnel syndrome. Following chapters provide recommendations, based on the literature evidence, on specific prescriptions to meet the pathomechanical uniqueness of each entity as well as several others.

Plantar Fasciitis

Plantar fasciitis is the common vernacular for mechanically induced subcalcaneal pain, presenting as pain and tenderness at the medial tubercle of the calcaneal tuberosity as a result of abnormal foot mechanics [9]. Today it could be the most common and persistent problem affecting the foot of athletes, regardless of sport. Foot orthoses are an accepted mechanical treatment for this pathology; however, the numerous variations in foot orthoses make it difficult to determine which variable is responsible for the change. One study showed that treatment with custom orthoses designed to prevent midtarsal joint collapse during gait resulted in 89% of subjects getting relief from their symptoms [10]. Kogler demonstrated that a wedge under the lateral aspect of the forefoot significantly reduced the strain on the plantar aponeurosis and suggested that this may be effective for the treatment of plantar fasciitis [11]. The following outcome studies provide additional evidence to support treatment with custom and prefabricated orthoses for plantar fasciitis.

The first study by Pfeffer [12] was a well-publicized study that compared the effectiveness of stretching alone to stretching in combination with one of four different shoe inserts in the treatment of plantar fasciitis. Shoe inserts included three prefabricated pads (silicone heel pad, $\frac{3}{4}$-length felt pad, and rubber heel cup) and custom foot orthoses. Though the conclusion states that prefabs along with stretching "is more effective than custom orthoses," an analysis of the statistics shows that all five treatment groups had an improvement in both pain scales, with no significant difference among the groups in the reduction of overall pain scores after 8 weeks of treatment when controlled for covariates. This misleading conclusion prompted a deeper look into the study details to determine why the authors would have made a statement that was not supported by their data.

A retrospective analysis shows that the device type was not consistent. Forty-five percent of the custom orthoses were rigid polypropylene (normal width, 14–16-mm heel cup, no posts or top covers). Another 38% were identical except that the flexibility was semi-rigid. The flexibility variance was not evaluated in this study, nor mentioned as a variable that could affect outcomes. The remainder of the orthoses (17%) varied dramatically. Variables other than shell flexibility that were altered included heel cup depth (range 8–18 mm), width (narrow–wide), use of a rearfoot post, and use of a top cover. The authors noted that patients were encouraged not to change their regular shoe wear. Did the authors believe that a narrow device with a 8-mm heel cup was equivalent to a wide device with a 18-mm heel cup for a patient with plantar fasciitis, or were they accommodating the patient's shoe choice as limited by their protocol? Improper footwear has been identified as a contributing factor in plantar fasciitis [13].

Another variable with the orthoses involves the negative cast. Custom orthosis studies generally allow only a single experienced practitioner to cast each patient, minimizing any effect of the casting process on orthosis outcomes. It appears that 13 different practitioners casted the 42 subjects, with these practitioners learning to cast by watching a video. Considering the number of uncontrolled variables in the custom orthoses group, it is unclear how the authors drew any conclusions about the efficacy of custom orthoses in the treatment of plantar fasciitis, or justified a comparison to the other treatment groups. Fortunately, there have been other outcome studies in the treatment of plantar fasciitis.

Another positive evaluation of custom orthotic therapy for plantar fasciitis by Lynch [14] evaluated the effect of three widely accepted treatments: anti-inflammatory (injected and oral NSAIDs), accommodative (viscose heel cup and acetaminophen), and mechanical (low-dye strapping followed by custom foot orthoses). This randomized prospective study found that 70% of the patients in the mechanical therapy group had improvements in pain and function, significantly better than the accommodative (30%) or the anti-inflammatory (33%) groups. Only 4% of the mechanical group had treatment failure, as opposed to 42% for the accommodative group and 23% for the anti-inflammatory group. The authors concluded that mechanical control with custom orthoses is more effective than anti-inflammatory therapy or accommodative therapy used in this study.

Martin [15] published a prospective randomized study that evaluated the effectiveness of three different mechanical modalities used in the treatment of plantar fasciitis including over-the-counter arch supports, rigid custom-made orthoses with a heel post, and night splints. Though all three devices were effective as initial treatments for plantar fasciitis after 12 weeks of use, "there was a statistically significant difference among the three groups with respect to early patient withdrawal from the study due to continued severe pain, noncompliance, or inability to tolerate the device. Patient compliance was greatest with the use of custom-made orthoses."

Langdorf [16] conducted a randomized trial that evaluated the short-term and long-term effectiveness of foot orthoses in the treatment of plantar fasciitis. The three treatment arms were sham orthosis made of soft, thin EVA foam molded over unmodified plaster cast, prefabricated foot orthosis made from firm density polyethylene foam, and Root functional custom foot orthosis. Both the prefabricated orthoses and the custom orthoses produced statistically significant improvements in function at 3 months. The authors noted that more participants in the sham group and the prefabricated group broke protocol than in the custom group.

Recently, Roos [17] evaluated the effect of custom-fitted foot orthoses and night splints, alone or combined, in treating plantar fasciitis in a prospective randomized trial with 1-year follow-up. The authors concluded that custom foot orthoses and anterior night splints were effective, both short term and long term, in treating pain from plantar fasciitis with all groups improving significantly in all outcomes evaluated across all times. "Parallel improvements in function, foot-related quality of life, and a better compliance suggest that a foot orthosis is the best choice for initial treatment of plantar fasciitis."

Although at first glance the data on the efficacy of orthotic therapy for plantar fasciitis in the athlete appears conflicting, every study supports the use of custom orthoses. Each study leaves little doubt that this pathology is mechanical in origin and effective treatment is accomplished through mechanical control by custom orthoses. Future research may shed light on which modifications of custom orthoses may be most effective in controlling the midtarsal joint motion to prevent stretching of the plantar fascia.

Functional Hallux Limitus

The inability to dorsiflex the hallux during sports or the forced dorsiflexion in the absence of adequate range of motion produces forces that create pathology including inflammation of the soft tissue, deterioration of the cartilage and subchondral bone, and proliferation of the osseous structures of the first metatarsal phalangeal joint.

Functional hallux limitus is defined by several authors as 12° or less of restricted hallux dorsiflexion in closed kinetic chain and 50° or greater motion in open kinetic chain examination. Functional hallux limitus is suspected to be the pathology behind the development of hallux abducto-valgus, hallux rigidus, hallux pinch callus, and subhallux ulcerations [18]. This section reviews functional hallux limitus (FHL) only, and not structural hallux limitus (SHL), since treatment of the latter, with orthoses, is seldom mentioned in the literature and is suspected to be ineffective.

Whitaker [19] established a definitive relationship between foot position and hallux dorsiflexion. This study used low-dye strapping for mechanical control and evaluated its effect in 22 subjects. The study demonstrated that the mean range of motion before application was 24.7° and 31.81° after application showing statistical significance. This provided quantifiable data demonstrating that changing the foot mechanics similar to that produced by an orthoses can reverse the joint restriction found in hallux limitus.

Grady's [20] retrospective analysis evaluated patients with functional hallux limitus treated with various surgical and nonsurgical modalities [3]. Hallux limitus was defined as less than 10° of hallux dorsiflexion. Forty-seven percent of the patients with symptomatic hallux limitus were successfully treated with custom orthoses alone.

The most recent evidence of the effect of orthoses on functional hallux limitus was published in 2006 [18]. This study evaluated the effect of a foot orthoses (made from a negative cast with the first ray plantarflexed) on hallux dorsiflexion in patients with functional hallux limitus of 12° or less. Forty-eight feet of 27 subjects were tested both in stance and in gait, with and without orthoses. The results demonstrated an increase in hallux dorsiflexion with orthoses in 100% of the subjects, both in stance and in gait. When the orthoses were used in stance, hallux dorsiflexion showed a mean increase of 8.8° or 90% improvement. The gait evaluation methodology used a reduction in subhallux pressure following heel lift as a determinant of increased hallux dorsiflexion. The functional orthoses resulted in a mean reduction in subhallux pressure of 14.8%. This study proved that in all subjects, orthoses reversed to some degree the joint restriction found in hallux limitus.

The mechanical origins of hallux limitus and hallux valgus have been debated for years, including the possibilities of genetic or shoe-related origins. We now have ample proof that the joint restriction is due to abnormal foot position and, most importantly, this limitation can be reversed by custom orthoses.

Tarsal Tunnel Syndrome

Most sports medicine health professionals always suspected a casual relationship between over pronator athletes and symptoms of tarsal tunnel syndrome. Apple [21] was the first to document that this entity was common to long distance runners and the first to recommend a custom orthotic device, especially before intervention with injection therapy or surgical decompression.

Keck [22] first described tarsal tunnel syndrome (TTS) as pain in the proximal medial arch and paresthesia along the lateral and medial plantar nerves. He noted that the foot was often excessively pronated at the subtalar joint in TTS. The etiology was hypothesized to be traction on the tibial nerve and compression of that nerve by the flexor retinaculum or compression of the medial plantar nerve as it perforates the fascia. No clinical outcome studies document orthotic effectiveness for TTS; however, three recent studies on the pathomechanics of TTS indicate why foot orthosis therapy would decrease symptoms.

Trepman [23] measured the tarsal tunnel pressure with the foot in various positions. The positions measured in this cadaveric study were neutral heel position with mild plantarflexion, everted heel position with mild dorsiflexion, and inverted heel position with mild dorsiflexion. They found increased pressure in the tarsal tunnel when the STJ was pronated and reduced pressure in the tarsal tunnel when the STJ was supinated and mildly plantarflexed.

Labib [24] evaluated 286 patients with heel pain over a 3-year period. The authors identified 14 patients who were diagnosed with the triad of plantar fasciitis, posterior tibial tendinitis, and tarsal tunnel syndrome (heel pain triad). The authors believe that the triad may be a stage of breakdown of the longitudinal arch and that failure of the static arch (plantar fascia) and dynamic arch (PTT) may result in a variable degree of arch collapse leading to TTS. They also postulated that the "lack of muscular support of the longitudinal arch produces traction injury to the tibial nerve and results in tarsal tunnel syndrome."

Kinoshita [25] developed a diagnostic test for TTS that sheds light on its etiology and treatment. The foot was passively held in maximal dorsiflexion and eversion for 5–10 s (with all metatarsophalangeal joints maximally dorsiflexed) to create nonweight-bearing STJ pronation. Patients diagnosed with TTS were tested preoperatively and postoperatively, with results compared to a control group. No symptoms were induced in the control group with this test. Preoperatively, 97.7% of patients with TTS had an increase in local tenderness, while 95.3% had an increase in Tinel's sign. The study confirms that this test is an excellent diagnostic tool for TTS and provides evidence that holding the foot in a non-everted position with an orthosis may improve symptoms.

This evidence shows, without a doubt, that tarsal tunnel syndrome is of mechanical origin. The activity of the long distance runner makes this pathology frequent and more intractable. The origin starts with eversion of the rear foot and lowering of the longitudinal arch increasing the pressure in the tarsal tunnel. Custom functional orthoses can be designed to reverse this mechanism by increasing the longitudinal arch plantarflexing the ankle and preventing rear foot eversion.

Knee Pain

The dynamics of internal rotation of the leg as a result of subtalar joint pronation and midtarsal joint motion is exaggerated in most sport activities. The ability of an orthotic device to limit either of these motions can have a dramatic effect on the pathology such as patellofemoral pain syndrome, medial knee pain, and medial knee osteoarthritis symptoms. Most of the kinematic and kinetic data suggest that there is a direct correlation between limiting STJ and MTJ motion and the reduction of symptoms. The exact mechanism of orthoses or the best material, additions, extensions, construction, and cast corrections have been yet delineated.

Saxena [26] was able to define and diagnose in a retrospective review of 102 athletic patients with patellofemoral pain syndrome. All subjects demonstrated an abnormal varus foot deformity. Seventy-six and one half percent of the patients were improved at their first follow-up visit and 2% were asymptomatic by that time. The group with improvement showed a statistically significant decrease in the level of pain related to the use of the orthoses.

Stackhouse [27] performed kinematic and kinetic studies to delineate the amount of internal rotation and adduction of the knee in athletes both with and without functional orthoses. The authors sought to identify a difference in the rearfoot strike patterns of the 15 subjects and relate the variance to foot orthoses. One segment of their analysis showed that orthosis intervention did not change the rearfoot motion but did change the internal rotation and abduction.

Rubin [28] investigated the effects functional orthoses with a lateral valgus wedge might have in patients who had significant medial knee pain and associated disability and osteoarthritis of the knee. Thirty subjects were confirmed to have osteoarthritis of the knee radiographically in the medial compartment. Each patient was casted for and dispensed a custom orthoses with a 5° lateral valgus heel wedge. The visual analog scale at dispensing, 3 weeks and again at 6 weeks, showed a significant reduction in pain. The reduction in pain was greater in individuals with less severe osteoarthritis, possibly suggesting that early intervention is an optimum treatment strategy. All of the subjects reported some reduction of symptoms at the 6-week threshold confirming the casual relationship of orthoses.

Patient outcome studies and kinetic studies confirm that custom functional orthoses may have a more proximal effect on symptoms and pathomechanics than just isolated to the foot and ankle. This is confirmation that the investigation of the effect of custom orthoses is far from complete especially in the athlete. Investigation has now begun to appear in the literature that demonstrates that these devices, if made correctly, may also have a positive effect beyond the knee, including the hip and back.

Summary

Jim Fixx and Harry Hlavac, four decades ago, saw a paradigm in sports medicine that has been realized today. Orthoses and orthotic therapy has now reached a level of scientific validity in many respects related to many pathologies. Orthoses not only have offered a proven treatment for some of the problems but have also reached a level of preventative medicine. Further investigation into pathology-specific and sports-specific orthoses may show an even greater efficacy and possibly performance enhancement.

References

1. Fixx J: The Complete Book of Running, Random House Inc. New York, NY 1977.
2. Hlavac, H F: The Foot Book: Advice for Athletes. Mountain View, CA World Publications 1977.
3. Frederick EC, Hagy JL, Mann RA: The prediction vertical impact force during running. J Biomech 14:498, 1981.
4. Frederick EC, Clarke TE, and Hamill CL: The effect of running shoe design on shock attenuation. In Frederick (ed.), Sport Shoes and Playing Surfaces. pp. 190–198. Human Kinetic, Champaign, IL., 1984.
5. McKenzie DC, Clement DB, and Taunton JE: Running shoes. Orthot Injuries Sports Med, 2:334–347, 1985.
6. Gross ML, Davlin LB, Evanski, PM: Effectiveness of orthotic shoe inserts in the long-distance runner. Am J Sports Med, 19 (4), 1991.
7. Kysgikn J, Wiklander J: Injuries in runners. Am J Sports Med, 15:158–171, 1987.
8. Sheehan GA: An overview of overuse syndromes in distance runners. Am NY Acad Sci, 301:877–880, 1977.
9. Scherer PR, Waters LL: How to address mechanically-induced subcalcaneal pain. Pod Today, 19(11):78, 2006.
10. Scherer PR: Heel spur syndrome. JAPMA, 81(2): 68, 1988.
11. Kogler GF, Veer FB, Solomonidis SE, et al.: The influence of medial and lateral placement of orthotic wedges on loading of the plantar aponeurosis. JBJS, 81–A(10): 1403, 1999.
12. Pfeffer G, Bacchetti P, Deland J, et al.: Comparison of custom and prefabricated orthoses in the initial treatment of proximal plantar fasciitis. Foot Ankle Int, 20(4):214, 1999.
13. Richie DH: Foot Ankle Q, 18(2):10, 2006.
14. Lynch DM, Goforth WP, Martin JE, et al.: Conservative treatment of plantar fasciitis. JAPMA, 88(8): 375, 1998.
15. Martin JE, Hosch JC, Goforth WP, et al.: Mechanical treatment of plantar fasciitis. JAPMA, 91(2): 55, 2001.
16. Langdorf KB, Keenan AM, Herbert RD: Effectiveness of foot orthoses to treat plantar fasciitis. Arch Intern Med, 166:1305, 2006.
17. Roos E, Engstrom M, Soderberg B: Foot orthoses for the treatment of plantar fasciitis. Foot Ankle Int, 27(8):606, 2006.
18. Scherer PR, Sanders J, Eldredge D, et al.: Effect of functional foot orthoses on the first metatarsophalangeal joint dorsiflexion in stance and gait. JAPMA, 96(6):474, 2006.
19. Whitaker JM, Augustus K, Ishii S: Effect of low Dye strap on pronation sensitive mechanical attributes of the foot. JAPMA, 93:118, 2003.
20. Grady JF, Axe TM, Zager EJ, et al.: A retrospective analysis of 772 patients with hallux limitus. JAPMA, 92:102, 2002.
21. Apple DF: End stage running problems. Clin Sports Med, 4 (4), October 1985.
22. Keck C. The tarsal tunnel syndrome. JBJS, 44–A:180, 1962.

23. Trepman E, Kadel NJ, Chisholm K, et al.: Effect of foot and ankle position on tarsal tunnel compartment pressure. Foot Ankle Int, 20(11):721, 1999.
24. Labib SA, Gould JS, Rodrigues-del-Rio FA, et al.: Heel pain triad (HPT). Foot Ankle Int, 23(3): 212, 2002.
25. Kinoshita M, Okuda R, Morikawa J, et al.: The dorsiflexion-eversion test for diagnosis of tarsal tunnel syndrome. JBJS 83A:1835, 2001.
26. Saxena A, Haddad J: The effect of foot orthoses on patellofemoral pain syndrome. J Am Podiatr Med Assoc, 93:264–271, 2003.
27. Stackhouse CL, Davis IM, Hamill J: Orthotic intervention in forefoot and rearfoot strike running patterns. Clin Bomech, 19:64–70, 2004.
28. Rubin R, Menz H: Use of laterally wedged custom foot orthoses to reduce pain associated with medial knee osteoarthritis: A preliminary investigation. J Am Podiatr Med Assoc, 95:347–352, 2005.

Chapter 12
Custom Foot Orthoses

Paul R. Scherer

A well thought-out prescription for custom foot orthoses (CFO) that takes into consideration the dysfunction of that particular athlete's foot and the activity of the athlete is a pre-requisite to a successful clinical outcome. Addressing the specific needs of the pathology producing the dysfunction as well as the symptoms the athlete is experiencing makes the difference between treatment success or failure and patient satisfaction or frustration. Dispensing the same orthosis for posterior tibial dysfunction and plantar fasciitis will not produce the same successful outcomes for both because these are different pathologies with different functional needs and different mechanical origins.

Clinicians should stop thinking about generic custom orthoses and embrace the concept of pathology-specific orthoses. Selecting custom orthoses with disregard for the particular pathology or foot type of an athlete is as effective as selecting an antibiotic without regard to the pathogen or the physiologic condition of a patient. Although there is adequate information in the literature to provide information about what type and modification of orthoses are best used for specific pathologies little information exists about what type and modification are best utilized for a specific sport.

A systematic approach to constructing the most effective orthoses for a patient's specific pathology takes only a little more time and effort than making generic orthoses. The following considerations help to select the various components for an orthoses. The steps include embracing the concept of pathology-specific orthoses and then prescribing correct material flexibility, positive cast modifications, posting, intrinsic accommodations, and special additions.

A review of the literature has shown that altering the position of the foot may contribute to improved function of some feet. Published research has described how an orthosis that is designed to invert the calcaneus can significantly reduce the pressure on the posterior tibial nerve in the tarsal tunnel syndrome [1]. Placing a greater

P.R. Scherer (✉)
Department of Applied Biomechanics, Samuel Merritt College of Podiatrics, 825 Vanness Ave, # 204, San Francisco, CA 94109, USA

M.B. Werd, E.L. Knight (eds.), *Athletic Footwear and Orthoses in Sports Medicine*,
DOI 10.1007/978-0-387-76416-0_12, © Springer Science+Business Media, LLC 2010

valgus correction on the forefoot portion of the orthoses dramatically reduces pull or strain on the plantar fascia as compared to varus correction on the rearfoot [2]. Repositioning the first ray both by casting method and by certain forefoot extensions can improve the range of hallux dorsiflexion in functional hallux limitus [3].

Knowing about the new concepts and still prescribing the same custom orthoses, regardless of pathology, is not providing patients with quality care that produces an optimum clinical outcome. Understanding what foot dysfunction caused the symptoms and focusing on a device design that works to reverse the dysfunction is the goal of pathology-specific orthotic therapy.

Material and Flexibility

Select material and flexibility for the body of the device that meets the needs of the patient's foot type and pathology. The two most common materials used in the United States and Canada are polypropylene and graphite composite. The comparative value of these materials is not as important as the concept that each material has several thicknesses or flexibility and each flexibility is specific to the needs of different foot types, pathology, and occasionally to the sport activity of the patient.

One prospective nonrandomized study did compare a thermoset material to the traditional polypropylene used to treat professional athletes. Subjects were able to perceive a significant difference of orthosis weight, resilience, and springiness. The subjects preferred the overall comfort of the thinner thermoset material [4]. The study did not determine a greater effectiveness related to the pathology, but assumptions can be made between comfort and patient compliance.

This chapter cannot provide the appropriate flexibility for every foot type and pathology, but a few examples will give the concept and the direction for improved outcomes. The ultimate combination of factors must be determined by the clinician for each individual athlete. The thinner the polypropylene, the more flexible the device will be, depending on the weight of the patient. There is a difference between milled and vacuumed polypropylene. A milled polypropylene device, since it was never heated for molding, is inherently more rigid at a particular patient weight. Conversely, the polypropylene in a vacuumed formed device has been essentially melted and develops a more flexible characteristic. Orthotic laboratories that use polypropylene will either ask for the desired flexibility, on the prescription form, or ask for the desired thickness. Orthotic laboratories that use graphite alter the formulation to make the devices more flexible or rigid for a particular patient weight.

The following two examples show how flexibility relates to foot types and pathology. Pathology related to gastroc-soleus equinus is difficult to control because the source of the deformity is such a powerful pronator and midtarsal joint deformer. Many clinicians use rigid devices for powerful pronators for better control, but actually this places the foot between the proverbial rock and a hard place, producing greater symptoms from the rigid orthoses than from the pathology. Compromising the rigidity of the device in this particular situation, by making it more flexible, maintains some but not total control of the deformity and allows the device to be tolerated. A runner with limitation of ankle joint dorsiflexion and compensation at the midtarsal joint needs a less rigid device. The opposite of this situation is controlling the extremely pronated foot with tarsal coalition or the peroneal spastic flat foot or adult acquired flat foot from PT dysfunction. Nothing but a rigid device will control this pathology and the more the patient weighs, the thicker the polypropylene must be to produce a rigid device.

Correction and Positive Balancing

Another important parameter of the orthosis prescription is orthosis shape and positive cast work. This section of the orthotic prescription includes heel cup depth, orthosis width, cast fill, medial skive, and positive cast inversion. Examples of how each relate to some pathologies can be described but obviously not how they relate to all foot pathologies.

Heel cup depth, from most orthotic laboratories, includes shallow (10 mm), standard (14 mm), deep (18 mm), and extra deep. The primary concept to remember when choosing a heel cup depth is the deeper the heel cup, the greater the surface area of plastic and the greater the control of the rearfoot. If the calcaneus is everted, a deep heel cup will provide greater control. The only reason to use a standard or shallow heel cup in the presence of an everted calcaneus is to accommodate the patient's athletic shoe selection, or because the pathology originates distal to the midtarsal joint. A rigid ski boot or hockey skate is so stable that heel cup depth is of little consequence. An attempt to treat posterior tibial tendinitis with an orthosis with a shallow heel cup is an effort in futility.

Orthosis width generally refers only to the width of the distal edge of the orthoses and the resulting breadth of the arch area. Width determines the stability of the orthotic in the athletic shoe during and after midstance and control over the first ray. The longest horizontal support against frontal plane motion of the orthosis in the shoe is the distal edge. The wider the orthoses, the less likely it will tilt with pronation at midstance. When treating pathology that involves excessive midtarsal joint motion, like plantar fasciitis and functional hallux limitus, a wider front edge withstands the deforming forces that are present in a dysfunctional foot. An orthosis raises the base of the first metatarsal to increase hallux dorsiflexion in functional hallux limitus. If the orthosis is narrow, it cannot create a force to hold the base of the first metatarsal up. A wide front edge is rarely an athletic shoe problem, with the exception of extreme styles like soccer cleats. Insisting on choosing orthosis width appropriate for the patients' pathology rather than allowing the orthotic laboratory to default to narrow so that the CFO fits in any shoe is essential.

Cast fill was originally introduced by Dr. Merton Root [5] as a technique intended to blend the forefoot correction into the arch of the positive. An orthotic laboratory should offer several cast fills to address the need of a specific pathology. An orthosis made from a positive cast with minimum fill will conform close to the arch of the foot. Minimum fill offers the most control over arch collapse and is essential for symptoms produced by cavus feet and hard to control pronated feet.

Standard fill lowers the arch slightly and makes the orthosis less "tight" against the foot in stance. This is useful when there are secondary issues with the foot, like limitations of motion secondary to osteoarthritis or intense sport activities, both of which require a more gentle control of the foot. Maximum fill for equinus, muscle spasm, or tarsal coalition is a strategy that allows for minimum control in situations where the least control can produce enough symptom reduction without creating other problems. Again, allowing the laboratory to select the arch fill without knowing the condition of the patients' foot could produce a clinical failure or a very uncomfortable orthoses.

It is critical that the practitioner control how much cast fill is added to the positive cast. Adding excessive cast fill is a common laboratory error practice since it produces a more forgiving CFO with less potential to cause arch irritation. Although somewhat less likely to cause arch irritation, an orthosis made from a positive cast with excessive fill will result in an orthosis with inadequate control, since the corrective forces that an orthotic device creates are ameliorated. Prescribing a minimum fill orthoses can be confirmed by matching it to the arch of the foot closely when the foot is held in casting position before dispensing.

The medial skive technique was probably one of the most significant and effective developments in orthosis design. This contribution to the custom functional Root-type design, developed by Kevin Kirby, D.P.M. [6], allowed for the manipulation of ground reactive force to provide better control of the rearfoot. Treating athletes with flexible flatfoot, plantar fasciitis with an everted heel, or PT dysfunction without this modification usually produces a less than optimal result. Most pathologies that include an everted calcaneus in stance are treated more successfully with this technique, which produces a rise in the medial side of the heel cup by 2, 4, or 6 mm. Clinicians who are introduced to this modification frequently discover significantly improved clinical outcomes when they add this modification to the prescription of patients with pathology related to an everted calcaneus. This modification is not effective with a shallow heel cup; it requires a deep or at least standard depth. Most laboratories don't charge for this additional modification.

Selecting the most appropriate rearfoot post is very important in the athlete. The original design, during the introduction of orthoses, included this hard plastic foundation for the rear portion of the device. Its purpose was to stabilize the orthosis in the shoe during midstance and not to invert the device nor correct for heel varus or valgus which is a common misconception. There is no other proven benefit or purpose for a varus rearfoot post and logically it doesn't make any sense to invert the front edge of the orthotic by increasing the rearfoot post varus.

Is a rearfoot post necessary for every pathology? No one knows. A prospective study to treat plantar fasciitis demonstrated a positive outcome in 85% of the patients treated with low-dye strapping and followed by functional semi-rigid orthoses [7]. None of the orthoses in this study had a rearfoot post. If you use a rearfoot post to stabilize the orthoses, a polypropylene post seems to be the most durable. Heel strike in some sports can significantly deform an EVA rearfoot post. Some laboratories offer a variety of shock absorbing materials, but today's athletic shoes are engineered to serve this purpose more effectively. Some laboratories offer soft posts, but within a few months the plantar surface of a soft post has rounded, losing its stabilization quality. Anecdotal evidence seems to indicate that for most pathology hard plastic rearfoot post stabilizes the orthosis by increasing the plantar surface area, reinforcing the shape of the heel cup and extending the life of an orthosis.

Orthosis Extensions and Additions

Selecting the forefoot extensions and special additions that make the orthosis specific to the needs of the particular pathology and the patient is vital to a positive outcome. Although there are literally hundreds of combinations of extensions and additions developed over the last 50 years, several are very important to understand if one treats by pathology, especially for functional hallux limitus, metatarsalgia, and posterior tibial tendinitis. Very little research is available on additions other than the metatarsal bar/pad and the reverse Morton's extension.

Functional hallux limitus has been accepted as the precursor pathology to the deformities of hallux valgus and hallux rigidus since it was first described by Pat Laird, D.P.M., in 1972 [8]. The contemporary concept is that some people have a decreased *stiffness* of their first ray which dorsiflexes in response to increased ground reactive force at the first metatarsal head, and this motion significantly decreases the dorsiflexion of the big toe joint. The purpose of an orthosis in this pathology is to reverse this by raising the medial column of the foot and plantarflexing the first ray. The reverse Morton's extension is an addition to custom orthoses that will dramatically decrease the ground reactive force under the first metatarsal head and allows the first ray to plantarflex and give greater range of motion to the hallux. This is a proven technique in non-sport experiments [3]. The reverse Morton's extension on a functional polypropylene device with a 4-mm medial skive is now classified as the pathology-specific functional hallux limitus orthotic device.

Posterior tibial tendon dysfunction (PTTD) or adult acquired flatfoot (AAF) following sports injury to this tendon has been successfully treated with foot orthoses. A study noted that in some cases the CFO worked as well as an AFO brace [9]. The orthoses stabilized the rearfoot and medial longitudinal arch in patients with chronic PTTD. A common complication of treating PTTD or AAF is the pressure placed under the navicular tuberosity by the rigid plastic of the orthosis resulting in pain. An addition called a sweet spot seems, in most cases, to solve this complication and reduce or eliminate the pain at this region in the medial longitudinal arch. A sweet spot is an orthotic implant of poron that is depressed into the body of the orthosis, while the plastic is still hot. This creates a soft cushion exactly where the navicular tuberosity touches the device. The clinician marks the area of the foot with a transfer marker, which identifies the area on the cast and allows the laboratory to implant the poron disk, of any size, in the exact area. This is also a useful pathology-specific addition for other problems like plantar fibromas and painful scars. The sweet spot can be placed wherever the clinician can draw a circle and be of any size, without disrupting the strength or integrity of the device.

The previously mentioned orthotic materials, construction technique, additions, and modifications obviously must vary according to age, sport, and intensity of the individual. Orthotic therapy for the athlete may have become more pathology-specific in the literature but because of the variations of age and sport a great deal of the decision making is left to the clinician with little evidence data to confirm any predictions of effectiveness.

So much remains unknown, even just considering orthosis flexibility. An average running sport requires 1000 foot strikes per mile [10]. The time of full foot strike is calculated in sixtieths of a second and is the only moment in time during the mile when the orthosis is effective. It is a very brief moment for the orthosis to have an effect, but according to many reports the positive effect on symptoms is more common than not.

Focusing treatment on a specific pathology rather than on a deformity can significantly improve clinical outcomes. An understanding of the pathomechanics that produced the athlete's symptoms allows the clinician to address the needs of the athlete more specifically and construct an orthosis more effectively. Considering the material flexibility, advanced positive cast modifications, posting, and special additions will enable the sports practitioner to make a better orthosis for the athlete. A prefabricated orthosis meets some of the needs of all patients. A generic orthosis meets some of the needs of all pathologies. But a pathology-specific custom foot orthosis should meet all the needs of a particular patient with a particular pathology.

References

1. Trepman E, Kadel NJ: Effects of foot and ankle position on tarsal tunnel compartment pressure. Foot and Ankle Int, Nov 20(11): 721, 2000.
2. Kogler G. Veer F. et al.: The influence of medial and lateral placement of orthotic wedges on loading of the plantar aponeurosis, an in vitro study. JBJS AM,81:1403–1413, 1999.
3. Scherer PR, Sanders J, Eldredge D. et al.: Effect of functional foot orthoses on the first metatarsophalangeal joint dorsiflexion in stance and gait. JAPMA, 96(6):474, 2006.
4. Richie DH Jr, Olsen WR: Orthoses for athletic overuse injuries. Comparison of two component materials. JAPMA, Sept 83:492, 1993.
5. Root M: Development of the functional orthoses. Clin Podiatr Med Surg, 11 (2), April 1994.
6. Kirby, KA: The medial skive technique: Improving pronation control in foot orthoses. J Am Podiatr Med Assoc, 82: 177, 1992.
7. Scherer P: Heel spur syndrome. JAPMA, 81(2): 68–72, February 1991.
8. Laird P: Functional hallux limitus, The Illinois Podiatrist, June 1972.
9. Chao W, Wapner K, Lee T. et al.: onoperative management of posterior tibial dysfunction. Foot Ankle Int, 17(12), December 1996.
10. Gordon GM: Podiatric sports medicine, evaluation and prevention of injuries. Clin Podiatr, 1(2), August 1984.

Chapter 13
Ankle Foot Orthoses for the Athlete

Douglas H. Richie

Ankle braces have emerged as a standard therapeutic modality in the treatment of the athlete. Over the past 30 years, more research has been published studying the treatment effects of ankle braces than any research on foot inserts or foot orthoses. Still, there remain many misconceptions and questions about the use of bracing of the athlete. This chapter provides an overview of the types, indications, and effects of braces used in the lower extremity.

Terminology

An *orthosis* is an apparatus used to support, align, prevent, or correct deformities or to improve the function of movable parts of the body [1]. The term *brace* is essentially synonymous with orthosis. The term *orthotic* is an adjective, i.e., "orthotic therapy" or "orthotic device." Yet, today most dictionaries list both an adjective and a noun usage of the term *orthotic* and consider an orthotic to be synonymous with the term *orthosis*.

An ankle foot orthosis (AFO) is any orthosis that covers the foot, spans the ankle joint, and covers the lower leg [2]. Thus, many popular ankle braces in use today would not qualify as true ankle foot orthoses simply because they do not cover a significant area of the foot.

Thus, for this chapter, the term *ankle foot orthosis* applies to the preceding definition, whereas the term *ankle brace* is used to describe an orthosis that covers a portion of the leg and spans the ankle joint, but that does not cover or support a substantial portion of the foot. The term *prophylactic ankle stabilizer* (PAS) is also found in the medical literature and should be considered synonymous with the term *ankle brace*.

D.H. Richie (✉)
Private Practice, Alamitos Seal Beach Podiatry, 550 Pacific Coast Hwy, Suite 209, Seal Beach, CA 90815, USA

M.B. Werd, E.L. Knight (eds.), *Athletic Footwear and Orthoses in Sports Medicine*, 119
DOI 10.1007/978-0-387-76416-0_13, © Springer Science+Business Media, LLC 2010

Types of Ankle Braces and Ankle Foot Orthoses

Ankle braces fall into three general categories. *Lace-up or gauntlet style braces* are usually made of canvas or nylon material (Fig. 13.1). Additional stabilizers made of metal or plastic are often provided which can be added to special pockets in the medial or lateral side of the gauntlet. *Stirrup ankle braces* are comprised of semirigid plastic uprights which are oriented along the distal fibula and tibia and extend across the ankle joint to the medial and lateral aspect of the body of the calcaneus (Fig. 13.2). Thus, stirrup ankle braces are also commonly referred to as *semirigid ankle braces*. The uprights are usually connected by a nylon strap which extends under the heel. The leg portion of the uprights is secured with Velcro straps in multiple locations. The limb uprights are usually padded with air bladder, gel bladder, or foam material. Stirrup style ankle braces can also be custom fabricated from plaster or other moldable materials for short-term use by the athlete.

A newer variation of the standard ankle stirrup brace is the *articulated stirrup brace*. Here a hinge connects a foot plate to the limb uprights at the level of the ankle joint (Fig. 13.3). The foot plate of an articulated stirrup ankle brace does not cover a substantial portion of the foot, usually extending from the heel to the proximal arch.

Ankle foot orthoses can take the form of both a custom and a non-custom (pre-fabricated) device. There are pre-fabricated AFOs gaining popularity for use in a non-ambulatory setting known as *night splints*. These devices are primarily used to prevent contracture of the gastrocnemius–soleus or the plantar aponeurosis during sleep.

Ambulatory ankle foot orthoses can take the form of both a custom and a non-custom (pre-fabricated) device. Pre-fabricated ankle foot orthoses include walking

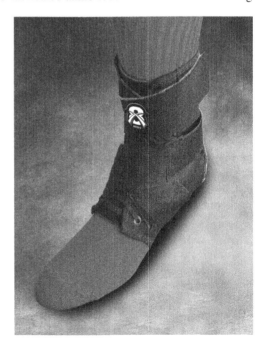

Fig. 13.1 *Lace-up or gauntlet style braces* are usually made of canvas or nylon material. (Courtesy of Swede-O Inc., North Branch, MN)

Fig. 13.2 *Stirrup ankle braces* are comprised of semirigid plastic uprights which are oriented along the distal fibula and tibia and extend across the ankle joint to the medial and lateral aspect of the body of the calcaneus. (Air-Stirrup Ankle Brace, Aircast, courtesy of DJO, Inc., Vista, CA)

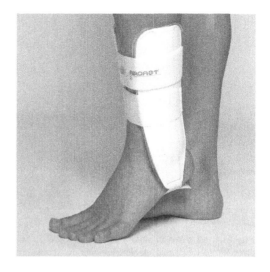

Fig. 13.3 A newer variation of the standard ankle stirrup brace is the *articulated stirrup brace*. Here a hinge connects a foot plate to the limb uprights at the level of the ankle joint. (Courtesy of Swede-O Arch Lok, Swede-O Inc., North Branch, MN.)

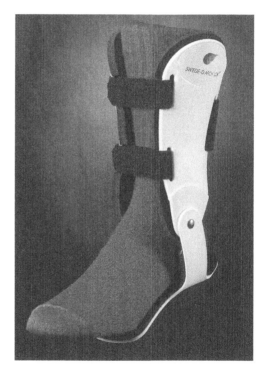

boots, solid and posterior leaf spring AFOs, and articulated AFOs with ankle joints (Fig. 13.4). Custom ankle foot orthoses can also use a solid and posterior leaf spring design, while articulated custom AFOs are generally a more preferred device for the active, athletic patient (Fig. 13.5).

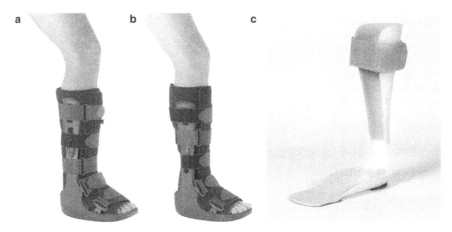

Fig. 13.4 (**A–C**) Ambulatory ankle foot orthoses can take the form of both a custom and a non-custom (pre-fabricated) device. Pre-fabricated ankle foot orthoses include walking boots, solid and posterior leaf spring AFOs, and articulated AFOs with ankle joints. (**A** and **B**, photos courtesy of Ossur Americas, www.ossur.com; C, courtesy of Douglas H. Richie, Jr., DPM)

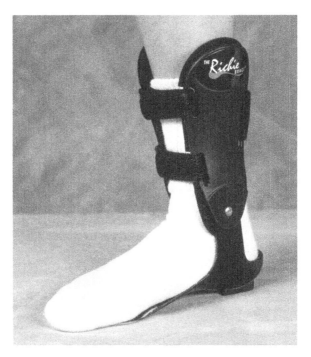

Fig. 13.5 Custom ankle foot orthoses can also use a solid and posterior leaf spring design, while articulated custom AFOs are generally a more preferred device for the active, athletic patient. (The Richie Brace, courtesy of Douglas H. Richie Jr., DPM)

Virtually all ankle braces and AFOs are worn outside the sock of the athlete. In many cases, the sock is vital in providing protection of the integument from friction and pressure of the orthosis. At the same time, compared to athletic taping, the ankle orthosis is usually never in direct contact with the skin which may compromise sensory stimulation and proprioceptive benefits.

Treatment Effects of Ankle Braces and Ankle Foot Orthoses

Studies of Kinetics and Kinematics of Ankle Braces

Most studies of ankle bracing have focused on the kinematic effects, or change in range of motion of the joints of the ankle and hindfoot. In most cases, these investigations have compared various braces, or have compared the results of bracing to athletic taping. Kinetic studies have focused on changes in ground reaction forces as well as displacement of center of pressure.

Kinematic studies have employed various methodologies which explain conflicting outcomes. In scrutinizing these studies, it is important to note if healthy vs injured subjects were studied. In some cases, subjects were evaluated soon after an ankle sprain, while other studies involved subjects with a history of chronic ankle instability. The majority of studies, however, used healthy, non-injured subjects.

When effects on range of motion of the ankle are studied, confusion may arise from the use of terminology. Most kinematic studies of ankle bracing measure effects on "ankle joint" range of motion. The axis of motion of the ankle joint, as originally proposed by Inman [3], is primarily a dorsiflexion/plantarflexion axis allowing almost pure sagittal plane motion. The subtalar joint axis, described by Manter [4], is an inversion/eversion axis, allowing motion primarily in the frontal plane. Thus, when kinematic studies document reduced inversion of the calcaneus, when wearing an ankle brace, the effects of the brace were really at the level of the subtalar joint, rather than the ankle joint. Other studies have measured effects of ankle braces on talar tilt, which is a true measurement of ankle joint inversion/eversion.

Finally, kinematic studies may measure displacement of the ankle during passive movements or during dynamic movements. Studies utilizing passive motion devices vary in terms of position of the ankle in either a plantarflexed or a dorsiflexed position. There is mounting evidence that ankle braces affect the ankle differently, depending on the sagittal plane position of the ankle. Dynamic studies simulating real sport movement, such as cutting maneuvers, may be more accurate methodology for assessing effects of ankle bracing.

Early studies of the effects of taping the ankle involved the use of varus stress radiography to measure changes in joint stability. Vaes and Lofvenberg used this technique to demonstrate that tape and a thermoplastic orthosis would be able to significantly reduce talar tilt [5, 6]. However, Vaes showed that the protective effects of taping reduced with exercise [5].

Similar results of taping were demonstrated by Gross [7]. Both taping and an Aircast stirrup significantly limited passive inversion and eversion of the ankle, but this range of motion increased after exercise in the tape group only. Greene and Hillman also compared the results of ankle taping to a semirigid ankle brace [8]. Again, both interventions significantly reduced inversion and eversion of the ankle. After 20 min of exercise, the taping intervention demonstrated a 40% loss of stability, which was not seen in the braced condition. Further studies have validated the finding that tape looses its ability to restrict ankle joint range of motion after as little as 10 min of exercise [9, 10].

Shapiro et al. studied the role of footwear on the effectiveness of taping and bracing the ankle in a cadaveric study [11]. High-top shoes alone and these same shoes combined with taping or bracing significantly improved resistance to ankle inversion compared to the low-top shoe. There was no difference between taping and any of the eight different braces studied.

Ashton-Miller et al. also studied the role of shoe design and found that a three-quarter-top upper allowed an athlete to develop an additional 12% voluntary resistance to inversion moment compared to a low-top shoe [12]. Also, a similar improvement was seen when the subjects wore a lace-up style brace, air-stirrup, or wore athletic tape. No differences were found among the protective devices.

Vaes et al. used an interesting dynamic measurement technique to determine both the speed and the magnitude of talar tilt in a braced and unbraced condition [13]. Patients with functional ankle instability demonstrated significant decreased range and velocity of talar tilt during a simulated sprain when wearing an air-stirrup ankle brace. A slower velocity of inversion was proposed to be an advantage for the athlete, giving more time for muscular activation to prevent a sprain.

Podzielny and Henning also studied restriction of inversion (supination) velocity with four different ankle braces, compared to the unbraced condition [14]. A "supination platform" was used to induce sudden ankle perturbation. Three of the ankle braces reduced overall supination range and supination velocity. No differences were found in plantar pressure distribution patterns.

Further kinetic studies of ankle bracing were conducted by Cordova et al. [15]. Ankle bracing did not change ground reaction forces during lateral dynamic movement. However, ankle bracing did reduce EMG activity of the peroneus longus during peak impact force.

Siegler et al. were among the first to investigate kinematic changes induced by ankle braces in all rotational directions [16]. Four braces (Ascend, Swede-O, Aircast, and Active Ankle) were studied to determine angular displacement of the segments of the ankle joint complex in three body planes with 6 degrees of freedom. The authors discovered that significant differences existed among the braces in terms of limitation of inversion–eversion, internal–external rotation, and plantarflexion–dorsiflexion.

Conflicting results of previous studies showing restriction of inversion with ankle bracing were reported by Simpson et al. [17]. Kinematic data were collected from 19 subjects with previous history of ankle sprain during lateral cutting movement.

Compared to wearing any of three different ankle braces (AirCast, Malleoloc, or Swede-O), the non-brace condition had a lower amount of ankle inversion. The authors speculated that the subjects may have used injury avoidance behavior in the no brace condition in order to prevent ankle inversion.

Gudibanda and Wang performed a similar study to Simpson, evaluating ankle position during cutting maneuvers, but using healthy subjects [18]. These investigators found that the ASO lace-up strap-reinforced brace did reduce maximum ankle inversion angle by 48% during forward lateral cutting which was significant. However, sideward lateral cutting, decreased inversion angle was only 3% with the brace which was insignificant. Also, the ASO brace decreased ankle plantarflexion angle significantly, by over 40% during both cutting maneuvers. The authors suggested that a reduced ankle plantarflexion angle was advantageous in reducing ankle sprain, citing previous studies by Wright and Neptune who showed that increased ankle plantarflexion resulted in decreased supination torque necessary to cause an ankle sprain [19]. Finally, ankle dorsiflexion was not affected by the ankle brace which the authors concluded would allow normal energy absorbing capacity of the ankle musculature.

Cordova et al. published a meta-analysis of 19 previous published studies comparing three types of ankle support (tape, lace-up, and semirigid) and kinematic changes before and after exercise. It should be noted that only studies of healthy, non-injured subjects were included [20]. The semirigid ankle brace provided the most significant restriction of ankle inversion initially and after exercise. After exercise, the semirigid ankle brace provided an overall decrease of ankle inversion by 23 degrees compared to the control condition. Conversely, the tape and lace-up conditions lost support over time, resulting in an overall restriction of inversion by 12 and 13°, respectively. For ankle joint eversion, the semirigid device was again more effective in reducing motion than either a tape or a lace-up brace. Dorsiflexion and plantarflexion range of motion was not affected by the semirigid condition but was most affected by the tape condition compared to the lace-up condition. Taping significantly decreases ankle joint dorsiflexion compared to a lace-up brace and a semirigid brace.

Nishikawa et al. studied shifts of center of pressure and foot pronation–supination angle in 12 healthy subjects in four conditions (semirigid, lace-up, taping, and no brace) [21]. Both the lace-up and the taping conditions were associated with greater pronation angle during static stance. During gait, the center of pressure was more laterally displaced with the lace-up and taping condition, increasing the ankle joint moment arm for pronation.

Eils and Rosenbaum studied subjects wearing 10 different models of ankle braces during free fall and maximum inversion during a trapdoor ankle perturbation maneuver [22]. Differences in the braces were found in maximum inversion angle which were dependent upon restriction of inversion velocity during free fall.

Spaulding et al. measured kinetic and kinematic variables in 10 healthy subjects and 10 subjects with chronic ankle instability [23]. Differences were noted in both kinetic and kinematic parameters between the two groups while walking on a level surface, up a step and up a ramp. There were no changes when the subjects wore ankle braces. The authors concluded that ankle braces did not alter selected gait parameters in individuals with chronic ankle instability.

Omori et al. performed a cadaveric study to determine the effects of an air-stirrup ankle brace on the three-dimensional motion and contact pressure distribution of the talocrural joint after lateral ligamentous disruption [24]. After severing of the lateral collateral ankle ligaments, inversion and internal rotation of the talus occurred. Application of the ankle brace only restored inversion displacement, not internal rotation. High pressure developed on the medial surface of the talar dome after ligament sectioning which was not corrected with the ankle brace. The authors concluded that the stirrup ankle brace functions to primarily restrict inversion. They also point out that ankle sprains also have a component of plantar flexion and internal rotation which are not controlled by this type of brace.

The role of footwear and its effect on performance of an ankle brace was studied by Eils et al. [25]. While an air-stirrup, lace-up, and taped condition significantly reduced passive ankle joint motion when worn in a shoe, this support was significantly compromised in the barefoot condition with the air stirrup only. The authors recommended a lace-up brace for activities which involve a barefoot condition such as gymnastics and dance.

Studies of Kinetics and Kinematics of Ankle Foot Orthoses

Kinetic and kinematic effects of ankle foot orthoses have been extensively studied [26–30]. However, most of this research has focused on the effects of ankle foot orthoses on patients with neuromuscular conditions. Few reports have been published on the effects of ankle foot orthoses in healthy subjects, and virtually no studies have been conducted on sport applications of these types of devices.

Kitaoka et al. studied the kinetic and kinematic effects of three types of ankle foot orthoses in 20 healthy subjects walking over ground [31]. In the frontal plane, all three orthoses (a solid AFO with footplate, solid AFO with heel portion only, and articulated AFO with footplate) significantly reduced maximal hindfoot inversion, but did not affect eversion. The solid ankle AFO design significantly reduced both plantarflexion and dorsiflexion of the ankle, while the articulated ankle AFO did not affect ankle sagittal plane motion compared to the unbraced condition. Midfoot motion was reduced with the articulated AFO, and increased with the solid AFO. Cadence was reduced with the solid AFOs. All three braces were associated with decreased aft and medial shear forces compared to the non-braced condition.

Radtka et al. studied the kinetic and kinematic effects of solid and hinged (articulated) ankle foot orthoses on 19 healthy subjects during stair locomotion [32]. A unilateral hinged ankle foot orthosis produced kinematic and kinetic effects which were similar to subjects wearing no orthosis. The unilateral solid ankle foot orthosis produced more abnormal ankle joint angles, moments and powers, and more proximal compensations at the knee, hip, and pelvis than the hinged AFO during stair locomotion. Subjects wearing orthosis walked slower during stair locomotion compared to the non-braced condition.

Hartsell and Spaulding measured passive resistive torque applied throughout inversion range of motion of the ankle in healthy subjects and those with chronically unstable ankles [33]. A hinged semirigid non-custom ankle foot demonstrated significant increased passive resistive inversion torque forces and restricted overall inversion motion better than a lace-up ankle brace.

In summary, the kinetic and kinematic effects of ankle bracing have been well studied with consistent results in several areas. Most ankle braces and ankle foot orthoses have been demonstrated to have an ability to restrict ankle joint inversion. Some braces affect ankle joint eversion, and little data are available to determine the effects of bracing the ankle in the transverse plane. In the sagittal plane, significant restriction of range of motion of the ankle joint and the midfoot can be accomplished, depending on the design of the brace, or use of simple taping.

What remains obscure is an understanding of the optimal range and plane of motion controlled by an ankle orthosis to achieve a desired treatment effect. There are clear indications that restriction of motion of any joint in the lower extremity will have negative effects in the neighboring joints, both proximal and distal. Of concern for the athlete is the effect of bracing on overall lower extremity function and sports performance.

Effects of Ankle Bracing on Sports Performance

Many forms of sport combine elements of running, jumping, and side-to-side movements. Speed and power of these movements are dependent upon an intact lower extremity which has efficient muscle firing and transfer of moment to the various joints for motion and subsequent displacement of the body to an intended direction. The range of motion and alignment of the joints of the foot and ankle are critical to the efficient movement of the entire body. Limitation of motion of any joint of the hindfoot complex could be an advantage if excessive motion were available. Conversely, limitation of motion could potentially have negative consequences if a joint is restricted to a less than optimal range.

Thus, many studies have been undertaken to determine the effects of bracing and taping on overall athletic performance. As seen in kinematic studies, performance studies of ankle bracing lack consistency in methodology and have given conflicting results.

One of the first studies of performance and ankle bracing was conducted by Burks et al. [34]. Thirty healthy collegiate athletes performed four performance events: the broad jump, vertical leap, 10-yard shuttle run, and a 40-yard sprint. The tests were performed with both ankles taped, or with both ankles wearing two types of lace-up braces. The results were compared to the no-tape, no-brace condition. Half of the subjects perceived that at least one device decreased their performance. All three conditions significantly reduced vertical jump. Shuttle run was not affected by the braces, but was slowed by the taping. Broad jump was affected by only one of the lace-up braces, not by taping.

Sprinting was affected by taping and one of the braces.

A different type of subject pool was utilized to study performance and bracing in a study by Hals et al. [35]. Twenty five subjects who had recent acute ankle sprain, but who had mechanically stable ankles with residual symptoms of functional instability, were studied. Performance tests included a shuttle run and a vertical jump, with and without an Aircast stirrup brace. Use of the semirigid ankle support significantly improved shuttle run time, but not vertical jump performance.

Jerosch and Schoppe also studied subjects with functional ankle instability to determine the effects of a flexible strap style ankle brace on dynamic movements [36]. In a side step running test, the ankle support produced a significant faster time than the unbraced condition. In addition, the authors found no negative effect after 3 months of brace use in terms of isokinetic strength as well as speed of side step running.

Cordova et al. performed a meta-analysis of 17 randomized controlled trials which used a cross-over design to measure effects of bracing on performance measures [37]. The studies included comparison of tape, semirigid, and lace-up braces. Of these studies, approximately 30% used injured subjects. In terms of sprint speed, the largest effect was found with a lace-up brace, which yielded a 1% impairment. For agility speed, the net effects of all three supports were negative, but only 0.5%. For vertical jump, a 1% decrease in performance was found in all three conditions. The authors concluded that these negative effects are trivial for most individuals, but may have greater significance for elite athletes. They also recommended that the benefit of external ankle support in preventing injury outweighs the small negative effects on sports performance.

Balance and Proprioception

Athletes with functional instability of the ankle have been demonstrated to have deficits in balance and proprioception [38–41]. Restoration of proprioception has resulted in reduced frequency of ankle sprain [42]. Research has shown that lower extremity orthoses can have a positive effect on balance and proprioception.

Functional ankle instability consistently causes deficits in postural control [43–45]. Studies of foot orthoses have shown positive effects in improving postural control in both injured and non-injured subjects [46–53]. Mechanisms by which foot orthoses can improve postural control include optimizing foot position, reducing strain and load on supportive soft tissue structures, and improving the receptor sensory field on the plantar surface of the foot [54].

Neuromuscular control of the ankle relies on afferent input to the central nervous system. In the lower extremity, the somatosensory system provides this afferent input. This system includes the mechanoreceptors in the ligaments of the ankle, the cutaneous receptors in the feet and lower legs and the stretch receptors located in the muscles and tendons around the ankle.

Feuerbach et al. determined that the afferent feedback from skin and muscle around the ankle joint was more important than ligament mechanoreceptors in providing proprioceptive feedback [55]. Their studies on healthy subjects showed that a stirrup ankle brace significantly improved accuracy of ankle positioning tasks performed off weight bearing. Other studies have shown improvements of ankle joint position sense when ankle braces are worn [56, 57].

Chronic ankle instability has been associated with delayed peroneal reaction time, which may be the result of proprioceptive deficits [58, 59]. Karlsson showed that athletes with unstable ankles had significant delayed peroneal reaction time when tested on trap doors which could simulate inversion ankle sprains [60]. When the subjects were taped around the ankles, peroneal reaction time significantly improved.

Improvements of the peroneal stretch reflex with ankle bracing were verified in other studies of healthy subjects [61, 62]. However, another study by Shima et al. showed that ankle taping and bracing would delay the peroneal reflex in both normal and hypermobile ankles [63]. They speculated that the effects of external support would limit ankle inversion and thus delay the peroneal stretch reflex.

The effects of ankle braces on postural control has been extensively studied. Baier and Hopf studied 22 athletes with functional instability of the ankle joint compared to 22 healthy athletes [64]. A significant improvement of postural control, as evidenced by reduced mediolateral sway velocity, was found in the instability group when wearing a both rigid and semirigid stirrup ankle brace. However, other studies, performed on both healthy subjects and subjects with functional ankle instability have failed to show any improvements of postural control with the use of ankle braces [65–68].

Studies of effects of ankle foot orthoses on balance have been performed on neurologically impaired subjects and have not been performed on athletes [69, 70]. Cattaneo et al. showed that AFOs would improve static balance in patients with multiple sclerosis, but would compromise dynamic balance during gait [70].

In summary, studies of effects of ankle orthoses on balance and proprioception do not provide consistent findings. Yet, studies of treatment effects of these devices commonly attribute any positive findings to improvements in proprioception. As with previous studies, investigations of proprioceptive effects show varied results because of the various types of subjects (injured vs non-injured vs symptomatic) and the methodology employed (static stabilometry vs dynamic posturography). Furthermore, ankle orthoses have not demonstrated the consistent improvements in postural control which have been previously demonstrated with foot orthoses in healthy subjects and subjects with chronic ankle instability. Further research is needed to determine the role of support of both the foot and the ankle in the treatment of athletes with chronic ankle instability.

Prevention of Injury

The ankle sprain is the most common injury in sport, comprising at least 20% of all traumatic episodes affecting athletes [71]. Braces are used more frequently for the prevention and treatment of ankle sprains, and for chronic instability of the ankle than any other musculoskeletal condition.

Several studies have validated the role of ankle braces to prevent sprain in various sports. However, the mechanism by which ankle braces and AFOs achieve positive treatment outcomes for ankle injury remains speculative despite a large volume of research on this subject.

The role of shoe design and athletic taping in basketball players was studied by Garrick and Requa [72]. The combination of a high-top shoe with taping reduced ankle sprains fourfold compared to standard shoes with no taping.

Rovere et al., in a retrospective study, compared the effects of tape to a lace-up brace in the prevention of ankle sprains in football players [73]. The lace-up brace was associated with one-half the number of ankle injuries as the taped condition.

Two prospective studies have been published comparing the effects of an Aircast splint to the non-braced condition in the prevention of ankle sprains. Sitler et al. followed 1601 cadets at the United States Military Academy while playing basketball over a period of 2 years [74]. There were 46 ankle injuries to this group during the time period, of which 35 occurred in the non-braced group. The braced group experienced 11 injuries, revealing a threefold increase incidence of sprain in the non-braced group. There was no statistical difference in injury rate comparing those athletes who had been previously injured prior to the study vs those who were not. The severity of ankle sprain was not different in the braced vs non-braced groups.

Surve et al. studied 504 soccer players randomized into two groups, braced with an Aircast vs no brace, and followed for an entire season [75]. The use of an air-stirrup brace reduced the incidence of ankle sprain by nearly fivefold, in the previous injured group of athletes only. The brace did not significantly affect injury rate in those athletes who had not been injured prior to entering the study. The severity of sprain was also significantly reduced with use of the brace in the injured subjects only. Thus, the benefits of the ankle orthosis was limited to those subjects with a previously sprained ankle.

Both studies by Sitler and Surve showed no increased incidence of knee injuries when wearing ankle brace. Sitler showed that bracing would not prevent severity of sprain, only incidence of sprain. They speculated that ankle bracing did not achieve its benefit by restricting joint range of motion, but rather by facilitating proprioception. Conversely, Surve showed a preventive benefit in severity of sprain by use of an ankle brace, but only in previously injured subjects. Olmstead et al. conducted a numbers needed to treat analysis of three previous studies (Garrick, Sitler, and Surve) to determine the cost–benefit of taping vs bracing in the prevention of ankle sprains [76].

To prevent ankle sprains over an entire season, taping was found to be three times as expensive as bracing. This cost was based upon supplies alone; the labor cost of repeated application of tape by the trainer was not included. The authors concluded that taping and bracing appear to be more effective in preventing ankle sprains in athletes with a history of previous sprain. Furthermore, the superiority of taping vs bracing in preventing injury has yet to be proven, but the cost–benefit analysis clearly shows an advantage for bracing.

Treatment of Injury

Ankle braces and ankle foot orthoses are commonly used in the treatment of injuries of the leg, ankle, and foot. There is no uniform consensus about the timing, selection, and criteria for use of ankle braces or ankle foot orthoses in the management of lower extremity injury.

Acute tears of the lateral ligaments of the ankle are best treated non-surgically with a functional rehabilitation program [77, 78]. Functional treatment of an ankle sprain utilizes early mobilization of the ankle joint to stimulate healing and improve the strength of ligaments after injury [79, 80]. Ankle braces have been recommended as a simple way to provide protection for the ankle after acute sprain, while allowing easy removal for range of motion exercises [78, 81, 82].

However, some researchers have suggested that simple ankle braces do not effectively stabilize the ankle after acute ligament injury, and long-term functional complaints can occur if weight bearing is allowed to early while wearing these devices [83, 84, 85]. Glasoe et al. recommend that a more protective "immobilizer boot" (i.e., pre-fabricated plastic ankle foot orthosis with soft liner and Velcro closures) be used for initial weight bearing in the treatment of Grade II and Grade III ankle sprains [86]. This report as well as others advocates early weight bearing, with protection around the ankle, to increase stability and stimulate ligament repair [87].

Pre-fabricated ankle foot orthoses such as walking boots appear to provide necessary protection of the ankle after acute ligament injury to allow early weight bearing, without the potential negative results that could occur with simple ankle bracing. In addition, these "walking boots" have been shown to be as effective as a cast in reducing soleus and peroneal muscle activity during the stance phase of gait, while actually significantly reducing gastrocnemius activity compared to a cast [88]. Thus, a walking boot may be preferred compared to a cast, in the management of trauma to the tendoachilles.

Progression from a walking boot to an ankle brace should occur sometime during the rehabilitation program for treatment of the ankle sprain. There is no consensus of opinion about the timing of this progression, and there are no accepted objective criteria for when to institute and discontinue bracing of the ankle during the recovery process. Since complete maturation of collagen does not occur until 9–12 months after ligament injury, many authorities advocate the use of some type of external orthosis for the treatment of ankle sprains until complete recovery has been attained [89].

Ankle foot orthoses are being increasing utilized, in favor of traditional ankle braces, in the treatment of tendinopathy of the ankle, degenerative arthritis of the ankle, and midfoot sprains [90]. Simultaneous control of both the ankle and the subtalar joint make ankle foot orthoses more suitable than ankle braces for the treatment of peroneal tendon injuries and posterior tibial tendon dysfunction [91]. In addition, ankle foot orthoses have demonstrated better recovery from syndesmosis sprain than a traditional lace-up ankle brace [92, 93].

Summary

1. Ankle braces have been thoroughly studied to determine the kinematic and kinetic effects on both injured and healthy subjects. These braces can limit the range and velocity of inversion, with less effects on eversion and plantarflexion.
2. Compared to tape, ankle braces are less likely to loose supportive benefit during exercise. Braces are more cost-effective than tape when used to prevent ankle sprains.
3. The effects of bracing on athletic performance are minimal and do not preclude the use of these devices for the prevention or treatment of injury.
4. There is some evidence that ankle braces will improve proprioception and sensory feedback, although studies of postural control do not show as positive of outcome as similar studies with foot orthoses.
5. Ankle braces have demonstrated a preventive effect for ankle sprain in subjects with previous sprain and may also prevent an ankle sprain in healthy subjects.
6. Ankle braces may not provide enough restriction of motion and support around the ankle joint for the immediate treatment of severe ligament injury of the ankle. Solid short leg walking boots (ankle foot orthoses) are preferred for this intervention.
7. Ankle foot orthoses support and control rotation of both the subtalar and the ankle joints and appear better suited for treatment of tendinopathy of the foot and ankle.

Chapter 14
Prescribing Athletic Footwear and Orthoses: The Game Plan

Matthew B. Werd and E. Leslie Knight

This book is focused on maximizing athletic performance and minimizing injury through the use of an appropriate prescription for athletic footwear and orthoses. Often neglected, overlooked, or misunderstood, this prescription should be the first step in the lower extremity treatment of the athlete. Overwhelming evidence is now available and has been presented which supports the use of custom foot orthoses in the athlete.

ACSM's Exercise is Medicine (TM) initiative recommends that physicians provide an exercise prescription to every patient on each comprehensive visit. Similarly, we should also provide that newly-exercising patient with an appropriate athletic footwear prescription.

This chapter presents a systematic approach – the game plan – for prescribing athletic footwear and orthoses, incorporating all facets to ensure maximal effectiveness. Each component of the prescription for athletic footwear and orthoses is broken down and discussed in depth in other chapters throughout this book. Please refer to the appropriate chapter for a more in-depth discussion of each component.

Barefoot running, or simulated barefoot running in minimalistic-type footwear, such as the Newton Running shoe, Nike Free, or Vibram Five Fingers, has gained some popularity. However, unbiased evidence-based research which supports or discounts the risks versus benefits of barefoot running is insufficient, and until valid studies are presented, recommendations for barefoot running should be made with caution. This statement is supported by a 2010 position statement issued by the American Academy of Podiatric Sports Medicine.

The Guidelines for a Customized Footwear Prescription

A 15-point sequential guideline, or checklist, customized for each athlete will be helpful in making decisions on athletic footwear; however, it is ultimately up to the sports medicine practitioner to choose which shoes and/or which orthotic devices are

M.B. Werd (✉)
Foot and Ankle Associates, 2939 South Florida Avenue, Lakeland, FL, USA

M.B. Werd, E.L. Knight (eds.), *Athletic Footwear and Orthoses in Sports Medicine*,
DOI 10.1007/978-0-387-76416-0_14, © Springer Science+Business Media, LLC 2010

Table 14.1 Prescription for athletic footwear and orthoses in sports medicine: A stepwise approach, "The Game Plan"

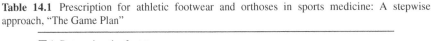

☐ 1. Determine the foot type
☐ 2. Determine the foot's function during gait
☐ 3. Consider any foot pathology
☐ 4. Consider size and weight of athlete
☐ 5. Consider the athlete's demands from their sport
☐ 6. Assess key features of the athletic shoe
☐ 7. Recommend athletic shoes
☐ 8. Recommend athletic socks
☐ 9. Recommend athletic shoe laces and lacing techniques
☐ 10. Recommend over-the-counter athletic shoe inserts
☐ 11. Recommend athletic shoe modifications
☐ 12. Referral for custom foot or ankle orthoses
☐ 13. Prescribe athletic custom foot orthoses and modifications
☐ 14. Prescribe athletic ankle foot orthoses and modifications
☐ 15. Follow-up re-assessment for possible modifications after wear-testing

most appropriate for each individual athlete (Table 14.1). This guideline provides a stepwise approach to each component of the athletic footwear prescription.

Determine the Foot Type

Foot type can be classified by the arch height, which will provide a starting point as to how the foot will function biomechanically during gait and which athletic footwear will be most appropriate. Historically, the "wet test" has been used as a quick and easy test for the lay athlete to determine arch type. A more contemporary and accurate determination of arch height and foot type can be made by either quantifying navicular drop or assessing the vertical forces beneath the foot.

The three basic categories of foot types are low arch (flat foot), normal arch, and high arch (cavus foot). In general, a low-arched foot is more flexible and will function with excessive pronation which will require additional medial support. A normal-arched foot will function with an appropriate amount of pronation and will not require additional medial support or excessive cushioning. A high-arched foot is more rigid foot and will function with limited pronation and will require additional cushioning and shock absorption.

Size of the foot must also be considered, as the foot size may affect proper fit of the shoe and may affect the choice of material and the size and thickness of a foot orthosis. Foot size can be categorized as large, wide, medium, small, or narrow.

Determine the Foot's Function During Gait

Gait evaluation is an important part of an athletic evaluation. Static examination of an athlete's foot type is a good starting point; however, a dynamic evaluation will provide more information on how the foot functions in real time. Based on the dynamic function of the foot, a more appropriate recommendation can be made regarding the biomechanical needs of the athletic footwear and orthoses.

Clinical evaluation of the amount of pronation during gait can be subjectively assessed by visualizing the athlete walk and run; however, a more objective and accurate gait analysis can be performed using hi-tech video analysis and force-measuring platforms or in-shoe pressure-measuring technology.

The amount of foot pronation noted during gait can be excessive, increased, biomechanically efficient, decreased, or absent (supinated). Examination of an excessively pronated foot during gait will demonstrate an internally rotated leg, an excessively everted calcaneus, a collapsing arch, and an excessively abducted forefoot.

It is important to observe not necessarily *how much* excessive pronation occurs but *when the excessive pronation occurs* during the gait cycle.

A complete biomechanical examination should note any asymmetries starting at the head and progress distally to the shoulders, back, hips, knees and patella, legs, ankles, and feet. The amount of core strength and stability should also be noted, as a weak core may predispose a lower extremity injury.

Consider Any Foot Pathology

Common foot pathology which may affect the choice of appropriate athletic footwear and orthoses includes (but is not limited to) posterior tibial tendon dysfunction, spring ligament strain, metatarsalgia, plantar fasciosis, calcaneal apophysitis, hallux valgus, hallux limitus, sesamoiditis, stress fractures, neuromas, sinus tarsi syndrome, lateral ankle instability, peroneal tendon pathology, tarsal tunnel syndrome, and Achilles tendon pathology.

Consider the Size and Weight of the Athlete

Physical size of the foot and the weight of the patient must be considered when recommending athletic footwear and orthoses. Shoe volume, width, and length must be adequate. Shoe and orthosis materials need to be sufficient to accommodate the athlete without breaking down prematurely.

Consider the Athlete's Demands from the Sport

Each sport has its own set of factors which may affect the choice of appropriate athletic footwear and orthoses, including the types of movement necessary. For example, distance running requires straightforward heel-to-toe motion while tennis requires side-to-side and front-to-back movements on the ball of the feet.

Sport surface also needs to be considered, whether it is a smooth court, a grassy field, artificial turf, or hard concrete.

Assess Key Features of the Athletic Shoe

Technologic improvements to athletic footwear and orthoses are ever-changing and the sports medicine specialist needs to be aware of advances and trends. In regard to running shoes, very few choices, features, or technologies were available during the early running boom of the 1970s – as evidenced by Dr. Subotnick on the cover of The Running Foot Doctor, published in 1977 – while a virtual explosion of athletic shoes, options, and technological advances has occurred since.

There has been a shift in focus from using cushioned materials in the 1970s and 1980s to using materials to help "control motion" in the 1990s – midsole materials are rated by durometer (hardness of material): the harder the midsole the more supportive the shoe – to a current focus on using materials in different locations within the shoe in order to help guide the foot through gait more biomechanically efficient.

The term *motion control* is ubiquitous among athletic shoe manufacturers when referring to a shoe which is produced to limit excessive foot pronation and is thus referenced in this book as well; however, it may not be the most appropriate term. An athletic shoe material or technology does not actually "control" the motion of the foot, but it may have the effect to guide the foot through a more biomechanically efficient pathway.

The term "preferred movement pathway" as proposed by Benno M. Nigg, Dr.sc.nat., Dr.h.c., and promoted by Australian sports podiatrist, and Academy Fellow, Simon J. Barthold, BSc (personal communication, 2008), may better reflect the intended function of athletic shoes which are produced to improve the gait of an athlete whose foot functions with an excessive amount of pronation during key moments of the gait cycle.

Athletic Shoes

Quarterly reviews of current athletic shoes are performed by the American Academy of Podiatric Sports Medicine (AAPSM) Shoe Review Committee (SRC) members. Athletic shoes are reviewed objectively, without any outside influence or bias. Reviews are categorized by their intended function and effect. The reviews are made available for review – without any fees or membership requirements – for sports professionals, athletes, and the general public on the Academy's website, www.AAPSM.org. Rating athletic shoes can be a difficult task, but reviews can be validated by implementing a consistent, reproducible, and objective rating system.

Although running shoes provide the bulk of the shoes which are reviewed by the Shoe Review Committee, most sport-specific shoes also are included. The sport-specific athletic shoe evaluation is based on a brief description and history of the sport, any necessary equipment, the demands on the lower extremity, available references and research, desirable design and construction features of the shoe, available shoes, specific shoe evaluation, shoe recommendations, a summary, and final comments.

Table 14.2 Objective features of a running shoe

Interior shoe volume
Toe box width
Seams and stitching
Insole
Last shape
Forefoot flexibility
Midfoot flexibility/ stability
Midfoot torsion
Midsole cushion at heel lateral and medial
Midsole firmness at heel
Heel counter
Heel contact shape
Rocker sole
Increased midfoot surface

Table 14.3 75-point rating scale for athletic shoes

Maximum motion control = 60–75
Moderate motion control = 45–60
Mild motion control = 25–40
Neutral or cushioned = 5–25

75 = maximum points possible; 5 = minimum points possible.

Multiple features of the running shoes have been identified as being integral to proper foot function and comfort, some of which are listed in Table 14.2. A 75-point scale (Table 14.3) rates each shoe based on criteria listed in Table 14.2, which documents the shoes' effect on pronation in the foot. A shoe with a higher score indicates that the shoe has more motion-controlling features and thus more suitable for an over-pronated foot. A shoe with a lower score indicates a shoe with less motion-controlling features and thus more suitable for a less-pronated (more rigid) foot. Table 14.4 shows examples of running shoes scored in each category.

Table 14.4 Example of ratings for running shoes scored in each category

Shoe A: Total 75 W/S (maximum motion control)
Shoe B: Total 50 W/SC (moderate motion control)
Shoe C: Total 30 W/SC (mild motion control/stability shoe)
Shoe D: Total 20 M/C (neutral or cushioned shoe)

W = multiple widths; M = one width; C = curved last; SC = semi-curved last; S = straight last.

Three basic tests for features of motion control in an athletic shoe can be performed quickly by the astute specialist or athlete. Figures. 14.1, 14.2, and 14.3 demonstrate the three basic tests that best define the stability and motion

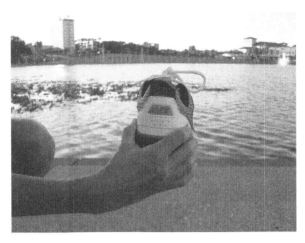

Fig. 14.1 Heel counter stability. Squeeze the heel to determine the amount of stability or flexibility

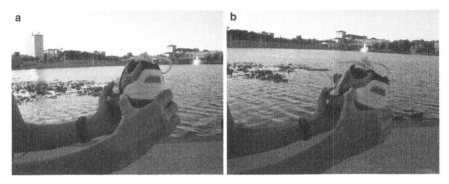

Fig. 14.2 (**a** and **b**) Midfoot torsional stability (shank rigidity). Twist the shoe while grasping the heel and forefoot to determine the amount of stability or flexibility

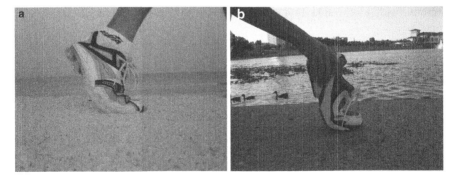

Fig. 14.3 (**a** and **b**) Forefoot flexional stability. Forefoot flexibility depends on both durometer of the midsole material and the depth of the flex grooves. Deeper grooves allow more flexibility of the shoe at the forefoot. The shoe should flex at the metatarsal–phalangeal joint, not further proximal through the midfoot

control in an athletic shoe. Assessing the shoes' heel counter stability, midfoot torsional stability (shank rigidity), and forefoot flexional stability can provide enough information to make an appropriate recommendation for or against the shoe.

Athletic Socks

Sport socks have evolved and many choices of materials, cushioning, and even sock length need to be considered, depending on the sport and application.

Athletic Shoe Laces and Lacing Techniques

Athletic shoe laces and lacing patterns are often not considered in the athletic footwear prescription, but should not be overlooked. Certain foot types and pathology may be improved by basic shoe re-lacing patterns, and shoe fit may be improved by using different shoe lace materials and lace-locking systems.

Pre-fabricated Athletic Shoe Insoles

Athletic shoe manufacturers invest very little technology in the inserts that come with shoes. Pre-fabricated athletic shoe insoles are helpful – in addition to the appropriate athletic shoe type – when additional cushioning (soft), support (stable, with additional arch padding), or pronation-limiting features (more durable, with hard plastic shell) are required.

Athletic Shoe Modifications

Athletic shoe modifications can further enhance athletic shoe fit and function and should be considered for certain athletic conditions.

Referral for Custom Foot or Ankle Orthoses

Referral for custom foot or ankle orthoses is the next step to be taken when all of the above steps have not fully resolved the athlete's condition. Evidence overwhelmingly documents and supports the effectiveness of custom foot orthoses in sports medicine.

Prescribe Athletic Custom Foot Orthoses and Modifications

The type of custom foot orthoses prescribed is dependent on a multitude of factors (Chapter 12). Custom foot orthoses have been proven to be an important adjunct in conservative care of the athlete, which function to decrease the risk of certain injuries and to potentially enhance athletic performance.

Prescribe Athletic Ankle Foot Orthoses and Modifications

Ankle foot orthoses have been proven to be an important adjunct in conservative care of the athlete. The type of ankle foot orthoses prescribed is dependent on a multitude of factors (Chapter 13).

Follow-Up Re-assessment for Possible Modifications After Wear-Testing

After each step above has been completed, a follow-up assessment of the athlete should be made after an adequate wear-test to assess effectiveness and to make modifications or adjustments if necessary.

Summary

Sports medicine specialists who are knowledgeable and comfortable in recommending appropriate athletic footwear and orthoses for their athletic patients will be providing the athlete with the greatest service. Having a solid game plan for recommending athletic footwear and orthoses for each athlete will be helpful in making critical decisions on athletic footwear. The sports medicine practitioner must ultimately decide which shoes or which orthotic devices are most appropriate for each individual athlete.

Part II
Sport-Specific Recommendations

Chapter 15
Walking and Running

John F. Connors

As more people strive to be fit, the popularity of walking and running continues to increase. It is imperative that the sports medicine practitioner has a basic understanding and knowledge of running shoes and custom foot orthoses. Walking and running shoes must have the ability to absorb shock (cushioning), guide the foot through each step (stability), and withstand repetitive pounding (durability). This chapter further reviews lower extremity walking and running biomechanics, running foot types and injuries, running footwear recommendations, and custom foot orthoses.

Gait Biomechanics: Walking vs. Running

The human gait cycle is complicated; it consists of a coordinated series of movements that involve both the upper and the lower extremities [1]. The gait cycle consists of a stance phase and a swing phase. During walking, the foot is in contact with the ground (stance phase) 60% of the time and off the ground (swing phase) 40% of the time. Both feet are in contact with the ground 20% of the time.

The running gait cycle does not have a period of double stance, but does have a period of *double float phase* in which both feet are off the ground at the same time. Running consists of only a swing phase and a stance phase. Impact shock with running is greater than walking, reaching 2–3 times body weight. Walking has a wider base and angle of gait than with running, and as running speed increases, the impact forces increase, and the center of pressure moves toward the midline. While running, the heel contacts the ground in a more inverted position than walking, and as speed increases, the amount of energy absorbed by the muscles increases as well.

J.F. Connors (✉)
Private Practice, 200 White Road, Little Silver, NJ 07739, USA

M.B. Werd, E.L. Knight (eds.), *Athletic Footwear and Orthoses in Sports Medicine*, DOI 10.1007/978-0-387-76416-0_15, © Springer Science+Business Media, LLC 2010

During running, the swing phase is longer compared to walking where the stance phase is longer. Stride length is longer with running and shorter with walking, and muscle activity is greater with running compared to walking.

Subotnick [1] has reported on the fundamental differences between walking and running. Subotnick and Cavanagh [2] report that during running, the base of gait approaches zero and that there is an increased functional running limb varus because the feet contact the ground directly under the center of mass of the body.

Video gait analysis allows the sports medicine specialist to assess the normal or abnormal mechanics of a walker or runner, assisting the practitioner to recommend appropriate running shoes and custom sport orthoses.

Classification of Running Foot Types

The Neutral Foot

This is the ideal foot type for long distance running. The forefoot is perpendicular to the rearfoot with no obvious forefoot varus or valgus. The foot is perpendicular to the leg at the ankle joint. The subtalar joint is neutral; neither pronated nor supinated; the midtarsal joint is maximally pronated; and the metatarsal–phalangeal joints are neutral [1].

The Pronated Foot

This is the flexible *loose bag-of-bones* low-arch foot that is excessively pronated. It is the most common of all biomechanical problems seen in a sports medicine practice. There is an increase in the range of motion at the subtalar joint and mid-tarsal joints which increases the parallel alignment on the midtarsal axis, permitting greater range of motion (abnormal motion). With the pronated foot during running, the key factor is for the foot to be neutral in the middle of midstance. When there is no sequential phasic resupination, torque and counter torque result, causing injury. Fatigue results when muscles work overtime against unstable fulcrums and when joints that should be stable and locked are unlocked and hypermobile [3].

The Cavus Foot

This is the rigid high-arch foot type which has decreased or limited pronation. A neutral foot has the normal amount of pronation and dissipates stress and helps protect bone and soft tissue supporting structures, while a cavus foot which lacks normal pronation is associated with excessive shock to bone and supporting structures. The cavus foot has a decreased range of motion, increased stiffness, and decreased pronatory compensation [3].

Classification and Selection of a Running Athletic Shoe

A runner's foot type (high arch, flatfoot, or normal arch) will help determine the appropriate type of running shoe. Shopping at a reputable running specialty store will also enable the patient to find the most appropriate running athletic shoe. Many running stores have a treadmill allowing the patient to try on different types of running athletic shoes.

Normal Arch

This is considered a neutral foot (normal pronator). This foot type is able to withstand the stress placed on the body while running. A stability running shoe is recommended for this foot type because it offers stability in the rear foot and flexibility/cushioning in the forefoot, thus allowing the normal motion to occur in the body.

Flatfoot Arch

Pes planus foot type, an overpronator which has too much motion within the foot. Over the course of training, the body will eventually breakdown leading to overuse injuries. This is the most common foot type seen in a sports podiatrist's office because this foot type leads to the majority of injuries seen by a specialist, plantar fasciitis, Achilles tendonitis, posterior shin splints, and runners' knee. This foot type benefits from stability plus or a motion control running shoe.

High Arch

Cavus foot type, an underpronator which is rigid and considered a poor shock absorber and is susceptible to overuse injuries with distance running. Patients with this foot type do well with neutral/cushioned running shoes. These types of running shoes encourage motion to occur, thus decreasing the stress being placed on the lower extremity.

A women's foot is shaped differently than a man's foot. Proper running athletic shoe selection for the female runner has been a problem. Carol Frey, a professor at The University of Southern California, studied 225 women aged 20–60 and found that more than half had narrow heels that caused problems when buying running shoes [4]. Running shoe companies are now making running and walking athletic shoes to accommodate this foot type. They are now making some running athletic shoes that are built narrower in the heel (rearfoot) and wider in the toe box (forefoot).

It is very important to note that the shape of the foot should match the shape of the running shoe. For example, a high-arched foot has a curved appearance, so

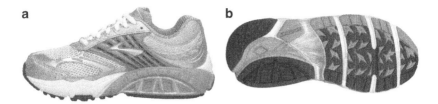

Fig. 15.1 (**A** and **B**) Brooks Ariel straight last running shoe for women. (Courtesy of Brooks Sports, Inc., Bothell, WA.)

a curved last type of running shoe would be most appropriate. A flat/overpronated foot type will have a straighter foot type and will need to get into a straight last running shoe (Fig. 15.1). It is important to examine both the foot type and the shape of the foot before considering which running shoe is recommended.

Stephen M. Pribut, a past president of AAPSM, practicing in Washington, DC, has recommended several factors to weigh when looking for a new running shoe, including [5] the following:

- Past experience with shoes
- Current Problems
- Biomechanical Needs
- Environmental Factors
- Running and Racing Requirements

Features to consider in the running shoe:

- Cushioning – The ability of a shoe to absorb shock.
- EVA (ethylene vinyl acetate) – Synthetic foam used in midsole.
- Heel Counter – Aids in heel support and rearfoot stability.
- Last – The form around which the shoe is built.
    - Board Last – increased stability, overall support.
    - Combination Last – improves stability, forefoot flexibility.
    - Slip Last – lightness, cushioning.
- Midsole Provides shoe cushioning. Considered the most important part of the running shoe as it is the cushioning and stability layer between the upper outsole. The most common materials for the midsole of a running shoe are ethylene vinyl acetate (EVA), polyurethane (PU), or a combination of the two.
- Outsole bottom surface of shoe. On running shoes the tread is designed for straight ahead motion.
- PU (Polyurethane) – Used in midsole. Firmer and more durable than EVA.
- Toe Box – Surrounds toes.
- Upper – The uppermost part of the shoe that encompasses the foot.

Types of Running Shoes

All running shoe brands such as Asics, Nike, Saucony, New Balance, Mizuno, Reebok, and Brooks classify their running shoe brands into categories (Fig. 15.2). For a complete and detailed list of current running shoe brands and models, please refer to the running shoe reviews by the Shoe Review Committee of The American Academy of Podiatric Sports Medicine posted at www.AAPSM.org.

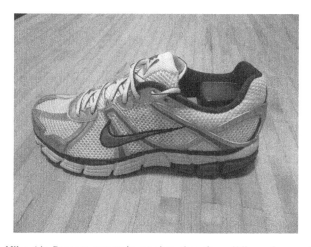

Fig. 15.2 A Nike Air Pegasus women's running shoe for mildly underpronated to mildly overpronated feet

Neutral (Stability): mild pronation control features

High Arch (Neutral Cushion): no motion control features

Flat Arch (Motion Control): maximal pronation control features

Light Weight Trainer (Recommended for fast training or racing): usually comes with a removable insole, so an orthosis can fit into this type of shoe. Light weight trainers and racing flats are discussed in more detail in Chapter 16 on racing shoes.

Racing Flat: only recommended for elite runners. Very light and offers very little support and shock absorption. For elite runners, these types of running shoes are often sent to the orthotic laboratory to make a custom running orthosis for their flats.

Trail Shoe: recommended for off road and trail running. This type of athletic shoe gives more lateral (side to side) support to prevent ankle sprains/strains and is constructed of higher durometer, more durable materials.

Running Socks

Running socks are designed to protect the foot while running and can contribute to overall foot health and performance. Socks also provide stability to the runner while wicking moisture away. Running socks are made of lightweight, moisture-wicking materials that help prevent blistering. Cotton socks should be avoided for running because cotton absorbs and retains moisture, which can cause blistering. A variety of running socks are available in different fabrics, shapes, sizes, and colors. The most important qualities to consider in a running sock are durability, thickness, breathability, and moisture-wicking capabilities. Please refer to Chapter 7, Athletic Socks, for a more thorough review and discussion of athletic socks.

Custom Running Orthoses

Please refer to Chapters 2, 11, and 12 for a complete and thorough discussion on custom foot orthoses. The majority of running injuries are due to biomechanical imbalances and/or improper training. Once the sports practitioner performs a biomechanical examination and finds that an overuse injury is due to a skeletal and/or muscle imbalance, then a custom running orthosis is essential.

The custom foot orthosis is an orthopedic device that is designed to promote structural integrity of the joints of the foot and lower limb by resisting ground reaction forces that cause abnormal skeletal motion to occur during the stance phase of gait [6].

Custom foot orthoses are classified as flexible, semi-flexible, and rigid. Examples of flexible and semi-flexible orthoses are polyethylene, polypropylene, and ortholene. Examples of rigid orthoses are carbon graphite, TL-2100, and Rohadur. The type of injury and the amount of instability determine which material and the amount of correction needed from the orthosis. It is imperative to have a good working relationship with an orthotic laboratory.

The more rigid a device, the more biomechanical control it offers compared to a flexible device. Conversely, a more flexible device has the ability to absorb impact shock but will offer less biomechanical control. It is up to the individual sports practitioner to decide what type of device is needed. Personal experience has been most successful using semi-flexible materials along with extrinsic rearfoot and forefoot posting. This type of device offers both shock absorption via the flexibility in the shell and biomechanical control via the amount of extrinsic posting. Factors affecting which type of running orthosis is prescribed include the runner's biomechanical needs, the weight of the patient, the number of running per week, and the amount of biomechanical correction necessary.

Shell modifications of a running orthosis include the following:

- Deep heel seat
- Medial flange
- Lateral flange
- First ray cut out
- Fifth ray cut out
- Navicular cut out
- Grinding the device wider

Posting of the rearfoot can be extrinsic or intrinsic. An extrinsically posted orthosis offers more stability. Posting of the forefoot can also be extrinsic or intrinsic, but an extrinsically posted forefoot will offer more stability. The biomechanical function of the forefoot will determine whether the forefoot is posted in varus or valgus.

Accommodations incorporated into a running orthosis include the following:

- Heel cushions
- Heel spur pads
- Metatarsal raise pads
- Metatarsal bar
- Neuroma pad
- Longitudinal arch pad
- Morton's extension
- Heel lifts
- Forefoot post to sulcus

Injuries That Influence Running Shoe Selection

Functional Hallux Limitus

Usually due to metatarsus primus elevatus. Recommend a stability running shoe with a semi-flexible functional orthosis with a kinetic wedge built into the forefoot posting of the orthosis.

Plantar Fasciitis

Usually due to an overpronated foot type. Recommend a stability running athletic shoe with a polyurethane midsole to aid in decreasing excessive pronation. Also recommend a semi-flexible orthosis with extrinsic rearfoot and extrinsic forefoot control to decrease overpronation and for shock absorption. If the runner has a high arch, cavus foot type then a neutral/cushion running shoe is recommended.

Achilles Tendonitis

Usually due to an overpronated foot type. Recommend a motion control running shoe with a raised heel counter. Also can recommend a stability running shoe and a semi-flexible orthosis with extrinsic posting and heel lift incorporated into the orthosis.

Anterior Shin Splints

Usually due to a high-arched cavus foot type. Recommend a neutral/cushion running shoe to allow motion in the foot and lower limb.

Posterior Shin Splints

Usually due to an overpronated foot type. A motion control running shoe is recommended with medial reinforcement with a polyurethane or dual density midsole to limit the amount of overpronation. A stability running athletic shoe along with a custom molded orthosis is also recommended. This type of orthosis is semi-flexible and has a deep heel cup along with extrinsic rearfoot and forefoot posting. This will also limit the amount of overpronation and provide shock absorption.

Runner's Knee

Usually due to overpronation. Again, a motion control running shoe with medial reinforcement in the midsole is recommended. Also a stability running shoe with a custom molded orthosis posted extrinsically in the rearfoot and forefoot will also limit the amount of abnormal pronation and provide shock absorption.

When prescribing a custom molded orthosis, keep in mind that every patient is different as far as their biomechanical needs. Shell modifications, posting (both rearfoot and forefoot) along with accommodations, are made on an individual basis.

References

1. Sports and Exercise Injuries: Conventional, Homeopathic and Alternative Treatments by Steven Subotnick, New York, North Atlantic Books, 1993.
2. Cavanagh PR: The running shoe book. Anderson World, 1980.
3. Subotnick SI: The biomechanics of running. Implications for the prevention of foot injuries. Sports Med, Mar–Apr2(2):144–153, 1985.
4. Frey C: Foot health and shoe wear for women. Clin Orthop Relat Res, Mar (372): 32–44, 2000.
5. Pribut SM. Current approaches to the management of plantar heel pain syndrome, including the role of injectable corticosteroids. J Am Podiatr Med Assoc, Jan-Feb, 97(1):68–74, 2007.
6. Valmassy RL. Clinical Biomechanics, St. Louis: MO, 1996.

Chapter 16
Racing, Cross-Country, and Track and Field

David Granger

In today's sport of running, there is a wide of variety of shoes for every type of race. Whether it is for a cross-country race, the high jump, or even steeple chase, there is a unique shoe to meet the demands of the race. Abebe Bikila, an Ethiopian runner, actually made barefoot running popular in 1960 when he won the Olympic Marathon in Rome. Since then, multiple African athletes have run barefoot, forcing many athletes and shoe companies to consider whether shoes are beneficial to running fast. Interestingly enough, Bikila returned in 1964 to set a world record in the Olympic Marathon while wearing shoes, only adding to the confusion of whether shoes are of benefit to racing.

The story of Nike co-founder Bill Bowerman – while working at his garage in Oregon and creating a legendary shoe tread with the help from a waffle iron – has been well documented. Fittingly, the name of that shoe was called the Nike Waffle. The year was 1971, and it was the beginning of a massive running boom, which produced some of America's top runners of all time. The shoe industry was trying to make a product lighter and faster to propel these athletes to faster times. In the past decade, there have been few changes to the technical component of racing shoes, whereas most of the emphasis is on fashion and lightweight polymers; both of which help companies to market their product.

Purpose of Specialized Shoes

A racing flat or jumping shoe's main purpose is to provide a covering to protect the foot. Of course, this is debatable when watching many competitors with bloody feet cross the finish line after being "spiked" by other harriers. Just as important is the interface between the foot and the competitive surface. Whether it be running on a muddy cross-country course or spinning on a platform to throw a hammer, the

D. Granger (✉)
Private Practice, York, PA, USA

M.B. Werd, E.L. Knight (eds.), *Athletic Footwear and Orthoses in Sports Medicine*,
DOI 10.1007/978-0-387-76416-0_16, © Springer Science+Business Media, LLC 2010

athlete must be able to achieve enough friction to stay on their feet. Every competitive track and field shoe has a specialized sole to meet this purpose. Finally, today's racing shoes are extremely lightweight, some of which weigh are a mere 6 oz! Who would have thought that the roots of today's science lay in a waffle iron?

Types of Racing Shoes

Lightweight Trainer

For most weekend warriors and many high school runners, this type of shoe is perfectly suitable for racing. The advantages of this type of racing shoe are numerous. Economically, it is a great option for the parents of high school athletes because the youngster can both train and race in this shoe. Once the decision is made by the adolescent to stick with the sport, it is reasonable to move into having both a regular training shoe and a more aggressive spike. It is also a very good shoe for marathon runners who are doing long tempo workouts and would like to get the light feel of a racing shoe, but still have support. On the opposite end of the spectrum, this shoe is also great for the masters' athlete who can no longer tolerate a super lightweight racing flat. Finally, a lightweight trainer is also marketed to a low mileage (less than 20 miles a week) neutral runner who simply wishes to not wear a heavier shoe.

Road Racing Flat

Perfect for the post-collegiate athlete making the conversion to road running, or the serious runner who wishes to have a competitive edge on the road racing circuit. This category has expanded in the past few years, as more shoe companies are applying dual density medial posting for the pronated runner and more cushions for longer races such as a marathon (Fig. 16.1). Shoes of this type have a minimal amount of material, including a mesh upper, minimally cushioned midsole, and a thin outer sole.

Runners may choose to wear a waffle type shoe or a rubber spike for shorter races such as a mile or 5K. A racing flat will be the most common type of shoe in this category. As noted above, this type of shoe can vary as to the amount of cushion and posting depending on the style and brand. This style of shoe will be common for a serious to professional runner from distances from the 5K to marathon.

Spike Plate

In order to understand the following explanation of shoes, one must become familiar with the term spike plate. This is simply an area in the forefoot of a shoe that houses spikes. There are, of course, different types depending on the race. In general, the shorter the race, the higher profile and less flexible the spike plate. Many

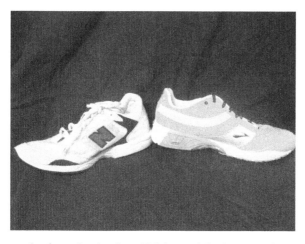

Fig. 16.1 An example of a road racing flat, which has a minimal amount of material, including a mesh upper, minimally cushioned midsole, and a thin outer sole

cross-country spike plates are rubber, and continuous with the midsole of the shoe, whereas sprint spike plates are hard plastic and add to the height of the forefoot. This, in turn, keeps the athlete on his toes for short distance races, while a more flexible spike allows a more natural heel to toe gait found in longer distances (Figs. 16.2a–d).

Cross-Country

Most serious high school athletes will choose a shoe with a rubber spike plate because it can be used for both cross-country and track. An alarming percentage of high school courses have pavement as part of the course and will make wearing a hard spike plate very uncomfortable. Another advantage of a rubber forefoot is that it is much more flexible than a hard plastic plate and does not have an aggressive negative heel. This eliminates many sources of injury for the novice runner. The runner can choose to screw either studs or different sized metallic spikes into the rubber spike plate for the variety of conditions encountered during a cross-country season.

Some high school and many collegiate athletes will choose a spike with a low-profile, hard plastic spike plate for their races. This type of shoe keeps the harrier on their toes more than the rubber spike plate to give them a faster feel and provides better footing. Most collegiate cross-country courses are all off road, so it is more reasonable at this level to have a more specialized spike. One must be aware that there is a greater chance for injury in a stiffer spike that keeps an athlete on his toes. This must be taken into consideration when treating an athlete, and a recommendation can be made to not race with an aggressive spike until he or she is pain free.

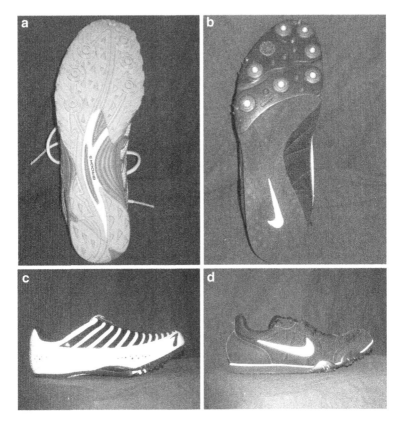

Fig. 16.2 (**a–d**) The spike plate is an area on the forefoot of a shoe that houses spikes

Track and Field

Sprints

When looking at a sprint spike, it is alarming to see how negative the heel is in relation to the forefoot. As mentioned previously, the purpose is to keep the runner on their toes for the entire race, typically between 60 (indoor track) and 400 m. Classically, the entire sole is plastic, since traction is only necessary in the forefoot. This hard plastic sole aids in rapid energy transfer necessary in explosive events such as a 100 m dash. All other components to the shoe are minimal, as to not add any unnecessary weight.

Middle and Long Distance

Variability exists in this group depending on athlete's preference. The main difference here will be in aggressiveness of the spike plate. Most shoes that are suggested for 800–10,000 m will have a plastic spike plate, with some type of rubber heel.

Many 800 and 1600 m runners prefer an aggressive spike plate, whereas the longer distance races cannot tolerate a negative heel for a longer period of competition. Conveniently, the latter is commonly the same spike that is used for cross-country races on smooth trails and golf courses. One must consider that a highly competitive athlete will run a 5K on the track at the same pace as a fast high school mile. Therefore, that particular runner may choose a more aggressive spike since they will be on their toes for the majority of the race.

Unique to this category is the steeple chase spike. The steeple chase is an event where the runner must overcome 35 barriers that are 36 in. high (30" for women) and do not collapse like a regular hurdle. Six of these barriers have a water jump that is 12 feet long, tapering from 3 feet at the base. A spike evolved for this event which has a water proof mesh upper in order for the spike not to gain weight during the race. Not all shoe companies make a steeple-specific spike since such a small percentage of runners can justify the purchase, so they may have to be specially ordered.

Jumps

The shoe designed for the triple jump, long jump, and pole vault are similar to sprinter's spikes in that they typically have a hard plastic spike plate with a negative heel. Some brands offer an extended spike plate, while others make a more flexible accommodating forefoot. The main difference is the rearfoot portion of the shoe. The sole has added traction and cushion needed for proper footing before jumping, as well as appropriate padding for landing in the triple jump (Fig. 16.3).

The high jump is fairly unique in that it is one of two shoes that may have spikes in the rearfoot. Traction in the rearfoot as well as the sides of the sole is necessary due to the tight, explosive turns seen in the approach to the long jump. In general, the sole is fairly rigid, in order for the jumper not to lose momentum on toe off (Fig. 16.4).

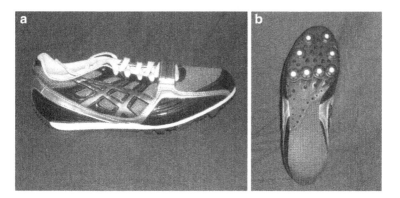

Fig. 16.3 (**a** and **b**) This shoe is designed for the triple jump, long jump, and pole vault

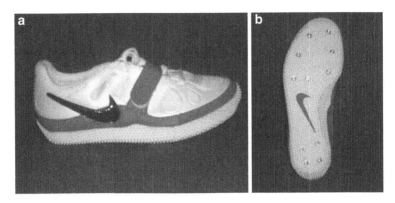

Fig. 16.4 (a and b) A shoe designed for the high jump may have spikes in the rearfoot

Throws

Shoes for throwing events are different in that they must endure both a heavier athlete and great rotational forces applied to the shoe. The outer sole of a throwing shoe is typically a smooth surface of synthetic rubber to aid in traction. This is necessary for events such as the discus, shot put, and hammer throw where the competitor is spinning in circles to propel their implement. Another specialized component of the throwing shoe is a dorsal strap to add stability to the upper. Again, there is a large amount of sheer forces generated through these athletes, which must be accommodated by the shoe in order to prevent failure (Fig. 16.5).

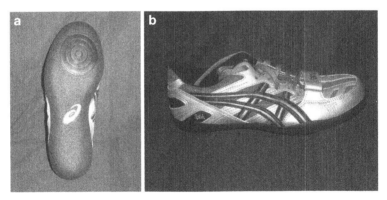

Fig. 16.5 (a and b) Shoes for throwing events must endure both a heavier athlete and great rotational forces applied to the shoe

The javelin shoe, like the high jump shoe, is unique as it is one of the only shoes with spikes in the rearfoot. In this event, it allows a proper foot plant in order to properly transfer momentum from the body to the javelin during the throw (Fig. 16.6).

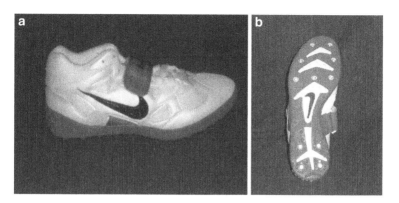

Fig. 16.6 (**a** and **b**) The javelin shoe, like the high jump shoe, has spikes built into the rearfoot

Putting It All Together

Spikes

The last important component to the racing shoe is the actual spike. Most shoes that have a spike plate come equipped with a spike wrench and $1/4''$ spikes. There are a variable number of spikes in a shoe, typically six for longer distance and eight for sprints. Most track surfaces allow $1/4''$ spikes, although the athlete should check with the facility before training or racing, as some may only allow $1/8''$. Similarly, cross-country courses on golf courses and field events such as the javelin may have regulations as to the length of spikes allowable, regardless of condition. For very muddy courses, some harriers will use as large as a $1''$ spike, assuming there are no paved areas to navigate. In muddy conditions where such a large spike is warranted, taping the shoe around the midfoot may be recommended, so it does not come off during the race. Similar to a large negative heel, caution is also given that the larger the spike, the more likely it is for posterior leg problems to arise (Fig. 16.7).

Training

Racing shoes may still have a place in the competitive runner's schedule outside of the race. While many runners choose to do all of their regular running and hard workouts in regular training shoes so can to feel lighter on race day, many athletes get injured in races because their legs are not used to being in competition shoes and in turn are prone to injury. A harrier's legs will better adapt to a shoe that has less cushion and possibly a negative heel if they are conditioned to do so through a series of workouts. Another advantage of wearing racing shoes for track interval sessions is they allow a faster cadence and rhythm that the runner will experience on race day. This is especially true in distances from 400 to 1600 m where interval

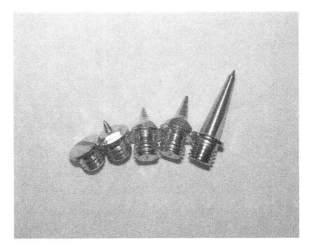

Fig. 16.7 Most shoes with a spike plate come equipped with a spike wrench and $\frac{1}{4}''$ spikes. The number of spikes and spike length depend on the event and field conditions

pace is close to threshold speed. In a sense, it is not practice that makes perfect, but perfect practice that makes perfect. Psychologically, runners will also be more eager to do a workout if they simply put on a pair of lightweight shoes.

Skin Issues

Most runners choose either not to wear socks or during competition or a very thin synthetic sock. When adding moist conditions to tight fitting shoes, the outcome is usually some type of skin or nail compromise. This is another advantage of wearing racing shoes for workouts – to prepare the foot for race day. Sometimes skin breakdown cannot be avoided, as race courses and conditions may be extreme, but in most cases, the athlete can be educated on how to prevent and treat such injury. This is accomplished by educating them on proper shoe fit and sock selection, and briefing them how to handle skin breakdown if it is to occur. For example, if a runner experiences blisters on the toes from rubbing in racing shoes, simple application of Vaseline® on race day may prevent serious problems during a marathon.

Support

Slightly modified standard low-dye technique for temporary support of the arch during competition when a standard orthotic will not fit into a racing flat can be effective. There are other taping techniques that are either very similar or just as effective; this method has been adopted over the years from trial and error (and many blisters). The taping itself is modeled after the original low-dye strapping for support, followed by an outer layer that allows flexibility to the runner and aids in skin protection.

Materials: 1″ athletic tape, 2″ Elastoplast, and pre-wrap spray.

1. Position the patient in a supine position at the end of an examination table with their heel hanging off the end. Make sure their ankle is held at 90° for the entire taping.
2. Pre-wrap adhesive spray may be applied before taping for longevity and support. Wax may also be applied to the plantar aspect of the taping to decrease sheer forces and add to the longevity of the modified low-dye strapping.
3. Place one piece of athletic tape starting at the second metatarsal head, around the lateral heel, to the medial side of the foot, and back to the third metatarsal head (Fig. 16.8a).
4. Place the next piece of athletic tape (if the foot is large enough) starting *proximal* to the first metatarsal head, around the heel, and ending between the fourth and fifth metatarsal heads:
   a. The first metatarsal head is not taped in order to mimic a first ray cutout as seen in many orthotic devices.

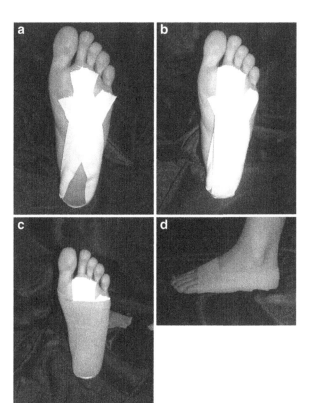

Fig. 16.8 Taping techniques. (**a**) Place one piece of athletic tape starting at the second metatarsal head, around the lateral heel, to the medial side of the foot, and back to the third metatarsal head. (**b**) Apply 1–2 "stirrups" from the forefoot (proximal to the sulcus of the toes) to the heel. (**c**) From proximal to distal, apply 2″ Elastoplast from lateral to medial, making sure not to wrinkle the athletic tape. The tape should end 1–2″ along the medial and lateral sides of the foot. (**d**) From lateral to medial, anchor all Elastoplast straps with another long piece of Elastoplast, including a strap across the dorsum of the foot

5. Apply 1–2 "stirrups" from the forefoot (proximal to the sulcus of the toes) to the heel (Fig. 16.8b).
6. From proximal to distal, apply 2″ Elastoplast from lateral to medial, making sure not to wrinkle the athletic tape. The tape should end 1–2″ along the medial and lateral sides of the foot (Fig. 16.8c).
7. From lateral to medial, anchor all Elastoplast straps with another long piece of Elastoplast, including a strap across the dorsum of the foot (Fig. 16.8d).

Teach the patient or the athletic trainer the technique so it can be applied the morning of the race. If the athlete does not have access to an athletic trainer or cannot tape his or her own foot, then recommend a low-profile prefabricated insole. An example of such a device is the Superfeet black or gray models. In the few cases where this will not provide the necessary support and the athlete still needs a custom foot orthosis, mold a low-profile device made from a thin, rigid material such as carbon fiber. Typically, the only patients requiring such devices are highly competitive athletes with extreme biomechanics, as most others will do well with other conservative measures.

If support is necessary during running outside of speed workouts, the athlete can be fit with either prefabricated insoles or custom foot orthoses for their training shoes. Typically, do not have the athlete wear orthoses with daily shoes unless they are severely pronated with either pain or instability. Proper gastroc-soleal stretching and intrinsic strengthening is instead emphasized for injury prevention. Arthur Lydiard, a pioneer of long distance running, had great insight into this concept many years ago. He once said, "You support an area, it gets weaker, you use it extensively, it gets stronger. Get on the grass and run barefoot and you don't have troubles. That's the first thing I did with all my athletes." With all of the technical advances in shoes, one must still consider fundamental concepts such as this in order to practice perfect.

Chapter 17
Triathlon and Duathlon

Kirk Herring

Historically athletic competition is ripe with epic contests, performances, and events. We need look no further than our own backyard to find some of the most heroic and compelling efforts. The Ironman Triathlon has evolved its own mystique becoming synonymous with epic physical efforts and stunning athletic performances. Many of these efforts have been sensationalized by the press and media motivating spectators, endurance athletes, and others to join and aspire to the ranks of multisport endurance athletes. Supporting this growth is an ever expanding array of highly technical equipment including bicycles and components, shoes, clothing, and nutritional systems geared to support novice, experienced, and professional athletes in their pursuit of personal glory. Regrettably, this surge of interest and participation has come at the price of injury; many endurance sport participants, whether first timer, novice, recreational, or professional, have suffered from an injury serious enough to require modification of training, rest and/or medical attention.

Technology alone cannot prevent the occurrence of an injury. Now more than ever, the ranks of triathletes are populated by midlife adults, many of whom are ex-athletes with dormant, hidden, and long forgotten musculoskeletal injuries. While the training required for these events offers the endurance athlete the benefits of cross-training, the long hours of rigorous training coupled with the demands of preparation for multiple sporting activities place the amateur and professional alike at risk of injury. With increasing frequency these athletes fall victim to a whole host of frustrating and sometimes devastating injuries, requiring weeks and sometime months for recovery. Overuse injuries account for up to 78% of injuries suffered by triathletes with injury exposure rates during the 6 months leading up to a competitive season estimated to be 2.5 injuries per 1,000 training hours and 4.6 injuries per 1,000 training hours during a typical 10-week competitive season [1]. A relatively recent

K. Herring (✉)
Private Practice, Inland Northwest Family Foot Care, 1215 N. Mcdonald Rd # 201, Spokane Valley, WA 99216-1557, USA

M.B. Werd, E.L. Knight (eds.), *Athletic Footwear and Orthoses in Sports Medicine*, DOI 10.1007/978-0-387-76416-0_17, © Springer Science+Business Media, LLC 2010

summary of injuries suffered by European triathletes estimated that 74.8% of long-distance triathletes suffered from at least one injury [2]. While some of these injuries can be considered acute in nature such as contusions, abrasions, and fractures, the majority of injuries would be classified as overuse injuries impacting the musculoskeletal system. Recent advances made in training systems, nutritional guidelines, endurance supplements/fluid replacements, cycling equipment, clothing, shoes, and foot orthoses have evolved to enhance performances, improve athlete comfort, and reduce the risk injury. Advising and educating the triathlete and the medical specialist providing treatment for the multisport athlete has become a cornerstone for the management of these athletes. In this chapter we will explore the indications, applications, modifications and role of athletic shoes, pedal systems, and foot orthoses for the treatment and/or prevention of lower extremity overuse injuries typically encountered by the triathlete, duathlete, and adventure race participant.

Overuse Injuries

Wolfe's law has had a profound impact on sport, training, medicine, and rehabilitation; it is generally accepted that tissues can adapt and remodel in response to applied stress. However, if the stress and frequency of its application exceeds the immediate or accumulative limits of the tissue and its ability to recover then cellular and tissue damage will occur and an injury will develop. Most frequently these injuries gradually evolve and would be classified as overuse injuries. Numerous circumstances are thought to be associated with overuse injuries including extrinsic and intrinsic factors. Multievent endurance activities are unique and blend several activities, typically swimming, cycling, and running. Each of these activities is associated with a key component of stress.

Cycling cadence and gearing resistance combine through long hours of training and competition can lead to tissue injury, failure, and the development of an overuse injury. Cycling over level terrain at a slow to moderate speed at a mid gear range (39/15) will offer minimal musculoskeletal stress. Most cyclists will generate power from the pedal and crank arm through the drivetrain from the 12 o'clock position to the 6 o'clock position, or during the down stroke of the pedal. A force–time curve for this activity would exhibit a single active propulsion peak of force corresponding to the midpoint between the beginning and end of each power stroke. Active forces are a result of a propulsion system generated by the cyclists' muscular effort, and when increased resistance is met such as during hill climbing or applied as would be the case with gear changes excess active forces will be dissipated in the joints of the lower extremity, hip, and low back. Supporting soft tissues thus serve to generate the power necessary for forward movement, to stabilize joints, and to dissipate excess and harmful stress.

Impact forces with the supporting surface at contact have been linked to the development of running overuse injuries. When running across a level uniform surface at a slow to moderate speed, most runners will exhibit a heel strike running gait. The resulting force–time curve reflects the impact forces generated from heel contact through toe-off and exhibits two peaks. The first, an impact peak represents heel contact and is associated with a steep upslope while the second peak represents an active propulsion peak with a more gradual upslope. Impact forces associated with overuse injury are dissipated through the joints and soft tissues of the lower extremity. Active propulsion forces resulting from the runner moving across the stationary supporting foot are also dissipated through the response of joints and adjacent soft tissues. Both forces have been associated with the development of overuse injuries.

Other forces act on the athlete and may contribute to the development of overuse injuries. While the exact cause for overuse running and cycling injuries is yet to be determined it is postulated that the etiology is multifactorial reflecting a diverse origin. Various factors have been discussed and can generally be organized into intrinsic and extrinsic factors. Training errors, anatomical abnormalities, and lower extremity biomechanics are widely accepted as common factors contributing to the development of overuse injuries. Careful selection of running and cycling shoes may help the athletes to reduce their overall risk of overuse injury and improve upon comfort and performances. Improper, damaged, and/or worn out shoes have been implicated in the development of overuse injuries. Additionally, the manner in which the foot is cradled within the shoe by way of an orthoses can contribute to enhancement of comfort, avoidance of overuse injury, and as treatment for an existing injury.

The Act of Running: Single Support and Double Float (Swing)

The act of running propels the triathlete forward during the running portion of training and racing. Running challenges the triathlete to coordinate simultaneously complex events through an as yet to be fully explained neuromusculoskeletal proprioceptive feedback system embedded in muscles, tendons, ligaments, joints, and skin to (1) establish a stable and adaptable base of support, (2) coordinate balance, minimizing unnecessary oscillations and excessive migration of the center of mass during forward progression, (3) coordinate foot placement to augment the establishment of a stable adaptable base of support, (4) regulate ground clearance of the foot during the swing phase, (5) generate the mechanical forces necessary to accelerate and maintain the forward propulsion of the runner, and (6) dissipate the mechanical energy (shock) resulting from impact and decelerate forward progression of the runner. While running gait is generally considered to be repetitive and predictable individual characteristics contribute to a high degree of individual specificity. Thus, injury changes to the running surface, shoes, orthoses, and even socks may trigger individually unique adaptations to the basic running form and gait cycle.

Running gait, although similar to walking, can be subdivided into two distinct phases: a *stance phase* and a *swing phase*. Because of inherent differences between individuals including stature, body proportions, coordination, joint range of motion, musculoskeletal strength, neuromuscular feedback pathways, proprioceptive abilities, previous injuries, and anatomical variations running gait patterns are unique. However, due to basic anatomic, physiological, and neuromuscular makeup running locomotion is accomplished in a similar manner for all individuals. The act of running is very cyclical, coordinating the alternating and rhythmic actions of the extremities and trunk through a highly automated series of movement patterns which rely on proprioceptive and neuromusculoskeletal feedback to coordinate the interaction of the trunk, arms, lower extremities, and feet to efficiently propel the athlete forward.

The *stance phase* of running gait represents the support period during which time the limb first encounters the support surface and ends when the limb leaves the support surface at toe-off. This phase encompasses approximately 40% of running gait cycle. Stance phase of running can be subdivided into five distinct phases:

1. Initial contact
2. Loading
3. Midstance
4. Propulsive phase also referred to as terminal stance
5. Preswing

The *initial contact phase* of running gait represents the commencement of the stance phase of running. This phase represents the initial contact of the swinging foot with the support surface. This phase may be described as a heel, midfoot, or forefoot contact moment. Most runners will consistently exhibit one of these contact patterns; however, variations may occur during any given run or between runners as a result of anatomical differences, running speed, stride length, cadence, running surface properties, and/or as a result of musculoskeletal fatigue. With increasing speed and certain anatomical or kinematic variations such as might be exhibited by a short limb, limited ankle joint dorsiflexion, tight gastrocsoleus muscle, or short Achilles tendon a runner may be more inclined to contact the support surface distal of the heel. With decreasing speed, reduced stride length, and musculoskeletal fatigue many runners will make initial contact with the support surface through heel contact. The *loading phase* of running represents that crucial period during which time the stance limb begins to dissipate the impact of the body with the support surface. These external forces can be as high as 3–6 times the body weight for the typical runner dependent on individual running kinematics, terrain, running surface properties, and even greater for the older runner. Knee and hip flexion as well as eversion of the heel acted upon by adjacent soft tissue also affects the dissipation of these forces. This phase is dominated by the effects of pronation of the STJ which serves to "unlock" the functional midtarsal joint (talonavicular and calcaneocuboid joints) of the foot and through a coupling action at the talo-crual joint to internally rotation of the lower leg. *Midstance* represents a crucial phase, one of transition; the stance phase limb continues to dissipate impact forces through pronation acting across the talonavicular joint while adapting to the support surface, shoes, or orthoses. This phase also marks the earliest signs of resupination of the foot.

Forefoot and midfoot contact running alters the loading response and midstance phases of running. This running style rapidly exerts a pronatory load across the oblique axis of the midtarsal joint and by way of pronation of the talonavicular joint indirectly acts to pronate the STJ. Impact is dissipated at the same time the posterior musculature of the lower leg is eccentrically loaded serving to both decelerate impact forces and store elastic energy in the musculotendinous structures.

During *midstance* the foot achieves full contact with the support surface. It is during this phase that the foot reaches its maximum level of pronation and with the assistance of the tibialis posterior muscle in addition to the momentum of the swing leg triggers the resupination of the foot, reversing the effects of pronation. This in effect permits the foot to achieve a stable foundation as the foot prepares to advance to the *propulsive or terminal stance phase of running. Propulsive or terminal stance* is established around a stable foundation of a supinating foot. This phase commences at the moment the heel of the stance limb is lifted from the support surface and ends when the finial propulsive forces are exerted through the big toe at toe-off. To achieve the most efficient transfer of energy the foot must be stable, a result of successful resupination of the stance limb. Resupination of the midtarsal joint and STJ is the cornerstone of foot stability; however, rotation of the pelvis generated by the swing leg and the influences of lower extremity muscles contribute to stabilizing the foot. The peroneal longus, flexor hallucis longus, and tibialis posterior muscles all contribute significantly to the establishment of medial column and forefoot stability while the tibialis posterior muscle reinforces the talonavicular joint and resupinates the rearfoot around the STJ.

Preswing phase of running gait is brief; many may even consider it to be nothing more than the terminus of the propulsive phase. Preswing serves to usher in a smooth transition, permitting the stance phase limb to shift its load to the contralateral limb and enter the swing phase of running with a minimal loss of forward momentum and or balance.

The *swing phase* of running is the period during which the foot and limb "unwind," becoming realigned in preparation for a new stance phase cycle. This phase should be considered as the period after the support limb leaves the support surface at toe-off and continues until the contralateral limb encounters the support surface at *initial contact*. This phase encompasses 60% of the running gait cycle. Swing phase of running can be subdivided into three distinct phases:

1. Initial swing
2. Midswing or double float (up to 30% of swing phase)
3. Terminal swing

Initial swing phase immediately follows preswing (toe-off). During this phase the foot continues its resupination and begins the realignment of the hip. However, the hallmark of the swing phase is *Midswing,* a period of *double float*. Unique to running, midswing represents a period when both limbs are suspended above the support surface as if floating. Depending on cadence, stride length, and the characteristics of the supporting surface this period may vary in its duration. During this phase the trailing limb is recovering from stance phase actions while the leading limb is preparing for initial contact. *Terminal swing* represents the finial resupination of the leading limb, initial contraction of muscles critical to dissipation of impact forces, and stabilization of joints critical to initial contact such as the hip, knee, ankle, and STJ.

The Act of Cycling: Spinning Through Power and Recovery Phases

Forward propulsion is typically generated by the cyclist through pressure applied to the bicycle drivetrain. The drivetrain is composed of the pedal, crank arm, bottom bracket, ring gear, chain, derailers, and rear sprocket (cassette). When seated or standing the cyclist will move the pedals and crank arm through a 360° circular path or *pedal cycle*. The typical triathlete will ride or *spin* (a high uniform cadence) at a cadence which repeats the pedal cycle from 60 to 100 revolutions per minute (RPM) generating up to as many as 6,000 pedal cycles per hour and 38,000 pedal cycles in a typical Ironman Triathlon. When the lower extremity is exposed to pedal cycle frequencies at this level even minor biomechanic abnormalities, musculoskeletal imbalances, and altered joint range of motion can manifest into overuse injuries.

The pedal cycle is divided into two phases: the *power phase* and the *recovery phase* [3]. When applied in sequence these two phases will generate the power necessary to propel the cyclist forward. The *power phase* is defined as the period which extends from the pedal starting position at "*top-dead-center*" (TDC) with the pedal at 0/360° and rotating clockwise to "*bottom-dead-center*" (BDC) with the pedal ending at 180°. It is during this phase that most cyclists will generate the majority of the power necessary to propel the bicycle forward. The *recovery phase* immediately follows the power phase and is defined as the period which extends from the pedal at BDC with the pedal at 180° and rotating clockwise back to TDC. During this phase the cyclist realigns the foot and leg and the power generating muscles are provided with an episode of rest or recovery before the next power phase. When cyclists use cleated shoes with a clipless pedal system, the recovery phase may also contribute significantly to recovery phase power transfer as the cyclist exerts an upward pull upon the pedal and crank arm through to the TDC position and the beginning of the next power phase. However, the primary biomechanical role of this phase remains one of realignment, returning the foot, knee, hip, and back to return to position which is more optimal for generating the next power phase.

A complex interaction of lower extremity joints and muscle activity act to provide forward propulsion for the cyclist. During the power phase the hip and knee extend, the ankle remains neutral or plantarflexes, and the foot pronates. Augmenting these joint actions are muscles of the lower extremity and back acting upon the hip including the gluteal muscles which extend the hip, the paraspinal muscles which stabilize the pelvis and low back, and the hamstring muscles which act to assist the gluteal muscle during extension of the hip [4]. The quadricep muscles act upon the knee to extend the leg, providing most of this effect in early power phase while the hamstring muscle continues knee extension in late power phase [4]. The ankle which typically oriented in a slightly dorsiflexed position at TDC begins to plantarflex in the power phase under the influence of the soleus muscle and is continued past BDC by the action of the gastrocnemius muscle and the flexor hallucis longus muscle [5].

The effect of the calf muscles and the deeper flexor hallucis longus upon the ankle joint is important to the transfer of power from the leg to the pedal and drivetrain of the bike [3]. These muscles perform to [1] resist hip and knee extension forces through a stabile ankle [4], provide propulsive power especially during the later stages of the power phase, and [5] place the foot in a neutral to slightly plantarflexed position at BDC augmenting the ability of the hamstring muscles to carry power across BDC into the recovery phase of cycling [3, 5, 6]. Gregor and Okajima observed that the most effective transfer of power from the foot to the pedal and drivetrain occurred when the foot (force) was applied perpendicular to the crank arm [7, 8].

Pronation of the foot occurs during the power phase of cycling. As force is applied by the extending leg to the foot the resistance of the pedal and drivetrain triggers STJ and MTJs to pronate [3]. This action leads to eversion of the forefoot, dorsiflexion, and inversion of the medial column and abduction of the forefoot. This may result in an eversion moment of the rearfoot at BDC.

Translocation of the knee in the transverse plane occurs as the knee extends through the power phase. This motion is dependent upon pelvic width, Q-angle, and the pedal–crank arm width. Typically as the knee extends it moves closer to the bicycle since the foot is fixed to the bicycle by the pedal. Excess Q-angles can further perturb the adduction of the knee during the power phase and may represent a significant contributing factor to overuse injury of the knee. Furthermore, abnormal function of the vastus lateralis and rectus femoris may further contribute transverse plane abnormalities by displacement of the patella too laterally when opposed by a weak vastus medialis muscle.

The recovery phase of cycling serves to realign the lower extremity. The limb moves from BDC to TDC as the hip and knee flex, the ankle dorsiflexes, and the foot resupinates. Cyclist that ride with cleated shoes and pedal systems may use the recovery phase as a power generating phase to augment forward propulsion of the contralateral limb. Under these circumstances the recovery phase limb is acted upon by the hamstring and gastrocnemius muscles [3]. Late in the recovery phase the anterior tibial muscle will begin to dorsiflex the ankle while the quadricep muscles continue to flex the hip and begins to extend the knee [5, 9, 10].

Biomechanic Role of the Foot

Root et al. proposed a Subtalar Joint Neutral Theory to classify the foot, basing this theory on subtalar joint (STJ) neutral position and a fully pronated midtarsal joint [3–5]. This system, although dated, classified structure, function, and functional relationships of the foot and the lower extremity; it remains the most comprehensive and widely applied system with which to classify the foot and its biomechanics [3–5]. This theoretical and conceptual model of foot function has undergone relatively little change since its first introduction; however, it has spawned several alternative theories which also strive to explain the function of the foot and more importantly the influence of foot orthoses upon the symptomatic lower extremity. These theories include the "Tissue Stress Theory," "Sagittal Plane Facilitation of Motion Theory," and "Preferred Movement Pathway Theory" [6–8].

Root et al. described the ideal or normal foot, its function, and based upon the STJ Neutral Theory a system of classification how the symptomatic foot should be supported with foot orthoses [11]. Central to the STJ Neutral Theory is foot function which is most efficient around a neutral STJ with the midtarsal joints "locked" in a maximally pronated position. By accomplishing this, the foot orthoses would (1) limit extraneous motion, control the foot around the STJ neutral position during gait, (2) minimize potentially harmful compensation(s) by the foot for lower extremity abnormalities, and (3) induce a strong "locking" action of the midfoot across the midtarsal joints [9, 10].

Unfortunately, this STJ Neutral Theory of function has not been adequately tested and limited evidence exists to support the concept that to remain injury free the foot must function around the STJ neutral position. (John Weed, 1985–1992, Personal communications) [11–20]. Yet, convincing clinical evidence exists to suggest that patients treated with foot orthoses constructed upon a model of the foot in the STJ neutral position tolerate the orthoses well and symptoms improve [21–41]. The lack of clinical and research evidence validating the STJ Neutral Theory has stimulated research to explain functional and mechanical action of the foot.

Alternative theories have been proposed in an effort to better explain foot function and the impact of foot orthoses. Each of these theories recognizes that a unique STJ axis of rotation exists and that foot orthoses directly or indirectly influences the motion at this joint. The *Tissue Stress Theory* proposed by McPoil and Hunt strives to associate treatment of injuries with orthoses as a process of assessment leading to orthoses management directed at the compromised anatomical unit or tissue [14]. McPoil and Hunt suggest that by utilizing the Tissue Stress Theory the clinician will have a better system from which to develop a system of examination and management of individual foot disorders [14]. The Tissue Stress Theory should allow clinicians the opportunity to more accurately develop a prescription for a foot orthoses which meets the anatomical/structural needs of an injured tissue rather than developing an orthoses prescription based upon unreliable measurements.

The *Sagittal Plane Facilitation of Motion Theory* described by Payne and Dannenberg hypothesizes that functional limitations of hallux dorsiflexion during the propulsive phase of gait may be responsible for abnormal foot function and complaints of pain [15, 42, 43]. Fundamental to this theory is the functional performance of the first metatarsal phalangeal joint; when hallux dorsiflexion is restricted during the propulsive phase of gait the foot will compensate by way of abnormal movement patterns which contribute to the development of injuries and complaints of pain [42–44]. Payne and Dananberg postulate that when the "sagittal plane" motion (dorsiflexion) of the hallux is reestablished through the introduction of foot orthoses a normalization of timing, movement patterns, and plantar pressures will occur throughout the lower extremity [15]. Recent evidence suggests that functional hallux limitus may trigger a retrograde response mitigated by other structural units or functional pathways [45]. However, central to this theory remains the limitation of hallux dorsiflexion at the first metatarsal phalangeal joint complex.

The *Preferred Movement Pathway Theory* proposed by Nigg et al. attempts to describe foot orthoses performance based upon a complex sensory feedback loop which serves to modify muscle activity [16]. A fundamental premise of this theory centers on the changes observed in muscle activity when foot orthoses were introduced. Nigg et al. observed that the joints and of the foot exhibited a preferred movement and activity pathway [46, 47]. However, when foot orthoses were introduced, joint movement pathways persisted but muscle activity was minimized [47]. Through a proposed sensory feedback loop the foot orthoses served to tune the muscles and thereby dampen potentially harmful soft tissue vibrations [46, 47].

In an attempt to explain the motion of the foot around the STJ Kirby [48] proposed a technique to illustrate the spatial location of the STJ. Kirby concluded that an abnormal position of the axis of rotation of the STJ had a significant influence upon the function and performance of the foot [48, 49]. Abnormality of the spatial position of the axis of rotation of the STJ may occur in the transverse and/or sagittal planes. Assuming planal dominance of motion, deviations of the axis of rotation in the sagittal plane will alter the magnitude of either the transverse or frontal plane components of the motion. Kirby, however, recognized that medial or the lateral shifts of the axis of rotation of the STJ in the transverse plane would significantly effect the function and performance of the foot [48–50]. The *Subtalar Joint Axis Location and Rotational Equilibrium Theory* of foot function was proposed to explain these effects and described three foot types: *medially deviated STJ axis, normal STJ axis*, and *laterally deviated STJ axis* [50]. This theory recognizes that the influence of weight-bearing activities upon the foot may vary dependent upon the spatial location of the STJ axis of rotation.

Anatomy of a Triathletes Running and Cycling Shoes

The Running Shoe

Since its inception over 40 years ago the modern running shoe has undergone an evolution of change driven by the needs of the athlete. Today's distance training and racing shoes are technically advanced with designs to suite nearly every foot type (pes cavus, neutral, and pes planus), anatomical circumstance (adducted foot, rectus foot, heavy runner, wide foot narrow foot, etc.) and running need (cushioning, neutral, stability, motion control, bare foot, and racing). Design characteristics of running shoes have been demonstrated to influence running kinematic variables of the rearfoot including foot position at contact, peak eversion, and peak eversion velocity [51–54]. While it is widely held that the potential for developing an overuse running injury is reduced with careful running shoe selection, no clinical data is available to date to support this hypothesis. However, the importance of selecting a well-designed running shoe is unequivocal; comfort, function, and fit are all enhanced when the triathlete selects a shoe based upon functional needs as well as training and racing demands.

The anatomy of a typical running shoe is composed of several coordinating components (Fig. 17.1):

> Upper
> Closure (Lacing) system
> Midsole
> Outsole
> Sock liner/foot-bed

The shoe *upper* which cradles the foot can be subdivided into a toe box, vamp, throat, collar, and heel cup. The *closure (lacing) system* serves to secure the shoe to the foot in a manner not to adversely impede function and comfort. The *midsole* acts to dissipate the forces of impact during the stance phase of gait and it acts to augment the transfer of stance phase forces through the lower extremity during the act of running. It is composed of a cushioning component which may include specialized stabilizing support units, thermal plastic units, and various specialized impact absorbing and force dissipating components. The *outsole* of the shoe is composed of a durable material with a sheet-like or modular pattern which promotes additional cushioning, support, and traction without sacrificing the transfer of stance phase forces through the lower extremity. The *sock liner/foot*-bed is the removable surface which serves to support the foot. It is typically composed of a fabric-covered and cushioned material molded to the shape of the foot which serves to promote

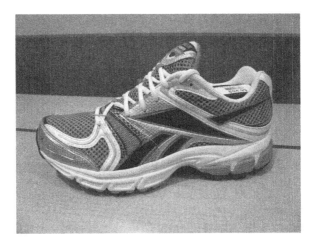

Fig. 17.1 Reebok women's running shoe

a comfortable fit while wicking moisture and dissipating friction. It may also act to augment midsole cushioning and the transfer of stance phase forces through the lower extremity.

The modern running shoe can trace its roots back over four decades to the innovations and design concepts first explored by Coach Bill Bowerman of Oregon; however, the modern running shoe now more adequately blends anatomical form with biomechanic function. The modern running shoe is built around a model of the foot or *last*. While each shoe manufacturer maintains their own unique lasts, all lasts can be organized into one of three general categories based upon the shape of the last. A *curve last* has a distinct *"C-shape,"* and when bisected by an imaginary line extending from center of heel through the forefoot more of the shoe will appear medial to the bisection. This is easily viewed when the shoe is examined from the bottom of the outsole. Curve-lasted shoes are best suited to runners with a normal to cavus foot type with adduction of the forefoot. A *straight last* is characteristically straight, and when bisected from center of heel to forefoot the shoe is divided into two nearly equal halves. These shoes are best suited to runners with a normal to pes planus foot type with a more abducted forefoot. A *combination last* represents a hybrid of a curve last and straight last; the rearfoot portion of the shoe is straight while the forefoot portion of the shoe is more curved. When bisected this shoe appears straight through the rearfoot and midfoot with a slight tendency to be adducted through the forefoot. This last best suits the widest range of foot types.

Running shoes can also be categorized by the method of construction. *Slip lasts* are constructed in a manner that secures the upper of the shoe at the midsole with a serpentine stitched line. These shoes afford the maximum degree of flexibility and the lowest level of overall stability. A *board last* shoe applies a fiber board from heel to toe which is glued to the upper where the upper joins the midsole. This construction is inexpensive and affords the greatest degree of heel to toe stiffing and overall resistance to longitudinal torque. A *combination last* blends the advantages of slip and board last construction by securing the rearfoot portion of the shoes upper to the midsole via a fiber board or stiffener leaving the forefoot serpentine stitching exposed. This construction is very popular and has undergone refinements which have integrated the rearfoot stiffener directly to the upper not by direct gluing but rather by stitching the stiffener perimeter directly to the upper at the union with the midsole. This shoe construction provides a reliable and stable rearfoot while maintaining forefoot flexibility without sacrificing longitudinal stability. These refinements to the classical combination last have permitted shoe designers to integrate the shoe upper with the lasting permitting a more effective coupling of upper to midsole.

The most visible component of the modern distance running shoe is the upper. The upper is composed of a breathable tough and lightweight material which is reinforced with various swatches of synthetic leather to promote structural integrity, medial–lateral sway stability, and to enhance forefoot flexibility at heel off through toe-off. A handful have improved lining designs to the point that all interior seams have been eliminated. This is a significant advantage for the athlete who is susceptible to blistering. Likewise shoe tongue designs have improved balancing padding without excessive bulk. Traditionally a U-shaped throat has been utilized;

this design is highly tolerant to a wide variety of midfoot anatomies ranging from the cavovarus foot to the low pes planus foot type. Various lacing systems have been employed but the variable lacing system is the most popular and functional. This system easily adapts to the introduction of a speed lacing system using elastic laces or a lace lock system.

The midsole of the distance running shoe has undergone the greatest evolution. The modern midsole is constructed from a variety of cushioning materials, stabilizers and support components, or *thermal plastic units* (*TPU*). The role of the midsole is to absorb and dissipate impact, stabilize the foot, and enhance the forward progression of the runner. Ethyl vinyl acetate (EVA), polyurethane (PU), sealed oil and gel chambers, and sealed air chambers represent the most common materials used. Each of these materials comes in a range of firmnesses, and unique placement into the midsole will impart specific cushioning, flexibility, and movement transfer abilities to the shoe. Typically softer cushioning materials are placed under the heel and forefoot for cushioning while firmer materials are positions under the medial heel extending into the midfoot and forefoot to promote enhanced stability. These materials are also frequently wrapped up onto the shoe upper at the transition zone between shoe upper and midsole to promote medial–lateral stability and to increase longitudinal stability. TPUs of various sizes and shapes are typical to most midsoles; these inserts serve to promote stability, act as a rearfoot to forefoot bridge, and guide the foot through the gait cycle.

Outsole technology is dominated by modular designs. Durability, traction, and grip are primary goals for shoe outsoles, especially given the variety of surfaces over which the distance runner will pass. However, the unique placement of outsole modules of different firmness, materials, and density can also enhance heel contact cushioning, guide the foot through midstance, and maintain forefoot flexibility at heel and toe-off.

The Cycling Shoe

The cycling shoe is unique among athletic shoes and serves to integrate the foot and lower extremity with the crank arm and drivetrain of the bike by way of the pedal. The typical cleated cycling shoe is designed around an adducted last which is comparable to a 2–4 in. dress heel [3]. The typical European designed cycling shoe also tends to be narrower than their domestic counter parts. However, the anatomy of a typical triathlon cycling shoe is standard and can be subdivided into four primary areas of importance:

Upper
Closure system
Sole/cleat anchor
Sock liner/foot-bed

Similar to running shoes, comfort and performance can be enhanced when triathletes carefully select training and racing shoes.

The *upper* of a cycling shoe is typically composed of leather, man-made synthetic leather substitutes (such as Lorica), synthetic fabric (nylons or polyesters), or a combination of materials. Backing materials may decrease irritation at pressure points but can also serve to increase internal heat and retention of moisture. The upper of the shoe should conform securely to the foot without excessive pressure points across critical anatomical structures (such as first and fifth metatarsal phalangeal joints) and promote adequate ventilation to avoid the buildup of excessive heat and moisture (perspiration) around the foot. The toe box and vamp shape should be adequate to fit the forefoot without crowding the toes unnecessarily, yet be adequately streamlined for efficient aerodynamics at higher speeds. Unlike running shoes most training and racing shoes suitable for triathlons will anchor the upper of the shoe directly to the sole. Additional stability may be achieved through the addition of TPU at critical stress points such as the forefoot and heel. The heel counter of the shoe will incorporate a firm heel cup composed of a thermoplastic material with light interior padding and a padded collar for comfort and to maintain a secure rearfoot fit.

Securing the shoe to the foot requires a *closure system* which is easy to use, adaptable to a variety of foot types, easy to use, and easily adjustable in transition and/or during training and racing. Multiple closure systems have evolved, one to three hook and loop straps and/or ratchet buckles are durable, secure, and easy to use. Strap systems which utilize hook and loop (Velcro) to secure the strap to the shoe have the advantages of reliability, ease of use, more adjustment possibilities, and speed of use. Unique to triathlon shoes are straps which are anchored laterally to the shoe and adjustable medially. This helps to keep loose "flapping" straps free of crank arms, bottom bracket, spinning wheels, and spokes.

The *sole* of the cycling shoe serves as the rigid link between the foot and pedal/crank arm and drivetrain. Typical outsoles are composed of a molded thermoplastic (nylon) material, carbon graphite, and molded thermoplastic reinforced with fiberglass. Rigidity, cleat mounting pattern, heel post, toe break angle, and stack height are all important characteristics to consider when selecting a cycling training or racing shoe. Carbon graphite soles offer the greatest rigidity while molded thermoplastic soles offer greater flexibility. While a rigid sole is important for efficient transfer of power from the lower extremity to rotational torque in the crank arms it may also prompt a more awkward running/jogging gait during triathlon/duathlon transition. Cleat mounting hardware is incorporated into the sole of the shoe and serves as the anchoring site for the pedal cleat. Anchor patterns may vary, some are unique to specific cleat–pedal systems while others may be more universal suitable for a wide variety of cleat–pedal systems. All anchoring systems approximate cleat placement at the metatarsal phalangeal joints and should permit cleat placement adjustment to suit the specific needs of individual cyclists. A heel post/pillar is typical to most shoes and serves to ease walking in cycling shoes, relieve strain on the Achilles tendon during walking, and provide limited protection to the sole. Running out of and into transition areas is awkward for the triathlete; to ease this brief run the triathlete may wish to consider a cycling shoe of a thermoplastic nylon or nylon reinforced with fiberglass sole to permit slight sole flex to ease an awkward run and to avoid running out the back of a more rigid sole shoe.

Toe break angle and *stack height* are two variables unique to cycling shoes. Toe break angle is the degree of rise of the forefoot of the shoe. Shoes with greater toe break angles may permit the cyclist to generate greater power during the power and recovery phases of cycling and ease muscular fatigue. A moderate toe break angle will permit the downward force applied by the extending lower extremity to the crank arm to remain closer to perpendicular to the crank arm, thereby achieving a more efficient transfer of force to rotational torque as the ankle plantarflexes through late power phase. However, high toe break angles will preload the plantar fascia and potentially increasing its intrinsic tension through excessive tightening of windlast mechanism increasing the potential for plantar (fascia) forefoot pain. Stack height of a cycling shoe may vary by brand, model, and design. It is the thickness of the sole of the shoe at the cleat attachment point measured in millimeters. By maintaining the foot close to the pedal axle power transfer during both the power and the recovery phases of cycling will be enhanced. Higher stack heights are more typical of molded thermoplastic nylon soles which require greater thickness to achieve sole rigidity. Carbon and carbon composite soles achieve equal to greater sole rigidity while maintaining low stack heights and can improve the overall shoe pedal–drivetrain efficiency. High stack heights may adversely impact the triathlete during run transitions in cycling shoes. During the brief run through transition, a high stack height can potentially dorsiflex the foot at the ankle increasing the concentric tension imparted upon the Achilles tendon and calf muscles. High stack heights can also increase the potential for lateral instability of the foot and ankle during run transitions.

A shoe *foot-bed or sock liner* is typically a thin and protective liner which separates the plantar surface of the foot from the interior of the shoe. This liner should be removable to permit replacement of the liner with a more efficient custom or prefabricated foot orthoses. However, when for those triathletes not requiring foot orthoses these liners should help to dissipate heat buildup, improve ventilation through sole, provide minimal cushioning, and carry moisture and perspiration away from the skin of the foot.

Classifying Running Shoes

Numerous guidelines for the categorization of running shoes have been circulated in the popular press. The following list of general categories is the most widely accepted and used for running shoes:

> Cushioning
> Neutral
> Stability
> Motion control
> Racing

Considerable overlap may exist; shoe authorities and manufactures may disagree on the assignment of a shoe to a category. However, based upon long-standing use and acceptance by the public this system provides a good starting point for the selection of an optimal training and racing shoe for the triathlete.

Shoes for *cushioning* represent designs which emphasize cushioning and flexibility. These shoes typically possess a uniform density midsole, limited shoe stabilizing add-in features, and an outsole which promotes flexibility while maintaining good traction with the support surface. These shoes promote an efficient running gait and rely on normal lower extremity and foot biomechanics. These shoes are best suited for the efficient lightweight runner with a normal to high-arched foot who demonstrates normal lower extremity biomechanics. The *neutral* shoe represents a design which promotes adequate cushioning, flexibility with the addition of limited stabilizing features. These shoes are best worn by a lightweight runner who exhibits normal lower extremity biomechanics. *Stability* running shoes are designed with the intent to augment the natural stability of the foot through all phases of gait. These shoes emphasize adequate cushioning and forefoot flexibility and enhanced motion controlling properties. These shoes are best worn by lightweight through normal weight runners with normal through moderately abnormal lower extremity biomechanics. Runners with normal foot biomechanics may elect to use this shoe to promote greater stability, especially during runs when fatigue influences normal running gait. *Motion control* shoes are intended to promote a maximum level of support and influence under the most extreme levels of excessive pronation of the foot during all phases of the running gait cycle. These shoes are better suited for runners with low-arched or a pes planus foot type and work well for individuals competing in the heavy weight class. These shoes are generally poorly suited for the lightweight runner due to the presence of very firm midsole materials which can promote excessive resistance to the normal foot function. *Racing* shoes represent a very special classification of running shoe; these shoes are intended to be lightweight and generally are poorly suited for the average triathlete.

Design innovations are frequently introduced to existing shoe models or shoe line-ups; however, rarely are entirely new design concepts introduced. However, Nike with introduction of the *Nike Free* brought to the running community an entirely new shoe classification. These shoes are designed as training or racing flats which intend to simulate the act of running barefoot while still proving adequate protection from foreign objects. These shoes do offer the triathlete with a training shoe to augment the strengthening of intrinsic musculature, otherwise not strengthened in a traditional shoe. However, these shoes provide little in the way of support for a foot which exhibits excessive pronation or for the runner which exhibits pronation of the foot through the midstance and propulsive phases of gait.

Finding the Perfect Triathlon Shoe

Finding the best training or racing shoe can be a formidable task. Numerous options exist; each shoe type and category is rich with near equal choices and each manufacture provides proprietary technology designed to enhance each run or ride;

considerable overlap exists between manufacturers promoting shoes within any given category. The process of selecting a suitable running shoe can be enhanced by following a few simple rules:

    Examine shoe for appropriate last shape
    Examine shoe for neutral position
    Examine shoe forefoot flexibility
    Examine shoe midfoot torsional stability
    Examine shoe heel counter rigidity
    Examine shoe upper side-to-side stability
    Examine shoe lacing system
    Examine shoe outsole traction
    Examine shoe last for orthoses fit

A few moments spent examining a new shoe can prevent the selection of a poorly constructed, designed, or possibly mismatched training or racing shoe.

To achieve an optimal fit, match the shape of the foot to the *shoe last shape*; fit an adducted foot and or cavus foot type to a curve-lasted shoe, a low/flat-arched pes planus foot type to a straight-lasted shoe, and fit the normal foot type to a combination-lasted shoe. The modern running shoe is built around a *neutral position* which places the heel counter of the shoe perpendicular to the support surface. Evaluate a shoe for neutral position on a flat and level surface; heel counters which are inverted or everted will impose an abnormal influence upon the foot through heel contact and can adversely effect the intended influence of foot orthoses throughout the gait cycle. Unnecessarily stiff or too proximal *forefoot flexibility* will increase the resistance to heel off leading to excessive momentary loads to the metatarsophalangeal joints and to the distal expansion of the plantar fascia. *Midfoot torsional stability* permits the rearfoot and forefoot to function independently in the frontal plain, yet provide resistance to sagittal and transverse plain movement. Excessive midfoot flexibility may increase the risks of overuse injuries linked to excessive and prolonged midstance and propulsive phase pronation of the foot. *Heel counter stiffness* relates to the rigidity or compressibility of the shoes rearfoot. Shoes with greater heel counter stiffness promote enhanced rearfoot stability at heel contact through midstance phases of gait. Heel counters with greater stiffness also provide a stabilizing influence to foot orthoses; enhancing orthoses heel cup influences directly to the foot and by providing a firm barrier against which the foot orthoses rearfoot posting may establish a predictable seating and a surface from which to establish leverage. *Shoe upper (vamp and quarter) side-to-side stability* is critical to maintaining the foot directly over the outsole and midsole of the shoe during all phases of running gait and under all circumstances of running surface and terrain. Excess shoe upper side-to-side movement will increase the risk of both chronic overuse injuries and even acute inversion (foot and ankle) injuries. Stable shoe uppers are well reinforced and exhibit minimal transverse plain (side-to-side) shift when stressed. Securing the shoe to the foot is the role of the *shoe lacing system*; important features for the triathlete to consider include adequate variability to the lacing system to suit the specific needs of the athlete, suitability of the lacing system to the introduction of elastic or speed laces, and a design which avoids pressure points across the dorsum of the foot. Triathletes train year round and under a wide variety of conditions. In many regions of the world training may occur on slippery, wet, or icy conditions providing far less than optimal footing and traction. Careful inspection of *outsole traction* design patterns and outsole composition should be considered when selecting a training/racing shoe. Bill Bowerman, Coach Oregon State University, was the first to introduce the waffle sole pattern which has given rise to a myriad of outsole designs. While waffle-type soles provided superb combination of flexibility and traction; its lack of surface area compromises its stability and traction on firm and slippery or icy surfaces. Mixed high–low horizontal and diagonal patterns with crisp edges and traction and flex channels will provide better traction on firm surfaces with poor traction but will become unsuitable when traction is required such as when running on trails. The firmness of the outsole will also influence flexibility, traction, and wear potential. Hard firm materials promote the greatest durability but may sacrifice traction, cushion, and flexibility while softer materials sacrifice durability. Most modern training shoes will accept foot orthoses; however, special considerations should be made for the *suitability of the shoe to accommodate a foot orthoses*. Shoes which will eventually be used with a foot orthoses should provide a versatile lacing system, alternatives to secure the rearfoot snuggly, adequately deep heel cup and rear quarter, removable sock liner, flat stable insole, torsional stability, minimal instep cut out, and adequate width and length. Many times the introduction of a foot orthoses will increase the shoe size need (length) by one half size.

When carefully selected, a well-designed cycling shoe can shave seconds off an athlete's finishing time and help the athlete to avoid injury. While overlap exists between running shoes and cycling shoes, such as *last shape*, *neutral position*, *heel counter rigidity*, *and orthoses suitability*, features unique to cycling shoes should be considered separately when selecting a cycling shoe:

Examine shoe upper for comfort
Examine shoe closure system
Examine shoe sole for stability
Examine shoe for cleat anchoring
Examine shoe toe break and stack height

The heart of every cycling shoe is a *comfortable upper* that snugly fits to the foot without contributing to pressure points, promotes good air flow through the shoe, and minimizes irritating internal seams. The triathlete should carefully examine the *closure system* for durability, ease of use, adjustability, and security. A stable sole is critical for the transfer of power from the lower extremity to the bike drivetrain; examine the cycling shoe for *longitudinal and torsional stability*. The sole should resist torsional flexion when a twisting force is applied especially during climbing and sprinting out of the saddle. While longitudinal flexion will ease running and walking through transitions zones too much flexion will sacrifice power transfer to the bicycle. Avoid cycling shoes that permit longitudinal flexion. Examine the shoe sole for proper *cleat anchoring*; a secure and adjustable anchoring site/system that fits to the intended pedal system is important to optimize power transfer, comfort, and minimize the potential for overuse injuries of the foot, knee, and hip. Examine the shoe sole for *toe break angle and stack height*; avoid excessive toe break angles which may enhance power transfer when pushing big gears but are not well suited for spinning in lower gears as is more typical to triathlon training and racing. Avoid excessive stack height, by keeping the pedal/cleat close to the shoe sole power transfer from the lower extremity to the bicycle drivetrain will be improved through all phases of riding.

Pedal and Cleat Systems

No discussion of cycling shoes should go without a brief discussion of pedal systems. Pedals serve as the link between the cycling shoe and the crank arms of the bicycle. Careful selection of a proper pedal system has been shown to reduce overuse injuries of the knee. *Float* is a terminology used to describe the ability of the cyclists foot to rotate in the transverse plain or for the shoe to be adjusted upon the pedal (in-toed or out-toed) to suite the structural/anatomical needs of the cyclists. *Clip-type* pedals into which the forefoot slips allow the foot to move side-to-side and to rotate in the transverse plane with limited resistance. However, this method of securing the foot to the pedal is inefficient and permits a significant loss of power during both the power and the recovery phases of the pedal cycle. *Clipless* pedals secure the foot directly to the pedal minimizing the loss of power during both phases of the pedaling cycle. Some clipless pedal systems permit the rider to adjust the angle of *float* necessary to achieve a neutral position of the lower leg (patella) to the pedal axle. Three basic systems are available and include unrestricted float, limited float, and fixed float angle; each permit transverse plane (in-toe or out-toe) adjustments of the shoe/cleat position in relationship to the pedal axle and when properly adjusted can reduce lower extremity overuse injuries resulting from transverse plane malalignment of the lower extremity. These pedal systems are especially effective when applied to reduce chronic overuse and torque strain exerted upon the knee and hip during the power phase of cycling. Common overuse injuries such as patellofemoral pain syndrome and iliotibial band syndrome will often respond favorably to a properly fit pedal system.

Socks for the Triathlete

Socks are often one of the most frequently overlooked pieces of sporting equipment/apparel; in our zeal to run and ride triathletes too often discount the potential benefit derived from the garment enveloping the foot. Over 30 years ago DuPont developed synthetic fibers which ushered in an era of *technical knitwear*. Today, this specialize off shoot of the sock and fiber producing industry has created wide variety of very specialized socks and sock fiber blends. When carefully selected the athlete is assured of a sock that will perform under the stresses of both running and riding.

The primary role of athletic socks is to protect the exercising foot from excess moisture accumulations, such as perspiration or extrinsic moisture (rain and spray/mist stations), promote padding, accommodate anatomical irregularities, reduce pressure, and reduce friction and torque forces. The military has long held to the recommendation of a two-sock system to minimize the occurrence of friction blisters [55]. The military has exerted a considerable effort to evaluate socks and boots in an effort to identify the best boot–sock system [56–58]. Herring and Richie observed that sock fiber-type and sock construction properties could be linked to the frequency, size, and severity of friction blisters among runners, and with careful sock fiber and construction selection the frequency of potentially disabling friction blisters could be reduced [58, 59, 60]. More recent evidence from the Office of Navel Research has associated the development of more serious lower extremity injuries including overuse injuries with military recruits suffering from frequent friction blister events [61]. Based upon these data alone the triathlete should carefully examine the intrinsic and extrinsic circumstances associated with running and cycling in an effort to select an optimal sock to reduce the risk of skin and thereby other musculoskeletal injuries.

Sock fibers can be grouped into two primary categories: natural fibers such as wool, cotton, and silk and man-made fibers such as acrylic, nylon, polyester, and polypropylene. Natural fibers have long been touted for their overall ease of handling, wearability, durability, and ease of cleaning. Man-made fibers (*synthetic fibers*) on the other hand offer a wider range of thermal and moisture management properties as well as providing fibers of excellent wearability, comfort, and durability. Each fiber possesses unique properties; the primary properties include fiber length, tenacity (strength), flexibility, extensibility, elasticity, and cohesion while the secondary properties include fiber resiliency, cross section, surface geometry, specific gravity, and moisture regain. When woven into yarns and knit into technical knitwear the resulting sock will exhibit characteristics consistent with the fiber content and fiber proportionality. For triathletes the properties of moisture and thermal management, cushioning, and the dissipation of friction and shearing forces are important attributes to seek in a technical sock.

The human foot exhibits a significant potential to produce perspiration. The human foot possesses approximately 3,300 eccrine sweat glands per square inch or approximately 200,000 eccrine sweat glands per foot. At rest the human foot is capable of producing approximately $\frac{1}{4}$ cup of sweat in a 12-h period. With vigorous activities, such as running and cycling, the triathletes' foot may produce vastly more perspiration in the same 12 h dramatically increasing the potential risk for friction blisters. This risk can be reduced by selecting socks which contain a high percent of *CoolMax* fibers; these *synthetic polyester* fibers are specially designed to minimize moisture regain (absorption) and possess a four-channel cross section which enhances the wicking potential of the sock. *Polypropylene* is another frequently encountered synthetic sock fiber used to manage moisture; however, due to these fibers' extreme *hydrophobic* tendencies it can trap excess moisture on the skin and limit the wicking of moisture away from the skin and increase the risk of friction blisters. *Synthetic acrylic* fibers are also excellent fibers from which to make athletic socks. These fibers offer the distinct advantage of a soft feel, comfort, durability, and excellent wearability, but due to the fibers' low moisture regain (absorption) and limited moisture wicking abilities they may leave the foot feeling slightly damp. *Merino wool* is an excellent natural fiber from which athletic socks are knit. Unfortunately, these wool fibers exhibit moderately high extensibility (stretch), poor overall elasticity (return to original shape during vigorous use), and moderately high moisture regain (absorption). The best sock would benefit from the properties of CoolMax, Merino wool, and acrylic blended together into one sock. This sock would exhibit the thermal benefit and moisture absorption properties of wool, the moisture wicking and low moisture regain properties of CoolMax, and the wearability and durability of acrylic.

Sock construction and design is as important to injury avoidance as fiber composition. Three basic design constructions are used and include *flat knit* construction, *Terry-loop* padded construction, and *double-layer* construction. A fourth construction, *Anatomically correct toe-socks*, is also available and may represent an excellent choice for a triathlete who suffers from frequent interdigital friction blisters. A flat knit construction offers only the advantage of a very low bulk sock, potentially an advantage in a tight-fitting cycling shoe; however, this design lacks the ability to absorb the friction and pressure forces associated with friction blister formation. Terry-loop padded construction provides the cushioning potential to dissipate friction and pressure, thereby reducing the risk of friction blisters. Socks of this design come in a range of padding bulks and anatomical alignment of the Terry-loop padding. Finally, double-layer sock construction utilizes two flat knit socks knit together at the cuff and toe to provide slightly greater cushioning potential and dramatically improved friction management without unnecessary sock bulk. For triathletes with a past history of friction blisters to the toes and feet the double-layer sock or lightly padded Terry-loop sock would provide the best potential to prevent an unanticipated skin injury.

Foot Orthoses Success

Foot orthoses for the triathlete can represent a diverse spectrum of externally applied devices, ranging from simple *over the counter* (OTC) arch supports to custom fabricated *ankle–foot orthoses* (AFO). The intended goal of any foot orthoses may be variable and dependent upon the specific needs of the athlete including (1) to enhance/achieve comfort during training and racing, (2) to limit abnormal lower extremity biomechanic events, (3) to enhance efficient running and cycling, (4) for the treatment/avoidance of injury, and (5) to improve shoe fit and performance. The most readily available foot orthoses are prefabricated OTC devices intended to replace the sock liner provided with a new running or cycling shoe. These devices come in a diverse array of designs and sizes intended to fit a generalized "average" foot. OTC devices are typically introduced to augment the properties of a shoe to enhance shoe fit, to improve local cushioning properties, and/or to improve the support of the foot. OTC devices are frequently beneficial and represent an important add-in to any new shoe fitting plan or as part of a more comprehensive plan of treatment for an injury or minor biomechanic fault.

Custom foot orthoses (CFO) are typically prescribed by a medical specialist and are created (fabricated) from model of an individual foot which has been balanced and modified to achieve a specific outcome. CFOs are typically an important part of a more extensive and comprehensive clinical plan of treatment for a previously diagnosed injury, biomechanic fault, anatomical/structural abnormality, and/or in an effort to alter the kinematics of running or cycling. The evidence supporting the clinical efficacy and benefits of these orthoses is growing [59–61].

The successful introduction of any foot orthoses should take into consideration the overall impact of the foot orthoses upon the athlete. This can be accomplished by examining the impact of the following constraints:

dysfunctional properties of the foot to be supported,
biomechanical properties of the foot,
unique morphology of the foot,
the injury,
pathomechanics of the injury,
intended sport shoe, and
intended sporting activity.

While the overall impact of one or more of these constraints may be dominant, considering each is critical to providing the most effective orthoses recommendation or prescription. When prescribing a CFO these constraints are most efficiently addressed by way of a *systematic approach* which integrates properties of the CFO with the athlete and injury. The prescription resulting from this approach would address

the need for a pathology-specific foot orthoses,
the creation of an accurate and functionally representative negative impression cast of the foot,
the importance of biomechanic-specific positive cast modifications,
an appropriate selection of orthoses shell construction materials,
the appropriate selection of rear post design, and
the contributing benefit of special additions, accommodations, extensions, and covering materials.

The resulting CFO would provide for the athlete the greatest potential for a device which is not only effective but also comfortable and well tolerated.

Pathology-specific foot orthoses have been shown to enhance the successful treatment of a variety of lower extremity injuries common to sporting activities [34, 36, 41, 62–68]. When implemented properly, the orthoses will diminish or counteract the occurrence of abnormal biomechanical forces which contribute to the injury of soft tissues, joints, and osseous structures during running and cycling. Thus the goal of pathology-specific foot orthoses is to identify the dysfunction of the foot relative to the injury and to direct specific device design characteristics to diminish the impact of the dysfunction upon the foot.

The creation of an accurate and functionally representative negative impression cast of the foot provides the first step leading to the fabrication of a CFO. While many techniques have been described this author prefers the suspension impression casting technique described by Root et al. This technique provides unique benefits not easily achieved by other commonly applied methods, such as ease of manipulation, intra-clinician cast consistency, ease of assessment for purposes of quality and casting position accuracy and ease of impression cast manipulation by orthoses making laboratories worldwide. While direct computer-based imaging technology has been available for a number of years its wide spread suitability for making of orthoses has been hampered by the proprietary nature of current imaging software, limited availability to the clinician, and the challenge to adequately miniaturize the imaging devices. However, any one of a number of modeling systems can achieve a satisfactory model of the foot from which to create a prescription foot orthoses as long as the clinician possesses the expertise and skills necessary to create a reliable and reproducible model of the human foot and recognizes the advantages and disadvantages of the modeling system being used.

Biomechanically specific positive cast modifications applied to CFOs can be categorized as either intrinsic or extrinsic in nature. Intrinsic cast modifications take place at the time the negative cast of the foot is "poured" to create a positive plaster model or scanned to create a positive computer model and typically includes balancing the bisection of the rearfoot to achieve an everted, perpendicular, inverted or Blake inverted positive model of the foot. Extrinsic cast modifications occur after a positive model of the foot has been rendered. These modifications generally are considered to include medial heel skive, cast fill, orthoses width, heel cup depth, fascial accommodations, and forefoot posting platform applications. The thoughtful combination of intrinsic and extrinsic positive cast modifications increases the potential that the resulting CFO will be effective.

Balancing of the impression cast at the time of "pouring" or scanning can impose a supinatory, pronatory, or neutral influence across the STJ and MTJ axis of rotation. When the posterior surface of the heel in the relaxed standing position is perpendicular and a mild or neutral supinatory influence is desired across the STJ and long axis of the MTJ a perpendicular or minor (2°–3°) inverted cast balance may be performed. While most orthoses making laboratories will default to a perpendicular balancing of the negative cast, many provide the opportunity to order other balancing positions. When the bisection of the posterior surface of the heel is everted in a relaxed standing position or when clear signs of heel eversion are noted during the late midstance or propulsive phases of gait are observed then an inverted balancing technique should be considered to increase the supinatory influence of the orthoses across the subtalar and midtarsal joint complexes. Up 6° can be tolerated; if a greater supinatory influence is required then a Blake inverted cast balancing technique should be considered. With this technique increased supinatory influence is directed across the subtalar joint. For every 5° of Blake inversion prescribed 1° of realized inverted positive cast position is achieved. Typical Blake inverted cast balancing for a triathlete would occur between 25° and 35° or a realized inverted influence of 5°–7°. Rarely would a clinician ever recommend an everted cast balance.

Kirby observed that the functional axis of rotation of the subtalar joint varied between individuals and he postulated that its anatomical location contributed significantly to the magnitude of the observed pronatory events effecting the foot [69–71]. He theorized that by directing a force against the plantar medial surface of the heel the functional axis of rotation of the STJ would be shifted laterally, thereby augmenting the role of stance phase muscles such as the posterior tibial, gastrocsoleus, and flexor hallucis longus muscles to resupinate the foot. The resulting *medial heel skive technique or Kirby technique* was developed. Typically a 2–6 mm skiving of the plantar medial aspect of the heel is accomplished on the balanced positive cast. Increased skive results in an increased supinatory effect; typically a combination of inverted cast balance and medial heel skive is used to achieve the desired results. Caution should be taken when the triathlete exhibits atrophy of the medial calcaneal fat pad, a laterally displaced plantar fat pad, a prominent cicatrix, or a robust medial calcaneal tubercle spur.

Cast fill is a technique whereby the positive model of the foot can be "smoothed" to enhance comfort and performance without sacrifice to function. Potential areas of impingement including the medial arch and lateral column are overfilled smoothing transitions without altering contours. Typically cast fills are considered to be no fill, minimal fill, standard fill, and over fill. Use minimal fills to achieve the tightest contours. However, minimal fills will increase the risk of orthoses intolerance including excessive local pressure points, impingement, and even blister formation. Apply minimal fills when maximum influence of the orthoses is desired such as the hard to control foot or cavus foot. Use a standard fill when limited joint motion is suspected to arise out of osteoarthritis or when diminished sensation is present. A maximum fill, although rarely indicated, is useful when fitting an orthoses to a triathlete with chronic intrinsic muscle spasms, equinus, tarsal coalitions, midfoot fusions, or under any other circumstances where minimal orthoses influence can achieve symptomatic relief.

The distal balancing platform which extends across the forefoot is critical for support of the forefoot to rearfoot relationship. A "light fill" or "no fill" may be applied under circumstances where additional rigid support of the distal metatarsal phalangeal joints is desired. However, excessive light fill tends to lead to separation of the anterior edge of the CFO from the interior of the shoe. This can potentially be made worse by cycling shoes which possess a slightly concave medial to lateral profile.

Orthoses width traditionally has referred to the anterior width of the orthoses shell immediately proximal to the metatarsal phalangeal joints. A variety of widths can be selected depending upon the magnitude of influence the clinician desires from the orthoses shell. The widths include extra wide, full width, wide, standard, narrow, and extra narrow. For most triathletes wide, standard and narrow shells widths should be selected dependent on the injury and forefoot width of the running or cycling shoe. Many cycling shoes, however, will not accommodate a wide shell; this author has increasingly prescribed a narrow or standard width shell with a medial flair. This effectively places greater orthoses surface area directly under the talonavicular, navicular medial cuneiform, and medial cuneiform articulations without compromising shoe fit. This technique is also beneficial when a wide or extra wide shell design restricts the natural plantar flexion of the medial column contributing to first metatarsal phalangeal joint dorsiflexion motion during the midstance and propulsive phases of running. This technique should also be considered when a tight or prominent central band of the plantar fascia is present.

New considerations for *heel cup depth* are now important as CFOs integrate heel skives and inverted balancing such as the Blake inverted. Shallow heel cups (12–14 mm) offer the advantage of ease of fitting into hard to fit shoes, especially cycling shoes or running shoes with narrow heel cups. While deep heel cups (18–24 mm) dramatically improve the surface contact area of the orthoses to the foot they also enhance rearfoot control critical to the application of various inverted balance techniques. Unfortunately, deep heel cups also increase the difficulty fitting an orthoses into shoes used by triathletes, especially cycling shoes. All heel cups require the application of an expansion, especially along the lateral and posterior lateral surfaces which serves to separate the foot from the orthoses shell minimizing the potential for heel soft tissue impingement such as edge irritation and blister formation. Herring and Green provide strong and compelling evidence that the expansion of heel soft tissues upon weight bearing can be accurately predicted from non-weight-bearing measurements [72, 73]. These authors measured the width of the heel under the conditions of non-weight bearing and weight bearing; reporting overall maximum and point of maximum heel soft tissue (heel fat pad) expansion for over 900 male and female individuals across a wide range of age classes. They observed that the point of maximum heel soft tissue expansion was individually specific and not directly linked circumstances such as gender, age, foot size, weight, or height, and this point of expansion occurs at a height which is well within the range used for deep heel cups (18–24 mm) [72, 73]. Too little heel cup expansion risks soft tissue impingement while too much expansion imposes shoe fit difficulty. Herring and Green encourage clinicians prescribing CFOs to send non-weight-bearing or weight-bearing heel width measurements taken at the level of maximum heel expansion to avoid too little or too much heel cup expansion performed by the orthoses making laboratory.

Fascial accommodations allow the clinician to relieve the potential for irritation of the plantar fascia against the dorsal surface of the orthoses. Typically this represents an increased selective positive cast fill placed medial and lateral to the prominent margin of the plantar fascia and rising above the cast adequate to produce a channel in the resulting orthoses to accommodate the plantar fascia. This addition is especially important for athletes with a plantar fascia which becomes prominent during the propulsive phase of gait or when the plantar fascia exhibits fibrotic changes resulting from previous trauma. This addition will alter CFO longitudinal shell rigidity; through a "girder and beam effect" the introduction of a longitudinal trough designed into the dorsal surface of the CFO will increase resistance to longitudinal flexion of the resulting device under weight-bearing load. While this effect may be desirable in concept, it will be difficult to control and only promote a locally beneficial resistance to device deformation, influencing the medial aspect of the CFO more dramatically than the unaltered lateral surfaces.

Other accommodations may be added when prominent plantar anatomical features are present and would result in unnecessary pressure points during running and cycling. Typically, these additions accommodate a potentially sensitive plantar fibroma, a prominent styloid process of the fifth metatarsal or an accessory navicular. However, under conditions where a pressure dampening effect is sought in addition to accommodation the orthoses making laboratory may be asked to fill the accommodation on the device with a cushioned material to form a "sweet spot." This CFO addition should be designed in such a manner that size of the "sweet spot" is larger than the anatomical structure to be accommodated to avoid edge impingement during running and cycling activities. An application for this addition may be on the medial flare of the CFO to augment the support and cushioning of the talonavicular joint and related soft tissues.

A diverse array of materials are available for the fabrication of CFOs. The *selection of orthoses construction materials* is critical to the overall comfort, function, and performance of the CFO. For triathletes three general materials are frequently used for the construction of the typical CFO and include polypropylenes, graphites/fiberglass, and foams. However, under special circumstances other materials may be occasionally applied to the making of a CFO. While each of these materials offer the triathlete a unique assortment of advantages they also impose identifiable disadvantages that may out weight the advantages. Important similarities exist between each of the most frequently used materials including (1) a range of flexibility, (2) ease of initial molding, (3) resiliency of material, (4) ease of post-production modification, (5) durability under repeated and heavy use, and (6) availability of material making them more suitable for triathlete CFO devices. Foam materials are frequently used because of inherent cushioning properties and low weight to produce a CFO; however, the foams do not adapt well to post-production modifications and exhibit poor durability and require frequent replacement. However, with a wide selection of CFO materials, the clinician is able to better select the most suitable material of rigidity/flexibility of the finial device dependent upon the unique needs of the foot and the injury/pathology.

Polypropylene is the most universally applied material for running and cycling CFOs. This material is available in a variety of thicknesses and can provide the clinician with a wide range of flexibilities to select from especially if EVA arch fill is used to augment rigidity of the selected shell material. Dependent upon the degree of flexibility desired, select polypropylene thickness and EVA arch fill based upon the weight of the triathlete. The thinner polypropylene offers a greater degree of flexibility, while thicker polypropylene promotes greater rigidity. Intermediate levels of device flexibility can be achieved through the addition of an EVA arch or under fill. Further flexibility enhancements can be achieved by adjusting the firmness of the EVA material used to under fill the shell. Also influencing overall device flexibility is the manner in which the device is formed to the foot. CFOs that are heated and vacuum formed to a model of the foot are generally more flexible than a CFO directly milled to the shape of the foot and of identical thickness. When polypropylene is heated it looses some of its natural rigidity.

Polypropylene has the distinct advantage that it can be molded easily to unusual shapes without wrinkling. This is of particular importance when considering the use of a balancing technique that will use a deep heel cup or when the shell must accommodate a prominent plantar protrusion (exostosis, prominent navicular tuberosity, a taught central band of the plantar aponeurosis, or fibroma). Once molded, polypropylene will retain its shape during repeated loading events; however, this material will eventually deteriorate, flattening, and loosening its initial functional control. Polypropylene's reduced resiliency is often described by some triathletes during running activities as a trend of greater perceived flexibility when directly compared to other more resilient (graphite and fiberglass composite) materials of similar flexibility.

Graphite materials have been used in the making of CFOs for more then 20 years. A variety of graphites are available including graphite acrylic laminates and composites. Graphite offers the distinct advantage of achieving functional support (semi-rigidity and rigidity) without excessive shell thickness minimizing bulk and weight. Graphite shell materials are also known for durability, longevity, high levels of resiliency, predictable flexibility through out the materials flexibility range, and mold ability. Similar to other shell materials graphite shells can be under filled to alter the flexibility properties of the raw material. Under filling a graphite shell with EVA should only be considered when the shell thickness desired is less than what would be optimal for the triathlete's weight or when the triathlete's weight exceeds even the most rigid materials. However, due to the risk of shell breakage, including hidden micro-fractures leading to orthoses failure, EVA under fills should be avoided and an alternate shell material such as polypropylene should be selected. Also when prescribing heel cup depths of greater than 18 mm, special attention must be applied to minimize wrinkling of the graphite around the narrower radius of curvature. This problem is being overcome as refinements to graphite shell technology has lead to ever thinner, stronger, and more resilient shells with increasingly better resistance to breakage and moldability, while maintaining consistent control throughout the flexibility range of the material. Increasingly graphite is becoming the shell material of choice for the triathlete desiring an orthoses of minimal bulk and weight with optimal durability, flexibility, and functional control.

Rearfoot orthoses posts promote no known functional benefit over the benefit already achieved by the orthoses shell. However, their continued use is done so with the intent to stabilize the foot orthoses in the shoe, especially during the heel contact and midstance phases of gait. Unfortunately no evidence has been provided to substantiate this hypothesis. A recent pilot study examined pressure (FScan) data generated by three subjects walking and explored their response to four rearfoot posting conditions (no post 0°, 4°, and 6° of motion). The results of this limited data concluded that posting the orthoses promoted no significant change to the subject's gait; however, a 0° rearfoot post did increase the duration of the heel contact phase of gait for each subject. These results would generally support the general hypothesis that rearfoot posts contribute little to the overall effect of the orthoses and at best can only serve to stabilize the orthoses in the shoe but only during the heel contact phase of gait. Thus, the basis for the use of a rearfoot post is done so more upon personal preferences and bias and not on functional outcome. However, the use of a 0° rearfoot post may influence heel contact phase stability adequately to permit a triathlete to use a less stable running shoe than might otherwise be recommended.

The finishing touches to any foot orthoses may include *special additions such as accommodations, extensions, and covering materials.* In fact, these additions are generally what the triathlete first encounters, evaluates, and scrutinizes; first impressions can be lasting and lead to a highly successful outcome or a disastrous conclusion. These additions should be selected based upon the characteristics of the foot and the specific pathology which is being treated by the foot orthoses. Numerous accommodations have been described and an endless array of special addition combinations could be described, each intended to suite a very specific application. Many special additions could be perceived as uncomfortable and counter productive when applied to the triathlete versus the general population. Several accommodations and special additions are of particular importance when considering the treatment of triathlon-related lower extremity injuries.

Extensions are additions that can extend the influence of an orthoses beyond the midstance phase of gait. These extensions can provide cushioning and/or promote a functional effect well into the propulsive and preswing phases of gait. The first most obvious role of an extension is to augment the natural cushioning properties of the forefoot and the cushioning of the properties of the shoe. An assortment of materials is available coming in a range of firmnesses and thicknesses. Avoid excessively thick cushioned extensions, while these will feel "pillow soft" walking they will also increase the energy demands placed upon the triathlete during running; select materials which are 1.5–3 mm (1/16–1/8") thick.

An extension may be applied to the orthoses to influence forefoot function. Increasingly the function of the medial column and first ray has been suspected in the development of overuse injuries. During gait a stable first ray (first metatarsal and medial cuneiform) is a requirement for resupination of the foot and a propulsive gait pattern. When the first ray is unstable it will be dorsiflex until the metatarsocuneiform joint end point range of motion is achieved. "Locking" the first ray against the ground is important to minimize the development of functional hallux limitus and eccentric overload to the tibialis posterior, peroneal longus tendons, and the plantar aponeurosis. The application of a reverse Morton's extension to the foot orthoses will dramatically reduce the ground reactive force under the first metatarsophalangeal joint and reduce the potential of impact of functional hallux limitus. Varus extensions of 2°–4° can be applied to a foot orthoses to help relieve propulsive and preswing phase eccentric overload applied to the tibialis posterior muscle–tendon complex during running helping to reduce some of the symptoms associated with medial tibial stress syndrome (shin splints). When applying a varus forefoot wedge, a stable medial column is necessary since the introduction of the wedge will increase the ground reactive forces exerted to the first metatarsophalangeal joint complex. Valgus extensions of $2°-4°$ can be useful to reduce eccentric overload exerted upon the peroneal tendons. This extension can be applied in combination with a reverse Morton's extension to further enhance medial column stability, limiting functional hallux limitus, and augment peroneal longus functional role during the stance phase of gait. Clearly, a functional orthoses extension can extend the influence of the orthoses well into the propulsive and preswing phases of gait.

Accommodations applied to the orthoses shell can help to alleviate painful forefoot symptoms such as metatarsalgia, capsulitis and intermetatarsal neuritis, and Morton's neuroma. Locally applied metatarsal pads will serve to redistribute plantar forces from a symptomatic metatarsophalangeal joint or intermetatarsal space to less symptomatic adjacent structures. Generally these are applied proximal to the symptomatic joint of intermetatarsal space. Metatarsalgia is a common complaint of triathletes who log high mileage. The application of a soft poron metatarsal bar which extends across the distal one-third of the orthoses shell will serve to off-load the symptomatic metatarsophalangeal joints and spread ground reactive forces of running across the less symptomatic metatarsal shafts much like the application of a rocker bar to a shoe sole would accomplish. Finally, cutouts, apertures, and slots can be added to an extension to reduce ground reactive forces under specific metatarsophalangeal joints.

Accommodations built into the orthoses shell were discussed in the section discussing positive cast modifications. Accommodations such as "sweet spots" serve to reduce pressure and the potential for irritation across problematic anatomical sites such as navicular tuberosity, plantar fibroma, or a prominent central band of the plantar aponeurosis.

Covering materials may also vary and range from firm to soft cushioning. Vinyl, leather, soft EVA, and closed cell foam materials are the most common materials prescribed. Closed cell neylon or Spenco cushioned materials (Spenco Medical Corp. Waco, TX) offer the distinct advantage of providing cushioning as well as dissipating friction and torque which can contribute to friction blisters of the foot. These materials can also help to reduce the buildup of unwanted perspiration and moisture from around the foot further reducing the likelihood of friction blisters. Covering materials may be of various length, covering just the orthoses shell, or extending to the sulcus of the foot or out to the tips of the toes. Full-length top covers are better adapted and more comfortable for the triathlete.

When considering extension and top cover materials and pathology-specific needs carefully consider the shoe environment into which the foot orthoses will be fit. Over crowding the midfoot, forefoot, and/or toes can be as problematic and painful as the original complaint or problem. Cycling shoes will significantly limit the accumulative thickness of accommodations, extensions, and top covers. Running shoes on the other hand will be far more forgiving to these additions.

By focusing orthoses treatment and design upon the specific pathology needs of the triathlete and by avoiding treatment driven by a deformity orthoses outcome will be improved. Furthermore, an understanding of the triathlete's pathomechanics leading to the symptoms and injury, running gait, and cycling pattern will permit the design and development of orthoses that best meet the needs of the triathlete and symptomatic pathology. Unfortunately, there are no clear-cut rules that can guide the clinician to the development of the most effective foot orthoses and clearly multiple and different orthoses models may provide the desired outcome of reduced symptoms. Thus by approaching the development of an orthoses in a systematic step wise manner will dramatically reduce the likelihood of orthoses failure.

The Athlete and Overuse Injuries

The triathlete comes in all shapes and sizes, from lightweight runners to over 200-lb Clydesdales of both genders and most age classes. Overuse injuries are the most common injuries confronting the triathlete during the long hours of demanding training and racing. Structural abnormalities, poor strength and range of motion, poor overall conditioning, improper training plans, old and worn out equipment, and poorly adjusted/fit equipment are some of the most common causes leading up to the development of an overuse injury. However, with so many new and inexperienced endurance athletes joining the ranks of triathletes old long forgotten and dormant injuries of work, sports, and recreation can be triggered or contribute to the development a new injury. Each of the sporting components associated with triathlons and duathlons exposes the athlete to a unique physical stress and can lead to a unique group of overuse injuries. Many of these overuse injuries can be prevented and/or treated in part through the careful selection and application of foot orthoses and shoes.

Running typically exposes the triathlete to many hours of pounding out long slow distance miles on pavement. As conditioning improves so might the demands of training as the triathlete begins to add strength and interval training to their training program. Numerous overuse injuries can be associated with running including those shown in Table 17.1 Each of these injuries can be linked to abnormal pathomechanics of the lower extremity and can respond complete or in part to the introduction of proper shoes and foot orthoses.

Cycling exposes the triathlete to the stress of long hours of spinning at high cycling cadences for long hours. Climbing and the effort to spin in big gears increase the stresses exerted upon the soft tissues and joints of the lower extremity leading to the potential for overuse injuries such as those shown in Table 17.2 These cycling injuries as with many overuse injuries of the lower extremity can respond favorably to the introduction of foot orthoses, careful selection cycling shoes, and pedal/cleat system.

Table 17.1 Overuse injuries associated with running

Low back pain
Iliotibial band syndrome
Patellofemoral pain syndrome (inferior and medial)
Medial tibial stress syndrome (shin splints)
Achilles tendinitis, bursitis, and enthesitis
Tibialis posterior tendinitis
Tibialis anterior tendinitis
Peroneal longus and/or brevis tendonitis
Flexor hallucis tendinitis
Spring ligament strain
Plantar fasciitis
Baxter's nerve entrapment
Metatarsalgia
Capsulitis
Sesamoiditis
Intermetatarsal neuritis and Morton's neuroma
Stress fractures (tibia, fibula, navicular, and metatarsals)
Friction blisters and subungual hematomas (black toenails)

Table 17.2 Overuse injuries common in cycling

Low back pain
Patellofemoral pain syndrome
Iliotibial band syndrome
Calf cramping
Medial malleolar contusions
Achilles tendinitis, bursitis, and enthesitis
Peroneal tendinitis
Intermetatarsal neuritis/Morton's neuroma
Metatarsalgia
Capsulitis
Sesamoiditis
Bursitis (fifth MTPJ)
Stress fractures (tibia, fibula, navicular, and metatarsals)
Friction blisters and subungual hematomas (black toenails)

The Older-Aged Triathlete

Increasing age influences the musculoskeletal and kinematic response to the running and cycling phases of triathlon racing and training. During the running phase, variations to the stance phase of gait may occur with increasing age. The older-aged runner (55 years and older) may exhibit degenerative musculoskeletal changes that influence ground reaction forces and kinematics during distance running. Older runners frequently experiences loss of lower extremity joint flexibility and ranges of motion, progressive weakness to muscle and bone, diminished vascular supply to many lower extremity connective tissues, atrophy, and loss of elasticity to numerous lower extremity connective tissue structures such as the plantar fat pad, plantar aponeurosis, and Achilles tendon and frequently the loss of strength and contractile velocity of major lower extremity muscle complexes. These changes frequently contribute to an altered running gait. Older runners exhibit a shorter stride length with a higher cadence, smaller knee ranges of motion, higher vertical impact speeds, higher impact peak forces, and higher initial loading rates than their younger running peers. Intrinsic shock absorbing capabilities of the lower extremity are also compromised with increased age as elasticity of connective tissues is lost.

The cycling phase of triathlon racing and training does not appear to influence the older-aged triathlete with the same magnitude as that experienced during the running phase of racing and training. However, the cycling phase of training and racing may also adversely effect the older triathlete. As observed to the running phase, the aging triathlete is more susceptible to the development overuse injuries; these injuries can be linked to the loss of lower extremity joint flexibility, progressive muscle weakness, and loss of elasticity of connective tissues including tendons, ligaments, and articular cartilage.

While these changes are representative of normal aging they may also provide an explanation for the higher incidence of overuse injuries associated with running and for the potential that similar circumstances may influence the older-aged triathlete. Given these factors and the demands of multisport training the older-aged triathlete may require special attention to intrinsic factors such as range of motion and strength training as well as extrinsic factors such as equipment (gearing, cranks, pedals, shoes, and foot orthoses), bike-fit properties, and training modifications in and effort to reduce even minor yet abnormal musculoskeletal and joint stress.

Chapter 18
Cycling

Paul Langer

Bicycling is a sport that is unique in that the human body functions as the engine of a machine. The energy to propel the machine forward is generated primarily by the lower extremity muscles and transferred to the bike's drivetrain through the pedals. Cycling as a sport as well as a mode of transportation has become increasingly specialized. Subcategories of bicycling sports include road biking, mountain biking, track racing, cyclocross (a combination of road and mountain biking), fitness (stationary, spin) cycling, and triathlon cycling. Each of the subcategories of cycling can employ different cycling positions and footwear/pedal systems. In addition to recreational cycling, the number of bicyclists who commute has been increasing. According to the US Census, the number of bike commuters increased by 9% between 1990 and 2000. The number of commuters will likely continue to increase due to increased funding of bicycle infrastructure.

Cycling Biomechanics and Considerations

The lower extremity biomechanics of cycling is dominated by sagittal plane motion and has been referred to as a kinematically constrained task by some authors [1, 2] due to the restricted frontal and transverse plane motion. The lower extremity movement is primarily controlled by the predetermined circular path of the cycle's pedal and crank arm [3]. Walking and cycling share some commonalities; both are bipedal locomotor tasks which alternate between flexion and extension with most power generated in extension [2]. Unlike weight-bearing sports where running impact and direction changes place strain on joints, cycling is a nonweight-bearing sport without impact forces or ballistic movements. However, in bicycling,

P. Langer (✉)
University of Minnesota Medical School, 701 25th Ave. S, Suite 505, Minneapolis, MN 55454, USA

M.B. Werd, E.L. Knight (eds.), *Athletic Footwear and Orthoses in Sports Medicine*, DOI 10.1007/978-0-387-76416-0_18, © Springer Science+Business Media, LLC 2010

the repetition of motion is much higher than any other sport. Highly trained and competitive cyclists often ride at cadences of 80–110 revolutions per minute which means that each lower limb is subjected to 4,800–6,600 revolutions per hour of riding.

There are a limited number of studies on the biomechanics of cycling and much of what has been published focuses more on pedaling efficiency and performance than on overuse injury mechanisms [4–6]. Just as with human gait, cycling biomechanics can be difficult to study due to high intersubject variability.

The Pedal Cycle

The pedal cycle consists of a power generating phase which begins at 0° or "top dead center" (12:00 o'clock) and ends to just after 180° or "bottom dead center" (6:00 o'clock). The recovery phase then follows from bottom dead center back to top dead center. The power phase is marked by extension of the hip, knee, and ankle. Power is generated primarily by the gluteals, quadriceps, and gastrosoleus muscles. Gregor et al. found that the quadriceps and knee extensors were primary power sources in the first half of power generating stroke while the hip extensors and ankle plantarflexors were primary in the second half [7]. During extension, the knee adducts and medially translates as the tibia internally rotates and the subtalar joint pronates [8]. Pedal reaction forces cause the midtarsal and subtalar joints to pronate and the medial column of the foot to invert and dorsiflex which, in turn, contributes to internal rotation of the leg [9]. Loads on the joints of the lower extremity are highest during the last 2/3 of the downward pedal stroke. Cyclists with clipless pedals (discussed in a following paragraph) can extend the power generating phase by engaging the hamstrings to flex the knee and draw the pedal back as the foot passes through bottom dead center.

The recovery phase then follows the power phase. This phase is marked by flexion of the hip, knee, and ankle. With clipless pedals, the hip flexors, hamstrings, and tibialis anterior are active during this phase. Flexion of the hip and knee causes abduction and lateral translation of the knee as the pedal rises [9]. The ankle dorsiflexes and the subtalar joint re-supinates during the recovery phase.

Most competitive and serious recreational cyclists now use shoe/pedal systems that attach the rider's foot to the pedal through a cleat/binding interface. These systems are referred to as "clipless" pedals (Figs. 18.1 and 18.2). The advent of clipless pedals was initially heralded as an innovation that allowed the cyclist to generate power during the recovery portion of the pedal stroke, but recent research has shown that at best, even highly trained cyclists only partially un-weight the pedal during recovery – they do not truly generate power [10, 11]. However, a mechanical advantage of un-weighting the recovery phase leg may be that less force is required by the contralateral leg to "lift" the recovery leg. One study's conclusions suggest that the clipless pedals' greatest mechanical advantage may be not in allowing the cyclist to pull up during the last 180° of the pedal cycle but in pushing forward over top dead center and sweeping back at bottom dead center [12].

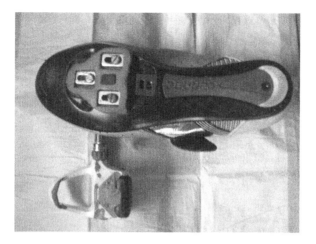

Fig. 18.1 Clipless pedal and cleat on outsole of shoe for road cycling

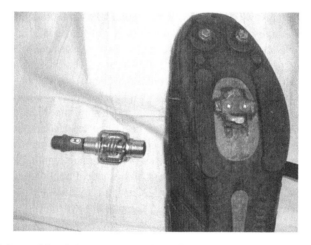

Fig. 18.2 Clipless pedal and cleat on outsole of shoe for mountain biking

Pedaling Technique

Competitive cyclists strive for an efficient circular pedal stroke that involves not just exerting a downward force during the first half of the stroke but also sweeping the foot backward at bottom dead center, pulling through the second half of the pedal stroke and then pushing the foot forward through the top dead center. This circular pedaling technique has long been presumed to be the most efficient; however, there is not any scientific data that confirms this presumption. In fact, one group of researchers after testing cyclists with four different pedaling techniques found that cyclists were most metabolically efficient when pedaling in their preferred pattern [13].

Pedaling technique is almost as varied as running technique. Some cyclists may be "mashers," meaning that they ride in low gears at a low (40–60) rpm and exert force only during the downward portion of the pedal cycle. "Spinning," a technique using higher gears and higher rpms (80–100+), has been advocated as a more efficient pedaling technique, but research does not confirm this. Some cyclists attempt "ankling" a technique where the ankle is plantarflexed during the power phase and dorsiflexed during the recovery phase. Just as runners and walkers self-select stride length and movement patterns to maximize metabolic economy and comfort [14], it has been suggested that cyclists will make technique, gearing, and cadence adjustments to alter pedal forces and maximize metabolic efficiency [15].

Pedaling Forces

Pedal forces acting on the foot are approximately half of bodyweight with seated pedaling and can approach up to three times bodyweight when standing, sprinting, or climbing [9]. Plantar pressures within the shoe are primarily localized to the forefoot and first ray while heel and arch plantar pressures remain low [16, 17]. Peak plantar pressure occurs between 90 and 110° of the pedal cycle [10, 18–20]. Researchers have shown that stiffer cycling shoes increase peak plantar pressures when compared to less-stiff shoes [17, 21]. Pedaling technique must be considered in injured cyclists as researchers have found that medial plantar loading increased with increased power output but decreased with higher rpm [16].

Much of what has been written on adjustments or modifications to address injuries or biomechanical faults has been described as trial-and-error processes. After selecting the proper frame size based on rider's height, parts of the bike can be adjusted to in accordance with a cyclist's body segment lengths. It is beyond the scope of this chapter to discuss the theory and practical applications of fitting the rider to the bicycle; however, those who regularly treat cyclists and triathletes should become familiar with bike fit.

Cycling Injuries and Risk Factors

Risk factors for overuse cycling injuries include training errors, poor pedaling technique, improper bike fit, anatomical malalignment, biomechanical faults, muscle imbalances, and inadequate cycling equipment. For all injured cyclists it is important to evaluate training distance and intensity, other athletic activities (many cyclists cross train and/or weight train), bike fit, anatomic factors such as muscle imbalances, lower extremity biomechanics, flexibility/rom, limb length asymmetry, and previous injury history. As with any athlete, activity modification and symptomatic treatment are important in addressing the injured cyclist.

There is a lack of evidence-based biomechanical treatment of cycling injuries. Many experienced cycling sports medicine specialists describe anecdotal and trial-and-error treatment methods. Most authors agree that addressing faulty biomechanics is important to prevent recurrence of injury in many cyclists. Excessive subtalar joint pronation has been linked to patellofemoral pain, iliotibial band syndrome, Achilles tendonitis, plantar fasciitis, metatarsalgia, and forefoot neuritis. Limited subtalar joint pronation and cavus foot type have been linked to sesamoiditis, Achilles tendonitis, extensor tendonitis, metatarsalgia, and forefoot neuritis as well [22].

Most research on bicycling injuries is focused on the area of traumatic injuries [23, 24]. Overuse cycling injuries are just starting to receive more attention from researchers. In a survey of 473 recreational cyclists researchers found that 85% had experienced an overuse injury [25]. The knee was the most commonly injured lower extremity site ranging from 35 to 65% or riders and females reported higher incidence of knee pain than males [25–27]. Foot injuries were reported in 15.6% and ankle/Achilles injuries in 7.3% of cyclists [25]. Many cyclists report chronic discomfort especially to the neck, butt, hands, and feet related to riding which they may not classify as an injury but more as a nuisance or discomfort.

Cycling Footwear

Cycling shoes, like other types of footwear, have become increasingly specialized. Since the shoe is only a part of the foot/shoe/pedal interface, this section will also discuss cleats and pedal systems.

The perfect cycling shoe transmits energy efficiently to the pedal, yet distributes forces evenly, dampens vibration, does not bind the foot, and allows heat/moisture dissipation while offering resistance to weather conditions. Sport-specific cycling shoes combined with a cleat and pedal system have been shown to increase pedaling efficiency [10]. Unlike many other sports where shoes are selected for fit, comfort, and biomechanical considerations, cyclists must select their footwear based on the type of cycling they participate in (road, touring, mountain), which type and brand of pedal system they will use, and then select the shoe with appropriate fit and comfort for their foot. For cyclists who choose to use a clipless pedal system, once they have purchased shoes they must then purchase cleats and attach the cleats to the shoes' outsole with bolts.

The unique structural features of cycling shoes are the stiff midsole/outsole and the cleat holes. Efficient energy transfer from the foot to the pedal is optimized with stiff materials [3]. Manufacturers of cycling footwear use rigid materials in the midsole/outsole for its ability to resist longitudinal as well as torsional bending. Less expensive and recreational cycling shoes are often made with plastics. More expensive and racing-oriented cycling shoes are made with carbon fiber composites which are lighter and more rigid. The more rigid materials have also been shown to increase peak plantar pressures in cyclists which has implications for those who experience foot pain [21].

The conflict that some cyclists encounter with cycling footwear is that structural features designed to enhance performance such as snug fit and stiff outsoles have also been linked to decreased comfort and foot pain. Some cyclists who experience significant foot pain or discomfort may benefit from less performance-oriented but more comfortable footwear. Some researchers have found that a lack of comfort negatively affects performance and increases the risk of injury [28, 29].

Cycling Shoe Fit

Much like skiers and skaters, competitive cyclists will fit their shoes to be snug so that there is minimal motion of the foot inside the shoe and maximal energy transfer to the shoe interface. Recreational cyclists are more willing to make performance allowances in favor of comfort and walkability. Ideally, the cycling shoe is snug in the heel and midfoot to minimize wasted motion and provides adequate forefoot length and width to minimize discomfort. Allowances in toe room are common to accommodate foot edema experienced in weight-bearing endurance sports like running, but research has shown that cyclists do not increase foot volume due to edema at shorter intervals of cycling activity [30]. As with any footwear there should be minimal side-to-side pressure at the widest part of the foot which usually corresponds to the first metatarsal phalangeal joint and fifth metatarsal phalangeal joints of the foot. The midfoot fit should be snug without creating pressure. Cycling shoes that are too loose in the midfoot will cause the cyclist to compensate by over tightening the closure system which may result in discomfort or dorsal foot injury. Heel fit of cycling shoes should not allow pistoning of the heel inside the shoe.

Some brands of cycling footwear are available in wide sizes and recently custom cycling shoes have become easier to find. Manufacturers are starting to introduce off-the-shelf shoes that can be heated and molded to the heel and arch. In addition, some manufacturers have started to offer shoes made on women-specific lasts.

Cycling Shoe Construction

Cycling shoe construction will be discussed below. Three general categories of cycling shoes will be described: road, sport, and mountain biking shoes (Fig. 18.3).

Road Cycling Shoe Construction

Like ski boots, road cycling shoes are not made for walking. The rigid sole and external cleat allow for only minimal walking. They are designed to be light, stiff, snug structures that allow the nonweight-bearing foot to transfer force efficiently to the pedal while minimizing wasted motion of the foot within the shoe.

> *Last.* Road cycling shoes are lasted much like track spikes, on a curved "performance" last with a board lasted foot bed. Performance lasts provide a low-volume, snug fitting upper and are narrower than conventional lasts. The board last combined with the stiff midsole/outsole provides rigidity for maximal energy transfer.

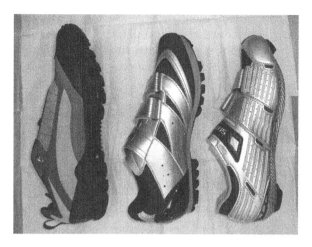

Fig. 18.3 Sport shoe, mountain bike shoe, road shoe

Upper. The road shoe upper is typically made of a fabric mesh, leather, and/or synthetic materials that allow for maximal ventilation. A rigid heel counter is incorporated to minimize rearfoot motion. The shoe's upper is secured to the foot with laces, ratchet-style buckles, Velcro straps, cable and rotary dials, or a combination thereof. The tongue is padded to distribute pressure of the closure system on the dorsal foot. High-performance racing shoe models will have a shroud or low-profile closure system to minimize wind resistance. Triathlon cycling shoes are road cycling shoes with simpler closure systems (such as a single Velcro strap) to allow for quick entry/exit. They usually have a seamless or fabric liner since some triathletes prefer to cycle without socks.

Foot Bed/Insole. Most cycling shoes are now made with removable insoles which can vary in quality and features. Many resemble the foot beds found in running shoes and may be made from closed cell foams or ethyl vinyl acetate and have a wicking fabric top cover. More expensive models may incorporate arch support, metatarsal support, or plastic shells.

Midsole/Outsole. In order to minimize weight and maximize stiffness, the mid-sole also serves as the outsole in road shoes. High-performance road shoes are made with the lightest, stiffest materials such as carbon fiber composites. Recreational road shoes use nylon which is still relatively stiff but heavier and less expensive than carbon fiber. Some cycling shoes incorporate the heel counter into a one-piece midsole construction. This helps lend signif-icant stiffness to the shoe while minimizing weight. One manufacturer has introduced shoes that incorporate a forefoot varus wedge of 1.5° into the outsole [31]. The performance road cycling shoe outsole typically curves in the sagittal plane. This outsole shape slightly dorsiflexes the digits and when the cleat is engaged with the pedal facilitates plantar flexion of the ankle

(Fig. 18.4). Most road cycling shoes are compatible with external cleats that attach the shoe to a pedal much like a binding attaches a boot to a ski. Road cycling shoes come with pre-drilled holes in the forefoot for placement of the external cleats. This exposed cleat design raises the foot off of the pedal and makes walking in road shoes difficult (Fig. 18.5).

Outsole. Some road shoes may have small rubber bumpers on the toe and heel for walking traction. In an effort to remove every last gram of unnecessary weight, racers often remove the bumpers.

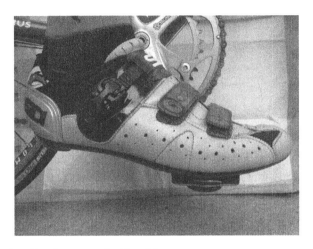

Fig. 18.4 Road cycling shoe engaged with pedal

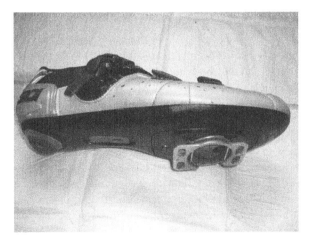

Fig. 18.5 Road shoe with external cleat

Sport Cycling Shoe Construction

"Sport," "trail," "fitness," "touring," and "recreational" are all terms used for cycling shoes that tend to be more comfortable than road shoes, yet also allow attachment of recessed cleats. They are designed with less emphasis on performance and more emphasis on comfort and walkability. Unlike road cycling shoes which are too rigid and have an external cleat which makes it almost impossible to walk, this category of cycling shoe is easier to walk in. Sport cycling shoes are usually heavier, less aerodynamic, more flexible, and may have little to no sagittal plane curve when compared to road shoes. This category of cycling shoe is popular with commuters, casual riders, cycle tourists, stationary fitness class participants, and those who simply cannot comfortably wear road shoes. Sport cycling shoes also may accommodate certain types of custom or those better than road shoes.

Last. Sport cycling shoes are lasted on semi-curved or semi-straight lasts much like walking and hiking shoes. The conventional last provides more width and volume than that found in road shoes. Most have a board last to provide some stiffness and torsional resistance.

Upper. Uppers are constructed of mesh fabrics, leather, or synthetic materials. Most sport cycling shoes use laces but some have Velcro straps, buckles, or a combination of closure systems. Plastic heel counters are incorporated into the upper along with a padded collar and tongue. The uppers often resemble hiking or walking shoes and in fact are often indistinguishable. The larger volume upper of recreational cycling shoes make them a better choice for those with exceptionally wide feet, or those who are uncomfortable in the stiff, snug road shoes.

Foot Bed/Insole. Like road shoes, most sport shoes now come with a removable insole that may incorporate padding, metatarsal, and arch support. Some foot beds offer minimal protection from the cleat bolts in the forefoot.

Midsole. Some sport shoes incorporate a polyurethane midsole to provide additional cushioning and walking comfort and may have a dual-density midsole as well. Some sport shoes will reinforce the midsole with fiberglass to lend more rigidity.

Outsole. Sport cycling shoes are constructed with carbon rubber outsoles and can be used with or without a recessed cleat (Fig. 18.6). The outsole is stiffer than a conventional hiking/walking shoe, yet provides traction and versatility when off the bike and is significantly less stiff than a road cycling shoe. Outsoles may come with pre-drilled bolt holes for cleats or may have a section under the forefoot that can be removed for placement of recessed cleats. The recessed cleat design protects the cleat from debris and makes walking much easier than road shoes.

Fig. 18.6 Outsole of sport
shoe without cleat

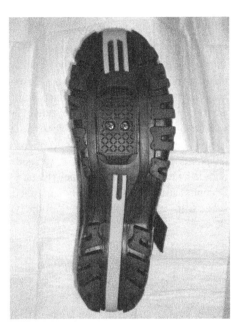

Mountain Biking Shoe Construction

Mountain biking (MTB) shoes are also popular for their comfort but have other unique features since mountain biking often requires cyclists to dismount their bikes to navigate obstacles such as logs, rocks, or streams. For this reason, MTB shoes have a more aggressive outsole traction design, a recessed cleat, and a rubberized sole for traction during walking. Some MTB shoes may be considered a hybrid of road and sport shoes – combining the performance features of the road shoes and for some the comfort features of the sport shoes. Within the category of MTB shoes there are shoes geared more for racing and competitive riders and those for more recreational MTB riders. Racing MTB shoes often resemble road shoes with recessed cleats and rubber outsoles while the recreational MTB shoes are more similar to the sport cycling shoes. The recessed cleat is protected from weight bearing and is less vulnerable to damage or to picking up debris such as mud like the external road cycling cleat would.

> *Last.* Competition MTB shoes are lasted on a performance board last like road shoes but recreational MTB shoes will offer a standard curved or semi-curved board last.
> *Insole/Footbed.* Like road and sport shoes, most MTB shoes now come with a removable insole that may incorporate padding, metatarsal, and arch support. Some foot beds offer minimal protection from the cleat bolts.

Midsole. The midsole of an MTB shoe may be made with stiff nylon, fiberglass, or carbon graphite. Some shoes will use a polyurethane midsole reinforced with a plastic or fiberglass plate for stiffness.

Outsole. Rubber sheet or studs. MTB shoes have threaded bolt holes drilled through the outsole for placement of a recessed external cleat (Fig. 18.7). Most MTB shoes have a rubber outsole with a rectangular rubber window that can be removed so that a cleat can be added to the shoe if the cyclist chooses. Toe and heel spikes may be found on the outsole of racing MTB shoes. The spikes resemble those found on soccer or football spikes and provide traction in mud. Some models have removable spikes.

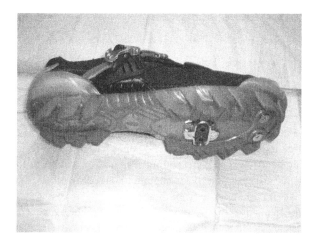

Fig. 18.7 Mountain bike outsole with recessed cleat

Selecting the appropriate type and model of shoes is only a part of the decision-making process for many cyclists. Many will then purchase a cleat and pedal system as well. The interface of the shoe with the bike is via the cleat and pedal system, and we would be remiss in a chapter on cycling footwear to ignore this important component of cycling. In many ways, cleats and pedals have become more technically sophisticated than the footwear.

Cycling Cleats

Cleats attach the shoe to the bike through an engineered pedal system (Fig. 18.8). The cleat/pedal interface is a single point of attachment at the ball of the foot. The cleat is attached to the sole of the shoe with bolts. The pedal is engaged by placing the cleat over the pedal and exerting a downward force until the spring-loaded pedal accepts the cleat. (One popular pedal/cleat system manufactured by

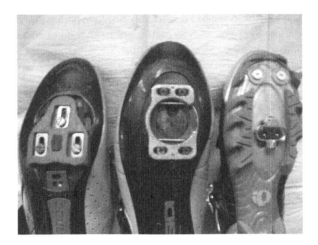

Fig. 18.8 Cleats attached to shoes' outsole, *left* two shoes are external, *right* shoe is recessed

Speedplay, Inc. [San Diego, CA], places the spring in the cleat instead of the pedal.) Most cleats are released from the pedal by externally rotating the heel. Some cleats can be released in multiple directions. Many pedals have adjustable tension so that the force required to release the shoe can be altered as needed. For example, newer cyclists may prefer a lower tension setting for ease of exit from the pedal while experienced cyclists, like aggressive mountain bikers, may set the tension higher to minimize the risk of early release from the pedal.

Road cycling cleats are usually made from lightweight plastics or metals while most MTB cleats are made from stainless steel. The plastic, externally mounted road cleats are more prone to wear than the recessed metal MTB cleats but both must be replaced regularly. Look Cycle (Salt Lake City, UT), is a company which introduced their cleat/pedal system in the mid-1980s that remains the most commonly used road cycling pedal system. Speedplay pedals introduced pedals with the highest degree of rotational freedom Shimano, Inc. (Irvine, CA), the maker of the recessed SPD (Shimano Pedaling Dynamics) pedal system is the most common MTB and commuter cyclist pedal system.

The first clipless cleat/pedal systems locked the foot in and allowed only sagittal plane motion about the pedal spindle, allowing 0° of internal or external rotation of the foot during the pedal cycle. But an innovation that has had implications on cycling injuries is the cleat/pedal system that allows internal/external rotation of the foot about the pedal's transverse axis. This rotation is referred to as "float" in cycling jargon and allows the cyclist varying degrees of freedom during the pedal cycle. Some performance pedals can be adjusted for the desired amount of float. For some pedal systems cleats are color coded to indicate how many degrees of float they allow. Pedals may allow up to 15° of float.

The location and alignment of the cleat on the shoe can be adjusted to address lower limb alignment or injuries. This is discussed in more detail in the sections on pedals and foot position.

Pedals

Pedals vary in shape and performance features. Bicycling pedals have evolved from a relatively large platform for conventional shoes to today's engineered pedal systems that attach a special cycling shoe to the pedal via a binding system. "Toe clips" were the first pedaling innovation which used a strap and cage over the forefoot to secure the foot to pedal, increasing pedaling efficiency, and minimizing the risk of the foot slipping off the pedal. While the strap secured the shoe to the pedal it still allowed some freedom in foot position. Disadvantages of toe clips include forefoot discomfort due to the tight strap and manually having to loosen the strap to enter/exit the clips. Some recreational cyclists prefer toe clips to standard pedals and to the newer "clipless" pedal designs.

In the 1980s clipless pedal systems were developed that used an external cleat on the shoe's forefoot that attached to a spring-loaded pedal much like ski bindings attach a boot to a ski. The pedals are engaged by placing the cleat over the pedal and exerting a downward force. They are released by externally rotating the heel. The spring tension of the pedal can be adjusted to make release easier or harder depending on the demands of the cyclist. Much like skiers and ski bindings, competitive cyclists will set the spring tension higher to minimize the risk of early release from the pedal. Recreational cyclists prefer an easier release and lower spring tension. In some pedal systems the spring tension can affect the rotational ability of the pedal. Clipless pedals allow the rider to increase pedaling efficiency by minimizing some of the "dead spots" in the pedaling cycle, allowing the rider to recruit more muscle groups and to un-weight the leg on the upstroke [32]. Clipless pedals also allow greater ankle plantarflexion and shear loads on the down stroke which helps to extend the power generating portion of the pedal cycle past bottom dead center [10]. One study found that clipless pedal systems were preferred by 57.1% of cyclists who had participated in an organized bike ride [25].

Multiple pedal/cleat systems are available today each with its own performance features. Injured cyclists or cyclists who are vulnerable to foot pain may have to consider whether a different pedal system may have features that are more appropriate for their needs. For example, some pedal systems have more rotational freedom which may be significant for those with knee injuries. Those with chronic forefoot pain may benefit from a pedal with a larger surface area to better distribute pressure.

An important cleat/pedal feature allows transverse plane foot rotation. Since cyclists exhibit varying amounts of in-toeing/out-toeing during different points of the pedal cycle it became necessary to allow some degree of adjustability and freedom in the transverse plane. More rigid cycling shoes and the fixed position of the cleat/pedal interface likely place undue stress on the knee [33]. Conversely some authors have implicated excessive rotational freedom as facilitating faulty knee and foot mechanics [34, 35]. Pedal/cleat systems that allow some freedom in the transverse plane are widely available.

Road cycling pedals are engineered to be lightweight and low profile. They are manufactured from plastic, aluminum, metal alloys, or titanium. More expensive pedals offer adjustable spring tension and adjustable degrees of float and are made from metals such as titanium. The weight savings has obvious energy saving benefits. The low pedal profile makes the pedal more aerodynamic as well as allowing more ground clearance in high-speed turns. The small surface area of some pedals concentrates the local plantar foot pressures. Some road pedals are double-sided allowing articulation with the cleat regardless of which side of the pedal is facing up.

MTB pedals are engineered to resist mud and debris, yet allow easy exit/entry. Most MTB pedals are double-sided, meaning that they have cleat receptacles on both sides of the pedal making it easier to clip in even if the pedal has rotated. Some MTB pedals combine the conventional pedal platform with the binding system. This makes the pedal easier to use for casual rides in conventional shoes as well. Most commuters prefer MTB shoe/cleat/pedal systems because of their versatility.

Foot Position on the Pedal

The cleat can be moved proximal/distal, medial/lateral, or rotated in the transverse plane. Most authors recommend placing cyclists in neutral lower extremity position to minimize risk of injury [36]. But there is not agreement on how to determine transverse plane neutral foot cycling position. One method of determining optimal transverse plane position of the foot on the pedal uses a device called a Rotational Adjustment Device (or RAD) (FitKit Systems, Billings, MT) and is placed on the pedal while the cyclist pedals on a stationary wind trainer. Some retail cycling shops or bike fit technicians use the RAD system when fitting bikes. Multiple authors advocate the benefits of this fit system [9, 37, 38]. Some pedal systems allow greater degrees of rotational freedom about the forefoot which makes for a larger margin for error or even obviates the need for setting the cleat in a neutral position.

Additionally, shims and wedges can be placed between the cleat and sole to address limb length inequality or forefoot varus/valgus as well as knee varus/valgus [34].

Cycling Insoles

Recognizing the benefits of comfortable foot beds, many cycling shoe manufacturers are now making their shoes with higher quality, removable insoles. The insoles often incorporate some medial longitudinal arch support and/or some transverse metatarsal arch support. The benefit of the removable insoles is twofold in that the insoles can be modified with additional arch support or metatarsal pads or replaced with custom orthotics to improve foot function.

Replacement insoles are also now more widely available. Some insole manufacturers are making an insole that is compatible with the lower volume last of the road cycling shoe and is often very similar to a replacement ice skate insole. Since touring and MTB shoes are lasted much like conventional athletic shoes, most prefabricated insoles will fit well. One cycling shoe manufacturer is producing replacement insoles that are sold with forefoot varus and valgus wedges that may be added or removed to address forefoot misalignment [39].

Cycling Orthoses

Custom foot orthoses have been used in cycling to correct biomechanical faults, reduce pedal/in shoe pressure, and balance limb length inequalities (Fig. 18.9). However, there is little research into the efficacy of orthotic management of cycling biomechanics and injuries. For weight-bearing activities custom orthoses have been shown to decrease peak plantar pressures and reduced foot pain [40, 41]. Additionally, custom foot orthoses have been shown to alter subtalar joint pronation, decrease internal tibial rotation, and decrease knee loads [42–44]. The snug fit and stiff soles of road cycling shoes and nonweight-bearing nature of the sport make intrinsic rearfoot posts and rigid shell materials the best choice [9, 45]. There are limitations to the amount of extrinsic modifications which can be made to the orthosis due to the snug fit and narrow last of most road cycling shoes. Touring and MTB shoes can often accommodate extrinsic rearfoot and forefoot posts and bulkier shell materials. Because the forefoot is the site of articulation with the pedal most orthoses and insole interventions are focused on this area. In addition, supporting the medial longitudinal arch and/or limiting subtalar joint pronation can improve foot mechanics, distribute plantar pressures, and increase comfort.

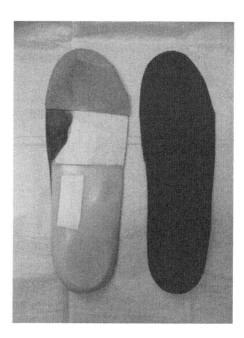

Fig. 18.9 Cycling orthosis with intrinsic rearfoot post on rigid shell, reverse Morton's extension, metatarsal pad, and full length top cover

Anderson and Sockler tested cycling subjects' oxygen consumption in three different shoe/orthoses states found that, while not statistically significant, there was a trend toward increased cycling efficiency with use of orthoses as workloads approached maximal loads [12].

Socks

Cycling socks are made from synthetic fabrics that wick moisture. Lightweight socks are used in warm weather and thicker socks are used in cooler weather. Some triathletes choose not to wear socks for cycling and many of the triathlon-specific cycling shoes are made with a flat-seamed fabric liner. In cold or inclement weather many cyclists wear a waterproof or insulated booty over their cycling shoes.

Footwear Recommendations and Modifications for Prevention and Treatment of Injury

Cycling shoes are selected based on type of cycling, pedal type, and fit. Unlike running shoes, there is not a significant variability in terms of lasts. Since sport and some MTB cycling shoes tend to have larger volume uppers, a more flexible outsole, and straighter lasts than road cycling shoes, they offer some versatility for treating cyclists with chronic foot pain/injuries or difficult-to-fit feet. Many of the most common shoe/cleat/pedal modifications used by cyclists and bike fitters have been handed down from the trial-and-error treatment methods used in competitive cycling for decades.

Knee Pain

Causes of knee pain include training errors such as pushing high gears or excessive hill training, bike fit issues such as improper saddle position or improper shoe/cleat position, and anatomical factors such as limb length inequality, overpronation, genu varum/valgum, ligamentous laxity, high-Q angle, and muscle imbalances among other causes [9, 22, 34, 38, 46, 47]. Common diagnoses of patellofemoral pain may be chondromalacia, patellar tendinosis, prepatellar bursitis, plica syndrome, and patellar subluxation. Other causes of knee pain include pes anserine bursitis and iliotibial band syndrome.

Faulty mechanics at the foot/shoe/pedal interface has been linked to each of these conditions by multiple authors. One group of researchers found that improper cleat alignment was the most common problem in those with patellofemoral pain [46]. Others found that both axial and varus/valgus knee moments were significantly reduced with pedals that allowed freedom in the transverse plane [48]. In addition seat position that is too high, too low, or too far forward has been linked to excessive patellofemoral loading by causing excessive knee flexion at the top of the pedal stroke [34]. Excessively long crank arms have also been implicated in increased forces acting on the patellofemoral joint [8]. The high pedal forces generated during the power phase of cycling have been implicated in increased subtalar joint pronation and chondromalacia [47].

Since excessive loads on the knee occur during the power generating stroke in cycling, optimizing alignment and minimizing torsional forces have often been the focus of biomechanical treatment. Foot/shoe pedal alignment and seat position changes may reduce knee strains. Spring tension of the pedals release mechanism can affect the rotational abilities of the pedal and must be considered in cyclists with knee pain. Much attention has been directed at controlling torsional forces on the knee by controlling STJ pronation with medial longitudinal arch support and forefoot varus wedging.

Custom foot orthoses can be used to correct functional foot disorders that may be contributing to knee pain. Correction of frontal plane deformities with appropriate forefoot and rearfoot posting has been used as an efficacious therapy for treatment of patellofemoral pain [49].

Using video analysis, Francis described decreased knee valgus in cyclists after introducing an orthosis [50]. Ruby and Hull, using a modified pedal that allowed eversion/inversion, were able to decrease varus and valgus knee moments [51] which suggests that forefoot posting of the shoe/foot/pedal interface such as with orthoses would have similar effect.

Iliotibial Band Syndrome

Inflammation of the iliotibial band (ITB) is commonly caused by anatomic abnormalities or poor bike fit which may contribute to friction of the ITB over the lateral femoral condyle during flexion and extension of the knee. Improper cleat alignment, limb length inequalities, excessive pronation, poor bike fit, and varus knee alignment are common contributing factors [8, 38, 46]. Shoe/pedal adjustments include using shims or spacers between under the cleat to balance limb length and/or orthoses to control hyperpronation. Cleats may need to be placed with more external rotation or a cleat/pedal system with more rotational freedom may benefit some cyclists.

Limb Length Inequality

For injuries that may be attributable to limb length inequalities, such as patellofemoral pain, hip/low back complaints, Achilles tendonitis, or iliotibial band syndrome, two methods of adjustment have been described. As is generally accepted anecdotally for weight-bearing activities, correcting approximately half of the suspected limb length is often a good starting point. Limb length can be compensated for by setting the saddle height to the longer limb and then adding a shim between the cleat and sole of the shoe on the short limb. An additional technique, for smaller limb length discrepancies advocated by Andy Pruitt, the former chief medical officer of US Cycling, involves shifting the cleat 1–2 mm distal on the short limb for measured limb length differences of less than 6 mm [52].

Achilles Tendon and Posterior Heel Pain

Rearfoot pain may be caused by Achilles tendonitis, retrocalcaneal bursitis, Achilles enthesopathy, and retrocalcaneal exostosis (Haglund's bumps). The heel cup and collar of the cycling shoe must be evaluated for proper fit. Seat height must be assessed for possible contribution to excessive dorsiflexion of ankle at top dead center of pedal cycle [38]. Appropriate shoe modifications include offloading pressure with adhesive felt padding to the inside of the heel counter, addition of a heel lift, addition of rubber heel cup, or permanent structural modification of the heel counter or upper by a skilled shoe repair shop. Insole modifications and orthoses that address biomechanical factors such as overpronation and/or equinus may be of benefit as well.

Plantar Fasciitis

While plantar fasciitis does not appear to be as common in cyclists as it is in weight-bearing sports, it is possible to address the symptoms in the cycling shoe. Low seat height can be a contributing factor [53]. Rubber or silicone heel cups may be added to shoes. In addition, the insoles can be modified with the addition of adhesive felt padding to support the medial longitudinal arch. Full length orthoses may be used to address any contributing biomechanical factors.

Forefoot Pain and Injuries

Foot injuries were reported twice as often as ankle and Achilles injuries in one study of recreational cyclists [25]. Because of the concentrated pedal reaction forces at the foot/shoe/pedal interface, cyclists are much more likely to suffer forefoot pain than midfoot or rearfoot pain. The small surface area of the pedal, stiff soled shoes, and plantar pressure generated by the pedal stroke can all combine to stress the soft tissue and osseous structures of the forefoot more than the rearfoot.

Ischemia has been proposed as an injury mechanism due to the constant pedal reaction force against the plantar forefoot [17] – cyclists often refer to this pain as "hot foot." Tight shoes, stiff soles, toe straps, high gears – low cadence pedaling technique, improper cleat position, and small pedal surface area have also been suggested as common causes of forefoot pain in cyclists [22]. In addition to ischemic paresthesias, forefoot pain may be caused by metatarsalgia, sesamoiditis, capsulitis, and Morton's neuroma.

Cleat position is important in addressing forefoot pain. Most riders will have their shoes positioned so that the cleat is directly under the metatarsal heads. This location has been suggested as the optimal location for energy transmission, but it can cause pain in some riders. Most cleats can be moved anterior and posterior as well as medial and lateral. A more proximal placement of the cleat has been suggested as a means of relieving many pressure-induced types of forefoot pain [35, 52].

Researchers have found that as power output increases pressure shifts to the medial forefoot. One study found that medial plantar loading increased with higher power outputs and decreased with increased cadence. This decrease was most pronounced under the first met head and toes and less under the fifth met head, midfoot, and heel [16].

Insole modifications for forefoot pain include forefoot cushioning, addition of metatarsal pads, aperture pads, use of forefoot extensions such as varus/valgus wedges, and addition of medial longitudinal arch support. The shoe's foot bed should be evaluated for protruding cleat bolts or manufacturing defects as well. As mentioned previously, many cycling shoes now are made with removable insoles which allow for modification or replacement. Metatarsal pads have been shown to decrease plantar forefoot pressures but their effectiveness is dependent on location and size [54, 55]. Metatarsal pads can be effective relieving pain due to Morton's neuroma, pressure-induced ischemia, metatarsal capsulitis, sesamoiditis, or metatarsalgia. Additional cushioning can be added to the forefoot with replacement insoles.

Orthoses for forefoot pain should use a rigid shell material, intrinsic rearfoot, and full length cushioned top cover [9]. Because of the high forefoot forces cycling orthoses should include metatarsal support in addition to control of biomechanical factors such as hyperpronation [8]. Metatarsal pads, extrinsic forefoot posting to sulcus, aperture pads, or Morton's extension/reverse Morton's extensions can be incorporated as needed. Road shoes will require a narrow shell to fit inside the performance lasted upper; sport and MTB shoes may accommodate a standard shell shape.

The Future of Cycling Footwear

Footwear manufacturers are increasingly moving toward the mass customization. The manufacturing infrastructure is slowly being adapted so that custom footwear can be measured, fit, ordered, and produced more economically and more quickly than ever imagined before. Custom-made cycling shoes and insoles will likely become more widely available and more affordable in the coming years. Performance enhancing and comfort enhancing features will likely continue to evolve.

References

1. Derksen T, Keppler J, Miller S: Chain reactions: the biomechanics of biking. Biomechanics, 11(4): 23–30, 2004.
2. Raasch CC, Zajac FE: Locomotor strategy for pedaling: Muscle groups and biomechanical functions. J Neurophys, 82(2): 515–525, 1999.

3. Faria IE, Cavanaugh PR: The Physiology and Biomechanics of Cycling. John Wiley & Sons, New York, NY, 1978.

4. Gonzales H, Hull ML: Multivariable optimization of cycling biomechanics. J Biomech, 22:1151–1161, 1989.

5. Hull ML, Gonzales H: Bivariate optimization of pedaling rate and crank arm length in cycling. J Biomech, 21:839–849, 1988.

6. Morris DM, Londeree BR: The effects of crank arm length on oxygen consumption. Can J Appl Physiol, 22(5): 429–438, 1997.

7. Gregor RJ, Cavanaugh PR, LaFortune M: Knee flexor moments during propulsion in cycling: a creative solution to lombards paradox. J Biomech, 8:307, 1985.

8. Asplund C, St. Pierre P: Knee pain and cycling. Phys & Sports Med, 32(4), 2004.

9. Sanner WH, O'Halloran WD, Biomechanics, etiology and treatment of cycling injuries. A Am Pod Med Assoc, 90(7):354–376, 2000.

10. Hull ML, Davis RR: Measurement of pedal loading in cycling I & II. J Biomech, 14: 843–872.

11. Redfield R, Hull ML: Prediction of pedal forces in bicycling using optimization methods. J Biomech, 19(2):523–540, 1986.

12. Anderson JC, Sockler JM: Effects of orthoses on selected physiologic parameters in cycling. J Am Pod Med Assoc, 80(3): 161–166, 1990.

13. Korff T, Romer LM, Mayhew I et al.: Effect of pedaling technique on mechanical effectiveness and efficiency in cyclists. Med & Sci Sports & Exer, 39(6): 991–995, 2007.

14. Hamill J, Derrick TR, Holt KG: Shock attenuation and stride frequency during running. Hum Mov Sci, 14, 45–60, 1995.

15. Pandolf KB, Noble BJ: The effect of pedaling speed and resistance changes on perceived exertion for equivalent power outputs on the bicycle ergometer. Med Sci Sports & Exer (5):132–136, 1973.

16. Sanderson DJ, Hennig EM, Black AH: The influence of cadence and power output on force application and in-shoe pressure distribution during cycling by competitive and recreational cyclists. J Sports Sciences, 18:173–181, 2000.

17. Sanderson DJ, Cavanaugh PR: An investigation of the in-shoe pressure distribution during cycling in conventional cycling shoes or running shoes, pp. 903–907. in Jonsson GB (ed.), BiomechanicsXB. Champaign, IL, Human Kinetics Publishers, 1987.

18. Broker JP, Gregor RJ: A dual piezoelectric element force pedal for kinetic analysis of cycling. Int J Sports Biomech, 6: 394–403, 1990.

19. Lafortune MA, Cavanaugh PR, Valiant GA, et al.: A study of the riding mechanics of elite cyclists. Med & Sci Sports & Exer, 15:113, 1983.

20. Lafortune MA, Cavanaugh PR: Effectiveness and efficiency during bicycle riding, pp. 928–936. In Matsui H, Kobayashi K (ed.), Biomechanics VIII-B. Champaign, Il, Human Kinetics Publishing, 1983.

21. Jarboe NE, Quesada PM: The effects of cycling shoe stiffness on forefoot pressure. Foot & Ankle Int, 24(10):784–788.

22. Gregor RJ, Wheeler JB: Biomechanical factors associated with shoe/pedal interfaces. Sports Med, 17(2);117–131, 1994.

23. Eilert-Petersson E, Schlep L: An epidemiological study of bicycle-related injuries. Accident Analysis & Prevention, 29(3):363–372, 1997.

24. Ekman R, et al.: Bicycle-related injuries among the elderly – a new epidemic? Public Health, 115:38–43, 2001.

25. Wilbur CA, Holland GJ, Madison RE, Loy SF: An epidemiological analysis of overuse injuries among recreational cyclists. Int. J Sports Med, 16:201–206, 1995.

26. Weiss B: Nontraumatic injuries in amateur long-distance bicyclist. Am J Sports Med, 13: 189–192, 1985.

27. Kuland DN, Bubaker C: Injuries in the bikecentennial tour. Phys Sports Med, 6:74–78, 1978.

28. Miller JE, Nigg BM, Liu W, et al.: Influence of foot, leg and shoe characteristics on subjective comfort. Foot & Ankle Int, 21(9):759–676, 2000.
29. Mundermann A, Stefanyshyn DJ, Nigg BM: Relationship between footwear comfort of shoe inserts and anthropometric and sensory factors. Med & Sci Sports & Exer, 33(11):1939–1945, 2001.
30. McWhorter JW, Landers M, Wallman H, et al.: The effects of loaded, unloaded, dynamic and static activities on foot volumetrics. Phys Ther in Sport, 7(2):81–86, 2006.
31. Specialized.com website June 29, 2007.
32. Tate J, Shierman G: Toe clips: how they increase pedaling efficiency. Bicycling, 18(6):57, 1977.
33. Holmes JC, Pruitt AL, Whalen NJ: Cycling knee injuries: Common mistakes that cause injuries and how to avoid them. Cycling Science, June:11–14, 1991.
34. Conti-Wyneken AR: Bicycling injuries. Phys Med & Rehab Clin N Am, 10(1):67–76, 1999.
35. Baker A: Bicycling Medicine. Fireside/Simon & Schuster, New York, 1998.
36. Balthazaar B: The effect of shoe/pedal interface position on knee injuries during cycling. Aust. J Podiatric Med, 43(4):118–124, 2000.
37. Burke ER: Serious Cycling, Human Kinetics Press, Champaign, IL 2002.
38. Mellion MB: Common cycling injuries. Sports Medicine, 11(1):52–70, 1991.
39. Specialized BG Insole product information, Specialized, Inc. 2007.
40. Novick A, Stone J, Birke JA, et al.: Reduction of plantar pressure with rigid relief orthoses. J Am Pod Med Assoc, 83(3):115–122, 1993.
41. Postema K, Burm PET, Zande ME, et al.: Primary metatarsalgia: the influence of custom molded insole and rockerbar on plantar pressure. Prosth & Orth Intl, 22:35–44, 1998.
42. Klingman RE, Liaos SM, Hardin KM: The effect of subtalar joint posting on patellar glide in subjects with excessive rearfoot pronation. J Ortho Sports Phys Ther, 25(3):185–191, 1997.
43. Cornwall MW, McPoil TG: Footwear and foot orthotic effectiveness research: A new approach. J Ortho Sports Phys Ther, 21(6):317–327, 1995.
44. Nawoczenski DA, Cook TM, Saltzman CL: The effect of three dimensional kinematics of the leg and rearfoot during running. J Ortho Sports Phys Ther, 21(6):337–344, 1995.
45. Denton JA: in Valmassy RL (ed.), Clinical Biomechanics of the Lower Extremities. Lower extremity function, pp. 455–456. Mosby Publishing, St. Louis, MN, 1996.
46. Holmes J, Pruitt A, Whalen A: Lower extremity overuse in bicycling. Clinics in Sports Med, 13(1):187–206, 1991.
47. Pruitt AL: The cyclists knee: Anatomical and biomechanical considerations, In Burke ER, Newsom MM (eds.), Medical & Scientific Aspecs of Cycling. Human Kinetics, Champaign, IL, 1988.
48. Ruby P, Hull ML: Response of intersegmental knee loads to foot/pedal platform degrees of freedom in cycling. J Biomech, 26(11):1327–1340, 1993.
49. Valmassey RL: in Clinical Biomechanics of the Lower Extremities. Mosby Publishing, St. Loius, MO, 1996.
50. Francis PR: Injury prevention for cyclists: a biomechanical approach, pp. 145–184. in Burke ER (ed.), Science of Cycling. Human Kinetics Books, Champaign, IL, 1986.
51. Wootten D, Hull ML: Design and evaluation of a mulit-degree-of-freedom foot/pedal interface of cycling. Int J Sport Biomech, 8:152–164, 1992.
52. Pruitt AL, Matheny F: Andy Pruitt's Complete Medical Guide for Cyclists. Velo Press, Boulder, CO, 2006.
53. Thompson MT, Rivara FP: Bicycle-related injuries. Am Fam Phys, 63(10):2007–2014, 2001.
54. Chang AH, Abu-Faraj ZU, Harris GF, et al.: Multistep measurement of plantar pressure alterations using metatarsal pads. Foot & Ankle Int, 15(12):654–660, 1994.
55. Holmes GB, Timmerman L: A quantitative assessment of the effect of metatarsal pads on plantar pressures. Foot & Ankle, 11(3):141–145, 1990.

Chapter 19
Racquet Sports: Tennis, Badminton, Squash, Racquetball, and Handball

Richard T. Bouché

Racquet sports make up an eclectic group of court activities that can be quite diverse. In this chapter we focus on the following racquet sports: tennis, badminton, squash, racquetball, and handball. Though it is beyond the scope of this chapter, it is paramount that readers become acquainted with certain background information on each of these individual sports including developmental history, rules and strategies, and necessary equipment. This information gives the reader "credibility" in dealing with racquet sport athletes and also provides a solid foundation for further study.

Court Design and Surfaces

Being familiar with court design and the various surfaces these sports are played on is paramount as this information will dictate the type and features of shoes that are recommended for each racquet sport [1–3]. Concerning court design, tennis and badminton are played on "open" courts (no walls) and handball, squash, and racquetball are played on "closed" courts with four walls, and in the case of racquetball and handball, a ceiling as well. Each of these courts has standardized dimensions. Concerning surfaces, tennis is played inside or outside on varied surfaces that can be generically considered hard, cushioned, or soft. Hard surfaces are most common and include asphalt and concrete that are usually covered by an acrylic coating that enhances appearance and provides protection from the elements. Cushioned surfaces comprise a hard surface covered with layers of resilient cushioned materials. Soft surfaces include grass (traditional surface), clay, and synthetic turf. Surfaces can also be considered fast and slow [1]. Fast surfaces include grass and synthetic turf and a slow surface would be clay. Other than the recreational "back-yard" game, badminton is classically played indoors on two types of floors, both are "sprung" floors (floors that are constructed to absorb shock and give a softer feel) with either

R.T. Bouché (✉)
Private Practice, The Sports Medicine Clinic, 10330 Meridian Ave N., Suite 300, Seattle, WA, USA

M.B. Werd, E.L. Knight (eds.), *Athletic Footwear and Orthoses in Sports Medicine*, DOI 10.1007/978-0-387-76416-0_19, © Springer Science+Business Media, LLC 2010

a vinyl absorbent covering or a hardwood strip covering. Handball, squash, and racquetball are played inside on a hardwood floor (usually maple). Traditionally, handball and racquetball floors have a urethane finish, and squash has an unfinished or partially finished floor [3].

Biomechanical Demands of Racquet Sports

One common denominator in all racquet sports is the biomechanical demands on the lower extremity. A variety of foot and body movements are required involving quick changes of direction. These sudden "stop-and-go" maneuvers involve specific movements depending on the level of play (novice versus advanced) and may include walking, running (forward/backward), sideward movements, hopping, jumping/landing, rotations, and stopping [4, 5]. These movements produce variable loads on the lower extremity and back that are often underestimated. For example, a tennis player who jumps up to hit a smash and lands on his/her heel (or in a "foot flat" position) may have up to six times body weight on their foot [6]. If the racquet sports player lands on their forefoot, they may have up to four times body weight on their foot [6] versus 2–3 times body weight with running [7].

One study looked at three specific factors in average versus advanced tennis players: (1) different types of motion, (2) location of foot where initial ground contact occurred, and (3) different directions of motion [5]. Various surface conditions were also considered (asphalt versus sand/clay). The differences in average versus advanced recreational tennis players were as follows [5]: (1) walking was the predominant movement in average players followed by running and hopping. In contrast, running occurs at the same rate as walking and hopping in advanced players. Significant sliding or sideslipping only occurred on sand (clay surfaces) and not on the hard asphalt surface tested in both groups; (2) initial foot-to-ground contact occurred mainly in the heel with average players and on the forefoot with advanced players. Contact with the inner and outer shoe edges also occurred with significant frequency in both groups; (3) direction of movement is predominantly forward for average players and lateral side-to-side movement becomes more frequent in advanced players. Lateral movements were commonly combined with landing on the forefoot. In a different study looking at side-to-side movements in court sport athletes, initial landing on the rearfoot was more common than initial landing on the forefoot in an approximate 3 to 1 ratio [8]. A reasonable deduction from these studies would be that specific design features need to be considered when manufacturing a racquet shoe, including the shoe/surface interface and how to best optimize foot support. Additional studies need to be performed on each individual racquet sport to validate these findings, and then apply that data to each specific sport shoe.

Common Injuries

A summary article regarding tennis injuries provided a systematic literature review since 1996 and suggested four principal findings that can be applied to all racquet sports in general [9]. (1) There is great variation in reported incidence of injuries; (2) most injuries occur in the lower extremities; (3) there are few studies that have clarified the association of risk factors and injuries; and (4) there were no randomized controlled trials investigating injury prevention measures. Anticipation of future studies to address injury patterns in each of these individual racquet sports will help dictate direction of treatment and prevention strategies.

Based on general trends from review of existing literature and the author's clinical experience, the following information on lower extremity injuries in racquet sports is summarized [9–19]. Overuse injuries which mainly affect the foot and ankle predominate including Achilles tendinopathy, plantar fasciitis, and stress fractures being most common. Ankle sprains and their sequelae, Achilles ruptures, and muscle strains are the most common acute injuries likely to be encountered. One notable prospective study on the epidemiology of 275 badminton injuries in one season provided the following valuable information: there was an injury incidence of 2.9 injuries/player/1000 badminton hours; men were more frequently injured than women; injury prevalence was 0.3 injury/player; type of injuries were overuse in approximately 75% and acute/traumatic in 25% [13].

The following injuries interestingly incorporate the word "tennis" into their name: tennis toe (subungual hematoma), tennis heel (intradermal bleeding), tennis fracture (fifth metatarsal base avulsion), and tennis leg (gastrocnemius myotendinous junction muscle strain). Though these injuries have been associated with tennis, their sports-specific incidence is unknown. In the author's experience, tennis leg is encountered frequently in court sports and is probably the most common muscle strain encountered in the lower extremity.

Racquet Shoe Design

Shoes for racquet sports can be considered part of a broader category of athletic shoes, that being court shoes. The foundation for present design of court shoes and athletic leisure footwear in general is based on the venerable sneaker which is perhaps the most significant design of all sports shoes. The sneaker has its roots in the Industrial Revolution and is of simple design, with a canvas upper and a rubber outsole. The earliest British version of the sneaker was the Plimsoll or sand shoe (1876) [20] and the earliest American version of the sneaker was Keds (1917), the first mass marketed athletic shoe [21]. The first racquet sports shoe was designed by Adidas for tennis in 1931[21].

Influenced by continued emphasis on fitness, popularity of racquet sports, injury patterns, and limited scientific research, court shoes have evolved from the basic canvas and rubber sneaker to highly technical, necessary pieces of equipment. A recent paper discusses the three most important functional design features for sport shoes, that being injury prevention, performance, and comfort [4]. This is in contrast to the non-functional design features of sports shoes (i.e., design, style, price, etc.).

Injury Prevention

For injury prevention in court shoe design, shoes should: be *generically stable* to counter excessive pronation and especially excessive supination involving sideward cutting movements, the later of which is common to court sports; *allow adequate cushion* in forefoot and rearfoot; provide *midfoot flexibility in the frontal plane* to allow uncoupling of forefoot on rearfoot as players are commonly on their forefoot but maintain *moderate sagittal plane stiffness* in the midfoot or shank of the shoe (Fig. 19.1); strive for *"ideal" traction* to avoid extremes of slipping versus foot fixation/"blocking," both of which can result in injury [4].

To reduce risk of injury from excessive supinatory motion, shoes with high/high–mid top quarter height and firm heel counters may help, in addition to external devices such as ankle bracing. But to be effective in reducing injury, these features must reduce inversion moments immediately after touchdown as shoe inversion takes place within 40 ms after touchdown [8]. Ironically, being barefoot is more stable than when wearing a shoe; the shoe sole increases the lever arm to impart an external inversion moment on the subtalar joint [8] (Fig. 19.2). Shoe sole stability is dependent on hardness, thickness, and torsional stiffness of the sole and therefore shoes which have softer soles of mild-to-moderate thickness, have torsional flexibility (frontal plane), and allow heel deformation of shoe sole medially and laterally may be best [8]. Excessive slipping of the foot inside the shoe has also been recognized as a potential problem for lateral instability and strategies to address this must be considered [8] including avoiding sock liners, insoles, and orthoses with slippery top covers. The shoe/surface interface (traction) plays a significant role in injury prevention and shoe choice. One study on tennis surfaces underscores this fact as most lower extremity injuries occurred on surfaces with high translational traction

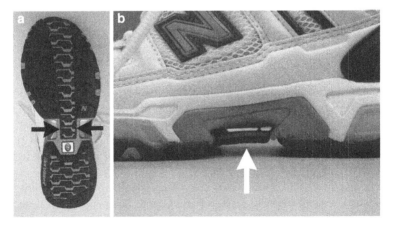

Fig. 19.1 Unique desirable design of a cross training shoe (rarely found in court shoes) with stiff, thin, longitudinally oriented outsole strut that provides sagittal plane midfoot/shank stability (**a**) (*black arrows*) but allows frontal plane torsional flexibility (**b**) (*white arrow*)

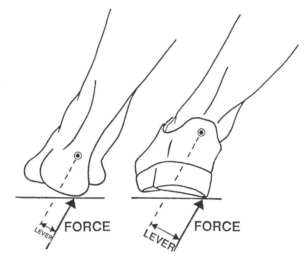

Fig. 19.2 Sideward (*lateral*) cutting movements barefoot (*left*) and with a shoe (*right*). The shoe sole imparts a greater external inversion moment on subtalar joint than when barefoot ([8], with permission of Lippincott Williams & Wilkins)

(asphalt, concrete, etc.) with few injuries on surfaces with low translational traction (grass, clay, etc.) [5]. The author feels that foot fixation/"blocking" is a major factor in the mechanism for ankle sprains and other injuries in the racquet sport enthusiast. In addition, increased rotational traction has been anecdotally associated with overload injuries therefore rotational resistance should be minimized [4].

Performance

Optimum *traction and minimizing energy loss* are factors that need to be considered for performance [4]. Matching shoe sole composition (solid rubber, gum rubber, polyurethane, etc.) and tread pattern [4, 22] (configuration, depth, orientation, etc.) to specific playing surfaces is the goal to prevent excessive sliding and/or foot fixation. From a performance perspective, players are willing to sacrifice injury prevention for increased traction which is a factor that must be considered. In many of the racquet sports (racquetball, squash and handball) gum rubber has been traditionally used as the outsole material of choice. When used on a finished hardwood floor, translational traction of gum rubber is high due to an increased coefficient of friction which results in problems with "foot fixation." This increases potential for ankle sprains and other injuries. The importance of tread patterns is underscored when appreciating specific tread patterns that are used for certain tennis court surfaces such as grass and clay. Grass courts mandate use of a "nub" outsole design (Fig. 19.3) whereas clay courts require a wide channeled herringbone outsole design (D.G. Sharnoff, 2007, Personal Communication).

Energy aspects of sports shoes include two issues: how to *maximize energy return* and *minimize energy loss* [23]. The influence energy return of sports shoes has on performance is probably minimal with one study finding a 30% loss of

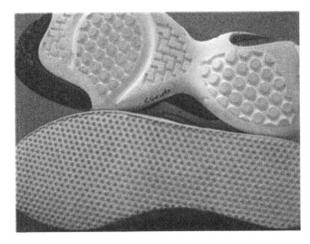

Fig. 19.3 Special "nub" outsoles on tennis shoes designed to increase traction on grass court surface

energy input with shoe midsole materials and poor timing, frequency, location, and direction of returned energy [23]. Minimizing energy loss appears to be a more realistic focus. This can be achieved by *reducing shoe weight* (lighter the shoe, less energy expended), *using appropriate cushioned materials* to minimize soft tissue vibrations (decreases need for muscle dampening), *stabilizing the ankle* (limits need for internal muscle stabilization), and *increasing midsole bending stiffness* at the metatarsophalangeal joints (improves running economy and jumping ability) [23, 24].

Comfort

The final functional design feature for sport shoes is comfort. Although this is the most important initial factor to consider when purchasing a shoe, there are few studies available that have addressed this issue [4, 25, 26]. If a sport shoe is not comfortable it can never truly function the way it was intended. Comfort factors to consider include fit, climate control, and various mechanical variables including skeletal alignment (heel eversion – more discomfort), torsional stiffness (stiffer – more discomfort), and cushioning (less cushion – more discomfort) [4, 24]. Comfort is not exclusive, as it can influence the other design features, injury prevention, and performance. An example of this is the positive role of internal heel counters which are used to control excessive rearfoot pronation/supination as well as improve shock absorbency of heel. This feature has been touted to prevent injury and improve performance as well as provide comfort [26].

Appropriate fit is paramount to achieving comfort in a shoe. Four phases of shoe fit include evaluation at rest (static), standing (weight bearing), while performing activity (functional) and after activity taking into account foot swelling [27]. Matching the athlete's foot to the appropriate shoe is based on the external shoe last (form or shape on which the shoe is manufactured) and proper sizing. Court shoe external lasts are usually straight or inflared to a variable degree. Proper sizing is dependent on length, width, and volume of the foot. For court sports, toe box shape, depth, and construction are paramount as well. Proper ventilation is dependent on hosiery used and a variety of breathable upper and insole materials presently available.

Desirable Features of A Court Shoe

There are specific features recommended for racquet sport shoes based on current court shoe design and research (Table 19.1). In addition to general shoe inspection, there are four simple tests that can be used for evaluation of court shoes: (1) midfoot sagittal plane stability (shank stability) – bend the shoe and appreciate the stiffness in the midfoot. It should be firm; (2) midfoot frontal plane flexibility– twist the shoe as if wringing a towel. There should be good flexibility (not too stiff); (3) rearfoot stability– grasp and squeeze the heel counter. It should be stiff and firm; (4) upper stability of the forefoot– put your hand inside the forefoot area of the shoe, splay out your hand, and move it back and forth in the transverse plane. The shoe upper should be firm and not extend over the midsole/outsole. If the shoe meets these criteria, it should be an acceptable shoe and likely a reasonable choice.

Table 19.1 Desirable features of court shoe

Durable outsole and tread pattern matched to surface
Plantar sole sub first MTPJ reinforcement
Full-length midsole cushion, especially forefoot
Sagittal plane midfoot stiffness (shank stability)
Frontal plane midfoot flexibility
Stable forefoot, midfoot, rearfoot, ankle
Forefoot – footframe support (midsole/outsole) w/"wrap-around" construction, medial and lateral flanges
Midfoot – nylon quarter support straps, stable tongue construction, external spats
Rearfoot – rounded outsole w/narrow heel; low heel height with recessed (low-to-ground) construction; firm heel counter w/reinforcement; stable top-line construction
Ankle – mid-high or high-top preferred
Variable width lacing system
Rubber toe cap/bumper for "toe drag"
Anti-shear, removable sockliner
Round/circular/squared toebox with ample width/depth
Breathable upper
Lightweight
Ability to fit insole, arch support, orthoses

Orthoses

It is the author's opinion that many court shoes available today are poorly designed and are generally disappointing in that many of the desirable features are missing. Due to this situation, the role of prefabricated insoles and custom foot orthoses has been critical in enhancing ability of shoes to prevent injury, enhance comfort, and increase performance potential. One notable example is use of orthoses to address the generalized lack of midfoot or shank stability found in most court shoes. An orthosis can provide this needed shank stability. Another factor to consider is lack of pronation/supination stability as court shoe design is usually generic and not specific to excessive pronators or supinators as many running shoes are. Custom foot orthoses can complement a generic court shoe to address excessive pronatory/supinatory problems and impact loading issues. A new paradigm has been introduced to explain the efficacy of orthoses based on muscle tuning and preferred joint movement pathways [28]. These new paradigms challenge the conventional thinking on impact loading and skeletal alignment, respectively [28]. Specific recommendations for court shoe orthoses fabrication can be helpful (Table 19.2).

Table 19.2 Recommended features for court shoe orthoses

Balanced/contoured/compressible (3.0–3.5 mm thick) polypropylene shell
Extra deep heel seat
Mild-to-moderate medial arch
Maximum lateral arch
Full-length, perforated, fine cell, medium soft, polyethylene foam (Ucolite, UCO International, Wheeling, IL) topcover
For excessive supinator consider other features to exert eversion moment on foot (i.e., lateral forefoot and/or rearfoot valgus wedge, extended lateral rearfoot post, etc.)
For excessive pronator consider other features to exert inversion moment on foot (i.e., medial forefoot and/or rearfoot varus wedge, rearfoot post, etc.)

Summary

This chapter has provided a succinct overview of important factors to consider when recommending court shoes and orthoses for racquet sports. It is important to appreciate the uniqueness of each specific racquet sport, demands on the lower extremity, common injuries, subject-specific anatomy (e.g., foot type), shoe/surface interface issues, desirable features for court shoes, and orthoses. Further study and research is needed on individual racquet sports to determine if these shoe and orthosis features truly prevent injury, enhance performance, and provide comfort as anticipated.

References

1. Miller S: Modern tennis rackets, balls, and surfaces. Br J Sports Med, 40:401–405, 2006.
2. Rheinstein DJ, Morehouse CA, Niebel BW: Effects on traction of outsole composition and hardesses of basketball shoes and three types of playing surfaces. Med Sci Sports, 10:282–288, 1978.
3. Chapman AE, Leyland AJ, Ross SM, et al.: Effect of floor conditions upon frictional characteristics of squash court shoes. J Sports Sci, 9:33–41, 1991.

4. Reinschmidt C, Nigg BM: Current issues in the design of running and court shoes. Sportverl Sportschad, 14:71–81, 2000.
5. Nigg BM, Luthi SM, Bahlsen HA: The tennis shoe- biomechanical design criteria. in, Segesser B, Pforringer W, (eds.), The shoe in sport, pp. 39–46. Chicago,IL: Year Book Medical Publishers, Inc, 1987.
6. Valiant GA, Cavanagh PR: A study of landing from a jump: implications for the design of a basketball shoe. in, Winter DA, (ed.). Biomechanics IX, pp. 117–122. Champaign, IL, Human Kinetic Publishers, 1983
7. Cavanagh PR, LaFortune MA: Ground reaction forces in distance running. J Biomech, 13:397–406, 1980.
8. Stacoff A, Steger J, Stussi E, et al.: Lateral stability in sideward cutting movements. Med Sci Sports Exerc, 28:350–358, 1996.
9. Pluim BM, Staal JB, Windler GE, et al.: Tennis injuries: occurrence, aetiology, and prevention. Br J Sports Med, 40:415–423, 2006.
10. Feit EM, Berenter R: Lower extremity tennis injuries. Prevalence, etiology, and mechanism. J Am Pod Med Assoc, 83:509–514, 1993.
11. Bylak J, Hutchinson MR: Common injuries in young tennis players. Sports Med, 26:119–132, 1998.
12. Maquirrianin J, Ghisi JP: The incidence and distribution of stress fractures in elite tennis players. Br J Sports Med 40:454–459, 2006.
13. Jorgensen U, Winge S: Epidemiology of badminton injuries. Int J Sports Med 8:379–382, 1987.
14. Jorgensen U, Winge S: Injuries in badminton. Sports Med, 10:59–64, 1990.
15. Kroner K, Schmidt SA, Nielsen AB, et al.: Badminton injuries. Br J Sports Med, 24: 169–172, 1990.
16. Hoy K, Lindblad BE, Terkelsen CJ, et al.: Badminton injuries—a prospective epidemiological and socioeconomic study. Br J Sports Med, 28:276–279, 1994.
17. Fahlstorm M, Bjornstig U, Lorenstzon R: Acute badminton injuries. Scand J Med Sci Sports. 6: 145–148, 1998.
18. Berson BL, Rlonick AM, Tamos CG, et al.: An epidemiologic study of squash injuries. Am J Sports Med, 9:103–106, 1981.
19. Chard MD, Lachmann SM: Racquet sports—patterns of injury presenting to a sports injury clinic. Br J Sports Med, 21:150–153, 1987.
20. Kippen C (last updated 12/2004): Sneakers and Trainers. Retrieved June 9, 2007, from History of Sports Shoes. Web site: http://podiatry.curtin,edu.au/sport.html .
21. SneakerHead (2001–2007): Retrieved June 9, 2007, from The Sneaker: A History- The History of Sneakers I (1800–1950). Web site: http://sneakerhead.com/sneaker-history-pl.html .
22. Li KW, Wu HH, Lin YC: The effect of shoe sole tread groove depth on the friction coefficient with different tread groove widths, floors and contaminants. Appl Ergonomics 37:743–748, 2006.
23. Stefanyshyn DJ, Nigg BM: Energy aspects associated with sport shoes. Sportverl Sportschad. 14:82–89, 2000.
24. Roy JPR, Stefanyshyn DJ: Shoe midsole longitudinal bending stiffness and running economy, joint energy, and EMG. Med Sci Sports Exerc, 38:562–569, 2006.
25. Miller JE, Nigg BM, Liu W, et al.: Influence of foot, leg and shoe characteristics on subjective discomfort. Foot Ankle Int, 21:759–767, 2000.
26. Llana S, Brizuela G, Dura JV, et al.: A study of the discomfort associated with tennis shoes. J Sports Sci, 20:671–679, 2002.
27. Rossi WA, Tennant R: Advanced principles of shoe fitting. in, Professional Shoe Fitting. New York, National Shoe Retailers Association, 1984.
28. Nigg BM: The role of impact forces and foot pronation: a new paradigm. Clin J Sports Med, 11:2–9, 2001.

Chapter 20
Football

Keith B. Kashuk, Maxime Savard, and Tanisha Smith

Football is a complex sport requiring rapid adaptation of the lower extremity to constantly evolving plays. It is a multidirectional sport encompassing several demanding movements such as running, sprinting, jumping, cutting, backpedaling, and kicking. Each movement induces a large amount of strain to the architecture of the lower extremity placing the athlete at risk for injury.

Running during a football game is visualized when the athlete breaks away from the rest of the pack with no fear of collision into another player. The athlete's position begins initially with a low center of gravity, wide base of gait, and increased angle of gait in preparation for rapid cutting, blocking, or collision [1]. As the athlete propels himself forward and accelerates he assumes a more upright position shifting the body's center of gravity to a more vertical direction. The lower extremity functions to maintain forward motion, resisting internal and external motion, and supporting the body's weight absorbing the impact at contact with the ground [2]. The ground reactive forces have been described to be 2–2.5 times greater during running compared to walking [3, 4]. Ideally during running the feet follow a line of progression directly beneath the center of gravity yielding essentially a zero base of gait [1]. The foot should be in a neutral position at midstance in order to balance the body over the supported foot for the single limb support phase. A narrow base of gait yields a longer stride length which enhances speed and efficiency during running. Deviation from the ideal running position results in rapid fatigue of the lower extremity and places the athlete at risk for injury. A wide base of gait and increased angle of gait require more effort from the muscles in order to stabilize the skeletal system against the ground reactive forces.

The base of gait may be altered by a pathological increase in the angle of gait caused by an excessively pronated foot. As the subtalar joint reaches maximum pronation the midtarsal joint is also unlocked and causes the foot to externally rotate allowing the foot to adapt to the surface of the ground. Excessive pronation does not

K.B. Kashuk (✉)
Department of Orthopaedics and Rehabilitation, University of Miami School of Medicine,
6350 Sunset Dr., South Miami, FL 33143, USA

M.B. Werd, E.L. Knight (eds.), *Athletic Footwear and Orthoses in Sports Medicine*,
DOI 10.1007/978-0-387-76416-0_20, © Springer Science+Business Media, LLC 2010

allow resupination prior to propulsion, and thus the extrinsic muscles of the lower extremity must work harder to stabilize the foot for push off [5]. Fatigue results when these muscles work for an extended period of time against an unstable fulcrum [1, 3, 6]. Therefore, supination during midstance returns the foot to a neutral position locking the midtarsal joint and providing a stable platform for propulsion.

A functional varus (calcaneal varus present during weightbearing) enhances pronation during the stance phase [7]. At heel strike the varus position of the heel forces the subtalar joint to compensate by producing excessive pronation to bring the heel in contact with the ground. Shoe wear is typically noted laterally, however, the rearfoot is noted to pronate excessively following heel strike [5, 8]. This condition is usually seen with running and may be associated with fatigue of the posterior tibial muscle resulting from compensation for the hyperpronation [5]. Excessive pronation may also be seen with a limb length discrepancy [5]. Compensation for a limb length discrepancy occurs at the subtalar joint by supination for the short limb and pronation for the longer limb.

Football places a large demand on the athlete's body especially when he is required to perform multiple sprints in a short period of time. A large amount of energy is expended by the lower extremity during propulsion in order to maintain a rapid momentum. Also the lower extremity is subject to greater forces during the breaking phase of sprinting in comparison to running. The center of gravity is noted to attain a more vertical position than during running due to the decrease in stride length but increased cadence of the lower extremity. The stance phase is substantially reduced and accounts for only approximately 22% of the gait cycle [4]. The base of gait and angle of gait increase in comparison to running, however, remain less than during walking. Therefore sprinting is less efficient than running and places a greater demand on the muscles of the lower extremity in order to maintain forward momentum and resist ground reactive forces. The gait cycle is substantially altered to accommodate the demands placed on the extremity. At faster speeds the athlete tends to land on the forefoot with less rearfoot purchase [3]. The foot is required to absorb a great deal of the ground reactive forces. Strain of the gastrocnemius muscle is seen commonly during the single leg support phase near the end of the gait cycle prior to push off [9]. The muscle is near its maximum length and is functioning to oppose ground reactive forces that tend to dorsiflex the ankle and extend the knee [10].

Jumping requires that the lower extremity generate a substantial amount of force in order to exceed ground reactive forces and propel the body in a vertical direction. It is characterized by several phases such as foot plant, takeoff, ascent, descent, and landing [3]. At foot plant the muscles causing plantar flexion of the foot generate the force necessary to neutralize the ground reactive forces. At foot plant forward momentum is resisted and the body is braced to prepare for takeoff. Initially there is flexion at the hip, knee, and ankle with a transition to extension of the joints as the body takes off and ascends [3]. As the athlete's body reaches his peak elevation, he begins to descend. Landing requires the combined effort of the abdomen, hips, thighs, lower legs, and feet with flexion occurring at the hip, knee, and ankle [3]. The lower extremity assumes a flexed position in order for the muscles to dissipate the ground reactive forces preventing excessive force transmission across the joints. Factors predisposing the athlete to injury include such factors as the jumping surface, training regimen, anatomical variation, and the angle and position of the back, hips, knees, and ankles during the movement [3]. These factors can play a vital role in placing the athlete at further risk for stress fractures and tendinopathies. Training programs that emphasize proprioception and muscular balance of the lower extremity specifically the hamstrings and avoid excessive knee extension and genu valgum at landing should be entertained in those athletes prone to injury [3]. Also training programs should focus their attention to implementing position-specific activities to reduce the injury rate during complex movements such as jumping [11].

The football player typically employs a low center of gravity and wide base of gait in order to adapt to or prepare for rapid cutting, blocking, or collision with another athlete. As the feet get further apart they tend to externally rotate increasing the angle of gait and lowering the center of gravity [12]. A wide base of gait provides the stability which is essential to collision sports such as football and also allows for a quick response in any direction.

Backward running or backpedaling also requires that the athlete employ a wide base and angle of gait [12]. Excessive force is endured by the forefoot as the athlete runs on the balls of the feet. A pronated foot is ideally suited for backpedaling because it allows the foot to adapt to different surfaces.

The biomechanics of kicking vary according to the type of kick required. Substantial strain is placed on the lower extremity during a field goal kick versus a punt. The kick is described according to three phases known as the back swing, leg-cocking, and acceleration phase of the leg [3]. A kick is initiated with the back swing phase when the foot initiating the kick leaves the ground and the leg moves into a position of maximum hip extension [3]. This movement is promoted by the hip extensors and hamstrings and slightly opposed by the hip flexors and quadriceps. The leg-cocking phase follows when the knee is flexed at the point of maximum hip extension allowing further posterior progression of the limb [3]. The force for the kick is generated during the forward acceleration phase of the leg with the forward drive of the limb generated by the hip flexors, and knee extensors until contact with the ball occurs [3]. The acceleration phase is antagonized by the hamstrings prior to ball contact to decrease the rate of knee extension [3]. This serves to protect the knee and prevent hyperextension. A good field goal kicker learns to have greater relaxation of the hamstrings during the leg acceleration phase producing a larger amount of force with ball contact [3]. The hamstrings and ACL function together to align the tibia and femur maintaining knee joint alignment [3]. Either structure possibly may be injured with knee hyperextension. Therefore it is essential that training programs focusing on strengthening the muscles acting on the knee and their proprioceptive response to end range of motion movements be implemented to reduce injuries associated with kicking.

Injured athletes require rehabilitation directed toward the specific phase of the movement that caused their injury. Commonly the calf muscle is injured during the late single leg stance phase of the opposite extremity maintaining the athlete's balance. During the single leg support phase seen with running, sprinting, or kicking, the gastrocnemius is strained excessively in order to counter ground reactive forces and resist internal and external rotation to maintain the body's balance [3]. The quadriceps is also commonly strained during kicking but no phase has been solely identified [3]. The hamstrings are most commonly affected during the acceleration phase of the leg with running, kicking, or jumping when they are placed under an eccentric load resisting hyperextension of the knee.

Foot Structure as It Relates Specifically to Football

The Rectus Foot Type

A "normal" foot or rectus foot type is described by one that is neither pronated nor supinated. The subtalar joint is in a neutral position with its total range of motion described as approximately 21–30° [5]. Inversion is described as utilizing approximately 30° of available subtalar joint range of motion with 15°° of eversion encompassing the remaining amount [5]. The forefoot to rearfoot relationship is also ideally perpendicular in the frontal plane and the forefoot to rearfoot angle is 10–12 adducted in the transverse plane [5]. This foot type is preferable for jumping and rebounding movements often utilized by receivers or backfield defensemen. Jumping requires a foot type that can act as a rigid lever for counteracting ground reactive forces and propelling the body into the air during propulsion. The foot must be able to also pronate and adapt to the surface of the ground and absorb the impact from the ground during landing.

The Pronated Foot Type

The pronated foot is ideally suited for a lineman in football because it allows for preparation for blocking and collision with another athlete. The foot is well adapted to the playing surface and provides a stable platform to absorb the high-impact forces associated with blocking. Also the forward lean position of the three-point or four-point stance increases dorsiflexion at the ankle, which may result in an anterior compression ankle spur [5]. The equinus component that develops secondary to the anterior ankle spur is further compensated by the dorsiflexion of the oblique midtarsal joint with pronation of the rearfoot [5].

Postural fatigue is commonly associated with a pronated foot type. Aching of the foot and posterior medial aspects of the leg are noted clinically [5]. During midstance excessive pronation prevents the midtarsal joints from locking and stabilizing the foot. The extrinsic and intrinsic muscles of the foot are activated to assist with stabilizing the foot which eventually leads to fatigue secondary to overuse. Once the muscles fatigue, the joints are placed through excessive range of motion producing an excessive amount of torque on the associated bones and joints resulting in injury [5, 6, 12]. Also as the foot excessively pronates the center of gravity and ground reactive forces are redirected lateral to the long axis of the foot further exacerbating the deformity [7].

The pronated foot may be seen unilaterally or bilaterally. It is important for the clinician to differentiate between the two and identify the etiology. A unilateral flat-foot in an adult is usually secondary to dysfunction of the posterior tibial tendon and may be further associated with arthritic changes of the subtalar joint [5]. Bilateral flatfeet may also be associated with posterior tibial tendon dysfunction or congenital ligamentous laxity [5, 6, 8]. Severe hypermobility and flattening of the medial longitudinal arch are associated with a hypermobile flatfoot.

Medial overuse injuries are commonly seen with increased pronation of the subtalar joint. Collapse and weakening of the medial longitudinal arch result in strains of the abductor hallucis and medial plantar fasciitis [5, 6]. There is also an increased incidence of hallux valgus associated with a hypermobile first ray secondary to hyperpronation [6]. Medial strain often results in anterior and posterior tibial tendonitis as the muscle becomes overworked attempting to resupinate the foot [5]. Stress fractures of the lateral malleolus of the ankle may be associated with overload of the medial column [5]. Medial shin syndrome is noted with increased use of the posterior tibial muscle inadvertently from its direct pull on the tibia [5]. Athletes often complain of pain along the medial aspect of the Achilles tendon [5]. A functional valgus of the knee is often observed and associated with patellofemoral symptoms from patellofemoral compression with mild instability and tracking of the patella noted [5, 10]. Furthermore medial quadriceps pain and pes anserinus bursitis may also be seen clinically with medial strain along the knee [5].

The pronated foot type often responds well to orthoses and rehabilitation of the lower extremity muscles. The orthosis supports the medial longitudinal arch and prevents its collapse limiting the function of the posterior tibial muscle and preventing excessive medial strain along the foot, ankle, and knee. Hyperpronation is essentially blocked by the orthotic device and prevents overuse of the tibialis anterior and posterior muscles in order to stabilize and supinate the foot during the stance phase. Strengthening and proprioceptive exercises directed at the lower extremity muscles aim to build endurance and prevent overuse of the affected muscles.

The Supinated Foot Type

The halfback position in football is best suited to a semirigid foot type that permits rapid cutting and maneuverability. The joints of the foot are locked and allow for rapid use as a stable platform for propulsion. The foot is, however, poorly adapted for shock absorption and is predisposed to lateral instability. Additionally the relative risk of injury to the lower extremity afflicted with a supinated foot type is generally six times that of a rectus foot type [3].

Rigidity and poor shock absorption characterize the supinated foot and place it at risk for stress fractures throughout the lower extremity [6]. The supinated foot is also poorly adapted for jumping due to its poor ability to absorb shock at impact. Sports, such as football, requiring frequent jumping further predispose the athlete to stress fractures and tendinopathies [3]. The forefoot is plantarflexed and in valgus during the rebound phase of the jump which limits available range of motion for shock absorption and places greater stress to the bones and joints of the lower extremity [3]. Increased rigidity of the midfoot predisposes the athlete to midtarsal bone stress fractures or ligament sprains [6, 12, 13]. Limited subtalar joint motion may make the athlete prone to stress fractures of the calcaneus from the pull of the plantar fascia and other attachments to the plantar calcaneus [5]. Plantar fascia tears or strains may also be seen. Stress fractures of tibia are seen proximally and are linked to a cavus foot type [5]. Decreased shock absorption of the entire lower extremity may also eventually lead to fractures of the femur and pelvis in high-contact sports such as football [5]. Furthermore anterior compartment or shin splint syndrome is observed due to an increased absorption of kinetic energy by the anterior muscle group of the leg [5]. Ground reactive forces are absorbed through the musculature of the lower extremity in an attempt by the body to dampen the loads placed upon it during locomotion.

Overload of the lateral column of the foot secondary to a supinated or cavus foot type results in several possible compensation patterns by the lower extremity. The athlete is prone to developing peroneal tendonitis or a peroneal cuboid syndrome [5]. Central and/or lateral strains of the Achilles tendon may also be observed due to the overload of the lateral column and varus position of the calcaneus [5]. An athlete with a rearfoot varus and cavus foot type may complain of retrocalcaneal bursitis or exostosis also secondary to the increased strain from the Achilles tendon [7]. Lateral instability may further cause lateral strain to the knee causing an iliotibial band syndrome or greater trochanteric bursitis at the hip [2].

Functional equinus is often associated with a cavus foot. There is an increased stress placed under the ball of the foot straining the plantar fascia and intrinsic musculature of the foot [7]. Stress fractures of the sesamoids are common due to increased stress placed plantar to the first metatarsal [7]. Anterior equinus places an increased load on the plantar aspect of the calcaneus by stretching the plantar intrinsic musculature and fascia as well as the gastrocnemius–soleus complex [7]. The foot is very rigid and does not allow for redistribution of the load medially during the stance phase. Therefore, such athletes are prone to lateral instability of the foot and ankle secondary to overload of the lateral column.

Lateral ankle sprains are commonly seen in football due to the repetitive side-to-side movements performed when an athlete is required to rapidly plant his foot and cut to change direction [12]. Furthermore high ankle sprains (tibiofibular syndesmotic tears), which are commonly seen in football, may be associated with symptomatic ossification of the syndesmosis following severe injury [14]. The astute clinician should be capable of diagnosing a syndesmotic tear and aggressively treating the athlete with immobilization and rest. Ossification of the syndesmosis may possibly be symptomatic in an athlete by hindering the force progression from the hip to the foot by blocking the internal rotation of the leg and also limiting pronation at the subtalar joint. A review of injury prevention strategies found that the risk of suffering from an ankle sprain was reduced with balance-training/proprioceptive exercises [13]. Orthoses were also found to be more effective than taping and that they should be implemented for at least 6 months following a moderate-to-severe ankle sprain [14].

Footwear Recommendations

Appropriate football shoe gear is essential for the ability of the foot to absorb high-impact forces and for injury prevention during this multidirectional sport. There are many different important characteristics of football shoe gear [15].

Astute football shoe recommendations can be made based on a vast knowledge of lower extremity kinematics, ground reaction forces, and an appropriate understanding of the varying positional demands on the field of the quarterback, kicker, as well offensive and defensive players [16]. Each position may at times engage in sprinting, stopping, and cutting movements, increasing friction that is created when ground reaction forces are increased thus and transmitted through the lower extremity increasing the potential for injury [17].

The correlation between modern football cleat design and athletic performance has generated scientific sports medicine research relating to the injury potential of traction aids. The incidence of lower extremity injuries is diverse and can be correlated shoe characteristics associated with cleat length and width, environmental factors and selected playing turfs (natural or artificial), and the torsional resistance sustained [18, 19]. Determining the efficiency of a shoe for football must encompass important facets including correct knowledge of the shoe–surface interface, release coefficients and minimizing excessive shoe fixation, and environmental conditions [12, 20]. Selection of the cleat design tailored specifically to a player's positioning and appropriate playing surface are injury preventative measures.

Historical Background

Athletic performance on the football field is enhanced when sharp quick internal muscular forces are coupled with traction and converted into motion. Historically, the association of rigid foot fixation and cleats inducing ankle and knee injuries led many proponents to challenge and further investigate and recommend alternative cleat designs back in the late 1960s and early 1970s [21]. Clinical implications of football injuries associated with excessive foot fixation were investigated initially, and then further propagated by Torg et al. [12, 20]. They developed an experimental design that replicated the necessary torque needed to disengage a shoe–surface interface and concluded that a safe release coefficient was 0.31 or less concluded after thorough investigation that football cleats should include a synthetic molded sole, have a minimum of 14 cleats, maintain a 1/2 inch cleat diameter and stipulated that the cleat should be no longer than 3/8 in. [12, 20]. After many observations of non-contact injuries to the lower extremity based on the above-mentioned study and other conventional research, cleat modifications and designs were made including plastic heel disks, lower profile oval cleats, and cleats attached to a rotation turn table as well as the evolution of a turf shoe designed specially for synthetic playing surfaces [19]. Scientific research continues and the development and evolution of the modern football cleat continue to motivate shoe-manufacturing companies.

Cleat Selection

While there are different facets of the modern football shoe to molded football cleats, turf shoes, replacement cleats, and kicking shoes. There are several cleat characteristics that should be determined when selecting the most appropriate shoe based on level of competition and player positioning. Each unique cleated shoe is made up of an upper, midsole, and outsole and can be selected based on its weight, color, and profile appropriate for the position and skill level [22]. Cleats can be mainly categorized by three main styles including high-tops, mid-cuts, and low-cuts dependent upon the positions [23] (Fig. 20.1a,b).

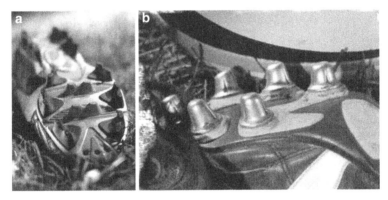

Fig. 20.1 (**a** and **b**). Newer evolved plastic lower profile oval cleats versus the traditional metal elongated cleats

Materials

Outsoles can include microfiber synthetic leather, kangaroo leather, or full grain leather all which known to be soft, lightweight, and tough. The outsole has a number of different stud configurations and shapes including circular studs specifically designed to provide perfect stud pressure reduction. Additionally, cleats with blades are designed to grab the field and provide comfort, whereas molded studs are ideal for firm ground with replaceable studs for softer ground [22].

The midsole is usually made from a foam that has been compressed using heat. Manufacturers use many different types of foam depending on the cleat being made. There are models which bring the foot closer to the ground, increasing agility, whereas certain models provide great comfort and stud pressure reduction and include a molded sockliner to provide an exceptional fit [22]. Internal lacing systems have also been implemented for various cleats which are suggested to help properly secure the cleat.

Overall, molded cleat patterns are suited for artificial or hard ground surfaces. Kicking shoes are created with a blunt nose and curved forefoot for power kicking. Replacement cleats consist of a set of interchanged spikes for detachable foot cleat shoes and are available in different types and sizes [22].

Lacing Techniques

Many cleat lacing patterns accommodate a variety of sizes and incorporate variable widths comfortably. There is prescriptive lacing that exists for each designated foot type including lock lacing, lacing for high insteps, narrow and wide feet. A locking lace helps accommodate for foot expansion and is performed using the extra two holes that may or maybe found at the top of the cleat inserting the lace back through the shoe. For players with a cavus-type foot stability can be added by performing a cross lace below the instep. Based upon the exact width of the player's foot, lacing techniques can be employed that use the specific lace holes that width to make the cleat fit narrow, whereas the exact opposite technique can be used for a wider foot [24].

Ankle Spatting

Ankle spatting or the technique of direct tape application over the shoe to enhance ankle stability is an attempt to counteract the 21% loss in the support of applied ankle tape. Whereas, the types of tape and the techniques used to apply it vary greatly, if done correctly, spatting will help maintain the shoe's proper position on the foot and ankle by reducing inversion for many players [7, 25].

Ankle Bracing

One of the most important proponents for preventing ankle sprains in the football player is the ability of the brace to restrict ankle inversion and eversion before landing from a jump. A semirigid pneumatic ankle brace provides a semirigid orthosis, provides support, and also functions to reduce ankle edema and ankle inversion. This provides the athlete a greater capacity to prevent frontal plane motion as well as to limit sagittal-plane ankle motion, and may help prevent lateral ankle sprains [26].

Orthoses

Because a linkage system exists within the lower extremity, questions should be raised about what effect an orthotic device will have, if any. As a general rule, a soft orthosis functions more to help absorb the impact of initial ground contact along with the shoe material [26]. For individuals engaged in football, a material that helps to absorb some of this impact could be beneficial if the athlete is having problems related to impact, such as heel pain, metatarsalgia, turf toe, or seasmoiditis [4]. On a more sophisticated level, the use of a varus heel wedge, whether in the shoe or within an orthotic device, may have some influence on the rotation of the subtalar joint. Because at the time of initial ground contact rapid eversion of the subtalar joint and flattening of the longitudinal arch occur, a buildup of material along the medial arch that prevents some of this rotation from occurring in theory would decrease the amount of internal rotation being transmitted to the lower extremity [27].

Sock Selection

Many different forces are placed upon the feet of an individual playing football due to the dynamic shearing forces that occur with running, sprinting, cutting, and in stance positions. The most appropriate athletic sock may be debatable, selection of a suitable sock fiber is a key element in the avoidance of friction blister formation a common injuries on the feet when dynamic shearing forces as present. Acrylic sock fibers have been associated with significantly smaller blister sizes as compared to cotton fiber socks [28].

Footwear Recommendations for Common Football Pathologies

Turf Toe

Football players are at greatest risk for this injury as they are tackled while landing from a jump or if another player lands on the back of their heel forcing the first MTP joint into hyperdorsiflexion. Usually, the plantar portion of the ligamentous complex tears, while the plantar plate becomes detached distal to the sesamoids [29, 30]. Turf toe injury is most commonly seen when an axial load is delivered to a foot that is fixed in equinus. This is a common occurrence in football lineman and involves the fixation of the forefoot on the ground in the dorsiflexed position with the heel raised [31].

Artificial turf surfaces and the use of poorly supported midsole shoes have increased the development of this condition. Shoe modifications incorporating a stiffer sole or an orthosis with a rigid forefoot section will help to limit hallux dorsiflexion and prevent hyperextension reinjury [4, 29].

Sesamoiditis

The tibial (medial) and fibular (lateral) sesamoids are important components of the first metatarsophalangeal joint complex and prone to injury in a football player due to the repetitive, excessive pressure on the forefoot [32]. Cleats with little insole

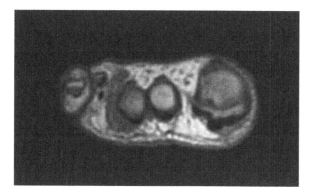

Fig. 20.2 Longstanding painful neuroma identified via MRI between the third and fourth metatarsal heads

padding can center excess stress on the first MTP or sesamoid and thus can facilitate the development of sesamoiditis. A player's sharp cutting movements and sudden deceleration with a high impact on the sesamoid bones can predispose a player to injury with hyperdorsiflexion. A custom-molded orthosis may be added into the insole to redistribute forefoot pressures [33].

Neuroma

A football player with an interdigital neuroma may complain of distinct symptoms of forefoot burning, cramping, tingling, and numbness in the toes of the involved interspace (Fig. 20.2). There are several accommodative devices that may be utilized including a forefoot pad with a metatarsal dome and a metatarsal lift pad. The metatarsal pad can also be incorporated into a custom-made full length semirigid orthosis within the shoe [6, 34].

Metatarsalgia

Many football players have previously complained of pain in the plantar aspects of the metatarsal heads, also known as metatarsalgia. Any biomechanical intrinsic or extrinsic circumstances that increase stress on the metatarsal heads may result in metatarsal head pain and the development of painful plantar keratoses [30]. An orthotic device, such as a metatarsal pad placed proximal to the painful metatarsal heads, may be helpful. Custom-made orthoses may also be molded specifically for the cavus foot to decrease load on the plantarflexed first and second rays in order to distribute weight evenly across the forefoot [27].

Lateral Ankle Sprains

Football predisposes many players to an inversion ankle sprain to the nature of cutting and pivoting which place the ankle at risk for inversion injuries. The mechanism for lateral ankle sprains can be described as a combination of inversion, plantar flexion, and internal rotation. The use of external support such as bracing or taping can decrease the incidence of lateral ankle sprains by limiting frontal plane ankle movement [15, 35].

Syndesmotic Ankle Sprains

The mechanism of injury for syndesmosis sprains has classically been ascribed to the ankle being subjected to an external rotation moment with the foot in a dorsiflexed, pronated position [36]. Management options can include a period of non-weightbearing with the use of crutches while in the acute phase with casting or bracing of the ankle including a semirigid pneumatic ankle brace of an individual [37, 38].

References

1. Thacker S, Stroup D, Branche C, Gilchrist J, Goodman R, Weitman E: The Prevention of Ankle Sprains in Sports A Systematic Review of the Literature. Am J Sports Med, 27(6): 753–760, 1999.
2. Bates B, Stergiou N: Normal Patterns of Walking and Running. in, Subotnick S, Strauss M, (eds.), Sports Medicine of the Lower Extremity, 2nd ed., 157–165. WB Saunders Co. 1999.
3. Fields KB, Bloom JO, Priebe D, Foreman B: Basic Biomechanics of the Lower Extremity. Primary Care: Clin Off Pract, 32:245–251, 2004.
4. McGuine T: Sports Injuries in High School Athletes: A Review of Injury-Risk and Injury-Prevention Research. Clin J Sport Med 16(6): 488–499, 2006.
5. Subotnick S: Sports-Specific Biomechanics, in: Subotnick S, Strauss M, (eds.), Sports Medicine of the Lower Extremity, 2nd ed., WB Saunders Co, 187–198, 1999.
6. Wu K. Morton's interdigital neuroma: a clinical review of its etiology, treatment and results. J. Foot Ankle Surg. 35:112–119, 1996.
7. Subotnick S: Clinical Biomechanics: Biomechanics of the foot and ankle. in: Subotnick S, Strauss M, (eds.), Sports Medicine of the Lower Extremity, 2nd ed., WB Saunders Co. 127–136, 1999.
8. Boerum V, Sangeorzan B: Biomechanics and pathiophysiology of flat foot. FootAnkle Clin 8(3):419–430, 2003.
9. Ochsendorf D, Mattacola C, Arnold B: Effect of Orthotics on Postural Sway After Fatigue of the Plantar Flexors and Dorsiflexors. J Athl Train. 35(1):26–30, 2000.
10. Davis I. Foot Structure, Mechanics, and Injury Risk. J Orthop Sports Phys Ther, 35(5): A15–A16, 2005.
11. Dick R, Ferrara M, Agel J, Courson R, Marshall S, Hanley M, Reifsteck F: Descriptive Epidemiology of Collegiate Men's Football Injuries: National Collegiate Athletic Association Injury Surveillance System, 1988–1989 Through 2003–2004. J Athl Train, 42(2): 221–233, 2007.
12. Mann, Roger A: Foot and Ankle. Section A: Biomechanics of the Foot and Ankle Linkage. in, DeLee J, Drez J, Miller M, (ed.), DeLee: DeLee and Drez's, Orthop Sports Med, 2nd ed. Philadelphia, PA: Saunders, 2003

13. McNerney J: Football Injuries. in, Subotnick S, Strauss M, (eds.), Sports Medicine of the Lower Extremity, 2nd ed. WB Saunders Co. 739–745, 1999.

14. Wetherbee E, Garbalosa J, Donatelli R,Wooden M: Dysfunction, Evaluation, and Treatment of the Foot and Ankle. in, Donatelli RA (ed.), Orthopaedic Physical Therapy, 3rd ed. St. Louis, MO: Churchill Livingstone, 2001.

15. Mullen J, O'Malley M: Sprains-residual instability of subtalar, Lisfranc joints, and turf toe. Clin Sports Med, 23:97–121, 2004.

16. Herbenick M, King J, Altobelli G, Njuyen B, Podesta L: Injury Patterns in Professional Arena football. Am J Sports Med, 36(1):91–98, 2008.

17. Cawley P, Heidt R, Scranton P, Losse G: Physiologic Axial Load, Frictional Resistance, and the Football Shoe-Surface Interface. Foot Ankle Int. 24(7):551–556, 2003.

18. Culpepper M, Nieman K: An Investigation of the shoe-turf interface using different types of Poly-Turf and Astro-Turf: Torque and release and release coefficients. Ala J Med Sci 2: 387–390, 1983.

19. Hedit R, Domer S, Cawley P, et al.: Differences in friction and torsional resistance in athletic shoe-turf surface interfaces. Am J Sports Med, 24:834–842, 1996.

20. Torg J, Stilwell S, Rogers K: The effect of ambient temperature on the shoe-surface interface release coefficient. Am J Sports Med. 24:79–82, 1996.

21. Bowers D, Martin B: Impact Absorption, new and old Astro Turf at West Virginia. Med Sci Sports. 6:217–221, 1974.

22. Football Cleats. http://www.weplaysports.com/football/shoes. 7/29/2008.

23. Football Cleats – 5 Things to Know. http://www.usafootball.com/articles/league-enhancement/center-articles/18-league-enhance.7/8/2008

24. Lambson R, Barnhill B, Higgins R: Football Cleat Design and Its Effect on Anterior Cruciate Ligament Injuries A Three-Year Prospective Study. Am J Sports Med. 24(2):155–160, 1996.

25. Prisk V, O'Loughlin P, Kennedy J: Forefoot injuries in dancers. Clin Sports Med, 27: 305–320, 2008.

26. DiStefano L, Padua D, Brown C, Guskiewicz K: Lower Extremity Kinematics and Ground Reaction Forces After Prophylactic Lace-Up Ankle Bracing. Journal of Athl Train, 43(3): 234–241, 2008.

27. Hoffman S, Peterson M. Foot Orthotics: An Overview of Rationale, Assessment, and Fabrications. In Donatelli RA (ed.), Orthopaedic Physical Therapy, 3rd ed. St. Louis, MO: Churchill Livingstone, 2001.

28. Herring K, Richie D: Comparison of cotton and acrylic socks using a generic cushion sole design for runners. J Am Podiat Med Assoc, 83(9):515–522, 1993.

29. Clanton T, Ford J: Turf Toe Injury. Clin Sport Med, 13(4):731–41, 1994.

30. Umans H. Imaging Sports Medicine Injuries of the Foot and Toes. Clin Sports Med, 25: 763–780, 2006.

31. Nelson A, Collins C, Yard E, Fields S, Comstock D: Ankle Injuries Among United States High School Sports Athletes. J Athl Train, 42(3):381–387, 2007.

32. Shapiro MS, Kabo M, Mitchell PW, et al.: Ankle sprain prophylaxis: An analysis of the stabilizing effects of braces and tape. Am J Sports Med 22:78–82., 1994

33. Hockenbury T:. Forefoot problems in athletes, Foot Ankle Clin Suppl, 31 (7), 1999.

34. Weinfeld S, Myerson S: Interdigital neuroma. J Am Acad Orthop Surg, 4:328–335, 1996.

35. Beynnon B, Murphy D, Alosa D: Predictive Factors for Lateral Ankle Sprains: A Literature Review. J Athl Train, 37(4):376–380, 2002.

36. Novacheck T: The biomechanics of running. GaitPosture, 7(1):77–95.

37. Smith M, Broker S, Vicenzino B, McPoil T: Use of anti-pronation taping to assess suitability of orthotic prescription: Case report. Aust J Physiother. 50:111–113, 2004.

38. Williams G, Jones M, Amendola A: Syndesmotic Ankle Sprains in Athletes. Clin Sports Med Update, 35(7):1197–1207, 2007

Chapter 21
Soccer

Robert M. Conenello

Soccer is, without question, the most popular sport in the world. It is easy to learn, relatively safe, can be played by those of all athletic abilities, and offers equal opportunities for boys and girls. Unlike other sports, soccer is a game of non-stop movement that requires a player to move quickly in all directions. It is also unique in that the players must use their feet to control and advance the ball. This chapter provides the reader with a resource for the variety of footgear available to the modern soccer player.

Lower Extremity Biomechanics and Considerations of Soccer

The soccer player is an extremely fit athlete who requires healthy lower extremities to succeed. The ability to move proficiently in all directions requires the feet to remain as close to neutral as possible. Running and sprinting in the forward and oblique directions are usually employed by all players, especially those positions attacking the goal. The skills of dribbling, maintaining control of the ball while running, and passing, as well as the inside of the foot pass, are essential at all levels of play. In order to pass, the player must balance on the non-kicking leg, bend the knee of the kicking leg, turn out from the hip of the kicking leg, look down at the ball and then swing the kicking leg [1]. Most high level soccer players need to be able to perform these motions equally well with both feet in order to be successful.

Soccer also requires players to maintain their balance while moving quickly and while backpedaling. Defenders use this skill by stabilizing themselves on the balls of their feet while moving backwards and side to side.

Jumping for a ball is also quite common during play. The player must be able to propel their body either up or side to side while having substantial proprioceptive abilities, while landing to prevent injuries. The goalkeeper is unique in that he/she

R.M. Conenello (✉)
Orangetown Podiatry, .450 Western Highway, Orangeburg, NY 10962, USA

M.B. Werd, E.L. Knight (eds.), *Athletic Footwear and Orthoses in Sports Medicine*,
DOI 10.1007/978-0-387-76416-0_21, © Springer Science+Business Media, LLC 2010

typically employs a low center of gravity with a wide stance ready to react in all directions.

A neutral or rectus foot type foot type is ideally suited for the ever changing demand that a soccer player encounters. The cavus foot type is at higher risk for inversion type injuries due to the constant cutting, as well as the possibility of entanglement with another player while challenging for a ball. A pes planus type foot will fatigue more quickly and leave the player more vulnerable for overuse injuries, such as plantar fasciitis and shin splints.

General Footwear Recommendations

The soccer shoe, or boot as it is commonly referred to, has evolved tremendously over the years. The surfaces on which the game is played on are varied, and as a result shoe manufacturers have created surface-specific shoes. The difficulty associated with playing soccer on different types of grounds has made it necessary for the shoes to offer proper resistance or ground traction.

Anatomy of a Soccer Shoe

In general shoes are comprised of two regions: the upper and the outsole. Different materials and technologies can merge to make a varied selection of shoes.

Upper Materials

The upper materials found in soccer shoes are composed of either leather or synthetic. According to Nick Romonsky, DPM, podiatrist for the United States national soccer team "The new uppers are now better mirroring the anatomical contour of the foot. Even the heel counter is contoured for a better fit and the overall shape helps provide comfort, stability, and better ball handling."

Leather uppers seem to be more popular with more experienced players due to their overall comfort. Carlos Alarcon of Eski's Sports in Ramsey, New Jersey, has been fitting players of all levels with shoes for the past seven years. He states "leather shoes will mold to the feet over time, and will allow for better feel of the ball by creating greater friction." True leather shoes are classified as either full grain or Kangaroo leather. Full grain is sturdy and offers better longevity than the more specialized leathers. The most expensive leather upper is K-leather or Kangaroo leather, which is a softer product that makes the shoe feel lighter and more form fitting. It is not as durable as full grain leather and wet weather will promote breakdown, so care should be taken to protect it.

Interestingly enough, many of the leading soccer shoe manufacturers are utilizing synthetic materials in their high end products. These shoes are manufactured with special microfiber technology. The Nike Mercurial Vapor uses Teijin fibers for this purpose. This fiber when exposed to sweat immediately becomes twice as thick for a smooth inflow of air [2]. This creates a good wear comfort depending on the condition of the wearer. The overall result of this adaptive material is increased comfort for the player.

On the opposite end of the synthetic spectrum are plastic type shoes seen in entry level cleats. These inexpensive shoes do not allow the release of moisture, which can lead to blisters. The plastic footwear may also form a fold or crease where the foot bends which may lead to potential hot spots or blisters. It is this author's opinion that these types of cleats should be reserved only for the very young player who is just being introduced to the sport.

Outsole Materials

Every type of outsole material is manufactured to perform under certain field conditions. The shoe must assure good contact with the playing surface, and the sole must adapt optimally to all types of surfaces [3]. The cleat should provide the player with enough traction to prevent from slipping and allowing the opportunity to turn, stop and accelerate easily.

Molded Shoes

These are the most common types of cleats and are best for use on firm natural playing surfaces. The rubber or hardened plastic projections provide traction control and support. These boots are ideal for beginning and intermediate players as they can be used on most types of playing surfaces. The traditional molded shoe contains a sole that has between ten and fifteen round studs (Fig. 21.1a,b). The bladed or x-grip design utilizes slimmer studs, strategically placed in different angles to offer a player better footing.

Detachable Cleats

These are cleats designed for unstable or usually slippery natural surfaces. They have fewer, longer studs than a firm ground shoe, and are usually made of hard

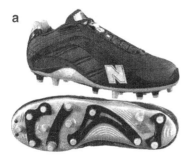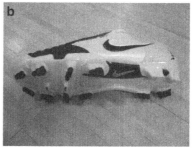

Fig. 21.1 (**a**) New Balance and (**b**) Nike soccer shoes showing molded cleats (a, courtesy of New Balance, Boston, MA)

plastic or metal tips. The type and length of the cleat can be changed depending on the weather and field condition. The reason there are fewer studs is so that mud and grass won't get trapped on the bottom of the footwear and make the soccer shoe become heavy [4].

Turfs

These types of shoes are commonly referred to as "turfs" as they are best suited for hard artificial playing surfaces (Fig. 21.2). The outside consists of multiple short rubber studs. This cleat pattern is more forgiving on the feet and body as it more evenly distributes pressure across the entire foot. These hard ground shoes are the author's choice for youth soccer players since they provide adequate traction but offer the most comfort for young feet.

Referees are an often forgotten population of the soccer world, that tend to be on their feet for many hours in a day. Dr. Paul Trinkoff, a Chiroprator and NCAA soccer referee, states, "Referees can be assigned to multiple games in a single day. The large amount of running puts a huge demand on the individual's feet, no matter what the surface. It is for this reason that the Turf, which is somewhat of a hybrid between a cleat and a sneaker, is the shoe of choice of most referees. The turf seems to accommodate well to all surfaces without compromising comfort or support."

Hybrid

The Adidas Tunit premium show is unique in that it is an adaptable system. It offers three upper soles, interchangeable chassis and all three sets of cleats for all playing surfaces and conditions.

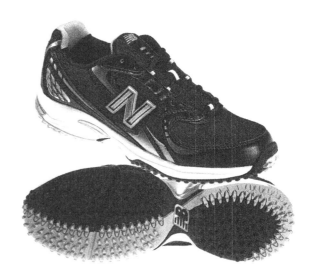

Fig. 21.2 Turfs shoes have many short rubber studs for hard artificial playing surfaces. (Courtesy of New Balance, Boston, MA)

Indoor

This type of shoe is intended to be played on hard flat surfaces such as gym floors. These low profiled shoes usually have gum rubber bottoms with a tread patters similar to traditional sneakers. Players will often opt for this type of shoe over a turf as the soles usually offer greater ball control.

Midsole

Unlike other sport shoes, soccer cleats are made very low to the ground with minimal midsole material. This design allows the player's foot to feel closer to the ground for optimal feel and aggressive maneuverability without sacrificing comfort. The problem encountered with this negative heel design is that it can cause a greater amount of traction on the heel through a pulling force of the Achilles tendon and the plantar fascia.

Manufacturers have created many proprietary technologies built to cushion and support feet from fatigue. Some of these include an insert of low density polyurethane or EVA placed in the sole below the heel. This feature aids in cushioning and helps protect the foot by absorbing and dissipating impact forces [5].

Lacing

Most soccer shoes incorporate a traditional lacing system as is seen in tennis shoes. Newer models utilize an innovative asymmetrical loop lacing system. These laces are oriented obliquely with a Velcro secured fold over tongue. The concept is to provide more foot to ball contact for better ball striking accuracy and ball spin.

According to Dr. Romansky, there could be potential problems associated with this lacing pattern. He states "There may be a decrease in the stability of the upper of the shoe which may shift to the side of the lacing system. Furthermore, a lacing system placed in such a manner may interfere with a player's ability to properly put spin on the ball."

Shin Guards

One other piece of equipment utilized by the soccer player is shin guards. These are small hard plastic guards that cover the anterior of the lower leg. Some styles of shin pads are incorporated into an anklet which also may have detachable ankle supports. The added bulk of these will affect the fit of the soccer shoe. It is for this reason that the player must be fitted for his boot with all game-related gear.

Orthoses

The use of custom molded functional orthotic devices in a soccer shoe can be quite challenging. The fit of a soccer shoe is different from that of street shoes as they are often designed with a more narrow upper and have overall smaller volume. This leads to a very neat fit for the player. Trying to add any sort of functional insert to this shoe design can be challenging.

A soccer device should increase contact surface area under the foot, stabilizing the rear-foot and mid-foot, which influences knee alignment during rapid deceleration [6]. Such a device consists of a co-polymer/crepe shell, posted with medium density crepe in the rear-foot. The heel cup is shallow at 5 mm. A 1/16" polyfoam top cover will mold to the foot and provide a nonskid surface, even in wet conditions.

Common Injuries and Preventions

The amount of time a soccer player spends in a game is minimal compared to the hours of practice and conditioning these athletes are engaged in. While repetitive drills, running and conditioning will make the player more proficient, it also increases the risk of injury. These ailments can be classified as either cumulative (overuse) or acute (traumatic) injuries. Overuse injuries may present as nagging soreness that is often overlooked, but can quickly manifest into a much more serious pathology. Acute injuries occur due to a sudden force or impact and can be quite dramatic.

Apophysitis

This is a growth plate disorder most commonly seen in the calcaneous (Severs Disease). It affects young athletes between the ages of 8 and 14 who are usually going through a growth spurt. This heel pain usually presents as a result of traction to the calcaneal apophysis from both the Achilles tendon and plantar fascia insertion. Clinical signs include compression tenderness of the growth plate on direct palpation and pain upon ambulation. The soccer cleat does not offer the player the same level of shock absorbency as a standard running shoe. It is also designed with a negative heel where the heel is lower than the toes. This causes pressure to be placed on the heel which leads to inflammation and pain.

Reducing the excessive motions of the foot in the cleat can help eliminate the player's symptoms. This is accomplished by adding a heel lift to reduce the tension on the Achilles and plantar fascia. As symptoms subside, a functional orthotic device may be fabricated to help prevent recurrence.

Plantar Fasciitis

This is an inflammation of the plantar fibrous attachment of the calcaneous to the ball of the foot. This is characterized by first step pain usually seen at medial aspect of the heel and arch. Fasciitis is exacerbated in the soccer player due to shoes with minimal arch support. An orthotic device that can decelerate pronation yet still fit comfortably in a soccer cleat will help alleviate the player's symptoms.

Achilles Tendonitis

Running and jumping on softer pitches can lead to excessive pronation. The flat soccer shoe is ill equipped to prevent these pathologic motions. As a result, increased motion above the calcaneous can cause an increased pull on the Achilles tendon. As a result, the tendon thickens and causes pinpoint tenderness proximally 4 cm above its insertion. A neoprene heel lift can be placed in the boot to decrease the tendon's pull. The player should also select cleats that have a rigid heel counter which can cradle the back of the heel. The counter should be rigid from the outside while affording sufficient internal padding.

Soccer Toe

This injury is a result of a painful jam or hyper-extension of the big toe. When a player tries to pivot quickly and utilizes the hallux to perform this motion, extreme pain may result. This condition is more common on artificial turf but can happen on grass as well. Treatment includes a stiffer, hard toe shoe that fits perfectly so that the entire ball of the foot is used for turning as opposed to only the large toes.

Inversion Injuries

These injuries include lateral ankle sprains and fifth metatarsal fractures. They are often seen by direct player to player contact while challenging for the ball. Usually contact is made when the foot and ankle are firmly planted in the turf. Improper cleat selection for the playing surface is often the culprit for these injuries. The player must select a stud pattern that will provide traction but will not sink deeply into the ground causing instability.

For patients with chronic lateral foot and ankle instability a custom molded functional orthotic device may be used. A low profile device with a rear-foot posted to neutral and a valgus posted forefoot may help prevent such injuries.

Conclusion

The dynamics surrounding soccer makes it imperative for the clinician to understand all of the variables involved in the modern game. A thorough evaluation of the player's shoe gear and fit and the surfaces they play on are all components that must be considered to prevent injury and increase productive participation.

References

1. Averbuch G, Hammond A: Goal! The Ultimate Guide for Soccer Moms and Dads. Rodale Press, New York, NY, 1999. p. 51.
2. Asian Economic News 8/1/2006
3. Masson M, Hess H: Typical Soccer Injuries – Their Effects on the Design of Athletic Shoes, in Segesser B, Pforringer W (eds.), The Shoe in Sport, pp. 89–95. Chicago, IL: Year Book Publishers, 1987:
4. www.soccerwebsite.org/cleats.html
5. www.soccergameinformation.com
6. www.biomechanics.com

Suggested Reading

1. Albert M: Descriptive three year data study of outdoor and indoor professional soccer injuries. Athl Train, 18:218, 1983
2. Auerbach G, Hammond A: Goal! The Ultimate Guide for Soccer Moms and Dads, Rodale Press Inc. 1999.
3. Braver R: Treatment solutions for common soccer injuries. Podiatr Today, Issue #10 2003.
4. Clonton T, Ford J: Turf toe injury. Clins Sports Med, 13(4):731–741, 1994.
5. Ekstrand J, Gillquist J: Soccer Injuries and Their Mechanisms: A Prospective Study. Med. Sci. Sports, 15:276, 1983.
6. Pribut S, Richie D: Separating the Buzz from the Biomechanics: A Guide to Athletic Shoe Trends and Innovations, pp. 85–97. Podiatr Manag, 2004
7. Romansky N, Soccer Injuries, in, Subotnick, S., Sports Medicine of the Lower Extremity, pp. 697–702. Churchill Livingstone Publishers, Philadelphia, Pensylvania 1999
8. Sullivan JA, Gross RH et al.: Evaluation of injuries in youth soccer. Am J Sports Med 8:325, 1980.
9. Torg JS, Pavlov H, Torg E: Overuse Injuries in Sports: The Foot. Clin Sports Med 6:291, 1987

Chapter 22
Skating

R. Neil Humble and Hilary Smith

Skating in all its various forms has shown increased popularity worldwide. Olympic speed skating champions are coming from areas of warm climate, and ice hockey teams are starting up in almost every populated geographical location. There are three major types of ice skating: hockey skating, figure skating, and speed skating. All these forms of ice skating have similarities and differences with respect to footwear and biomechanics. A close cousin to the three major types of ice skating is in-line skating. This is a similar biomechanical activity and an increasingly common recreational and fitness endeavor.

Management of all the various forms of skating with respect to both performance and injury reduction involves discussion of footwear. In general, all footwear functions to both improve performance and lessen the likelihood of injury. Skate boots also do this and depending on the demands of the type of skating being done the boot type and structure can change dramatically.

All skate boots function first to help protect the foot from acute external traumatic events, second to protect the foot within the boot by adding internal comfort, and finally to assist in performance-based outcomes and biomechanics of the sport.

Hockey Skate Boots

Anatomically there are three main parts of a hockey skate boot: the boot itself, the blade housing, and the blade (Fig. 22.1). First, the skate boot itself is generally rigid for protection and support. As with most athletic footwear the lasts vary from one manufacturer to another. Other than a good fit, one must carefully look at the pitch of the boot from heel to toe, which can vary from 5 to 9° and affect forward lean.

R.N. Humble (✉)
Department of Surgery, Division of Podiatry, University of Calgary, #308, 4935 40th Ave. NW, Calgary, AB T3A 2N1, Canada

Adapted from Humble RN. Podiatric management in ice skating. Podiatry Management November/December 2003, pp. 49–63, with permission.

M.B. Werd, E.L. Knight (eds.), *Athletic Footwear and Orthoses in Sports Medicine*,   247
DOI 10.1007/978-0-387-76416-0_22, © Springer Science+Business Media, LLC 2010

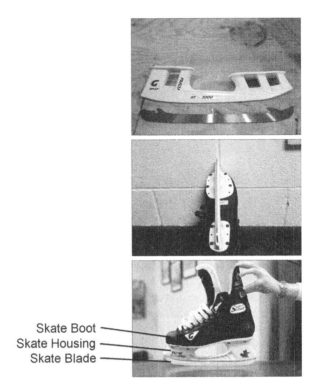

Skate Boot
Skate Housing
Skate Blade

Fig. 22.1 Skate anatomy. (From Humble RN. Podiatric management in ice skating. Podiatry Management November/December 2003, pp. 49–63, with permission.)

With respect to lasts the heel fit is the most important single fitting point. Boots can be stretched and adjusted in the forefoot, but if the heel does not fit well and without slippage, adjustments are difficult. The fit of a skate is slightly different than that for regular shoes. Sewn skates generally fit one to one and a half sizes smaller than one's regular shoe size. Skates need to fit snugly and toes should "feather" the toe cap. Interior in the boot is the liner of the heel counter. This portion of the boot is usually made with heat moldable materials, to allow for individual player differences and thus comfort adaptations. Also on the interior of the boot is a removable insole under which lies the skate blade housing rivets.

The exterior of skates was traditionally leather, but gradually have been substituted with synthetic materials. Graphite and polypropylene materials have been added for strength and protection of the boot with flex points added to allow proper ankle joint plantarflexion in the skating motion. The toe cap is always rigid for toe protection.

The next part of a skate is the skate blade housing. This portion of the skate is riveted or screwed onto the boot itself. The attachment of the blade housing to the boot can be a point of biomechanical input. This housing can be moved medial to lateral, or anterior to posterior on the boot. Its standard position is to hold the blade centrally under the heel and then to continue forward under the second metatarsal head and further forward through the second digit. The blade housing can also act as an attachment site for heel lifts and wedges as they are sandwiched between the housing and boot. The portion of the rivet inside the boot can be a potential source of irritation.

The last anatomic portion of a skate is the narrow skate blade itself. This portion of the skate is traditionally made of stainless steel and is a necessity given the surface of the activity but can be adjusted in many ways for specific biomechanical effect. It is rockered front to back and can be varied for desired performance. The rocker acts as a balance point with as little as 1 in. contacting the ice. A longer radius of curvature allows for more blades to contact the ice and thus can improve balance and speed. A shorter radius of curvature increases the ease of turning and improves maneuverability. The bottom surface of the blade is hollow ground to create a medial and lateral edge or bite angle (Fig. 22.2). This curvature of hollow can be altered at the time of sharpening to get a desired bite into the ice. The technology in skate blades is ever changing. One newer technology is disposable titanium blades that can be purchased with varying degrees of rocker and with varying curvatures of hollow. These blades stay sharper longer than traditional stainless steel blades and can be easily removed and replaced when worn out or damaged. An even more recent advancement in blade manufacturing is the ability to buy blades with varying bite angles. These blades are presently being tested to prove their expected capability to increase speed and turning ability.

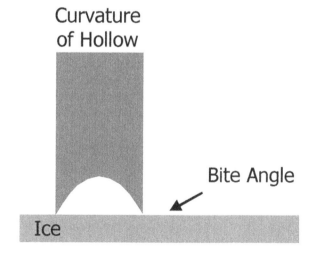

Fig. 22.2 Frontal plane blade–ice contact; surface is hollow ground along its length. (From Humble RN. Podiatric management in ice skating. Podiatry Management November/December 2003, pp. 49–63, with permission.)

Goalie Skates

Goaltender skates are similar to player skates, with some obvious differences specific to the requirements of the position (Fig. 22.3). The boot itself does not go as high up the lower leg as traditional skate boots. This is primarily due to the need for increased ankle mobility in this position. Also, the skate blade housing encompasses the entire lower portion of the boot to create a plastic housing of protection for the foot. The blade has a longer radius of curvature to help improve balance, as well as a wider width to avoid breakage. All the same adjustments that can be done in a player's hockey skate can also be done on a goalie skate.

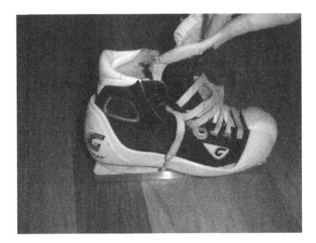

Fig. 22.3 Goalie skates

In-Line Skates

Two major components differentiate in-line skates form traditional hockey skates. The most obvious is that instead of a blade, wheels are attached due to the difference in sport surface. Just like skate blades can be changed for rocker and material, so can the types and sizes of wheels be altered. The second major structural difference is the ventilation systems used to accommodate heat transfer as most in-line skating is done in a warmer environment than traditional ice skating (Fig. 22.4).

Figure Skates

The design of figure skates as we know them today has changed very little in over a century. The biggest changes, like those seen in hockey skates, are with construction materials. Figure skating boots are designed to provide the foot and ankle with the stability necessary to perform difficult jumps and spins; however, this rigidity brings with it a myriad of lower extremity problems and injuries. The figure skate blades vary in that there are "picks" at the anterior end of the blade to help with function and maneuverability, and the radius of curvature is longer than that of a traditional hockey skate blade.

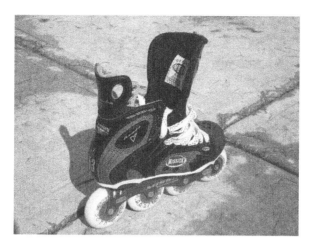

Fig. 22.4 In-line skates

Since 1990 the actual art of skating figures, also known as compulsories, has been eliminated from the sport, and has been replaced with increased emphasis on free skating, which includes jumps, spins, lifts, and throws [1]. The stiffness of skate boots has long been linked to lower extremity injuries in figure skating, and the increased amount of time spent practicing jumps may result in a greater frequency and degree of severity of these injuries [2]. Skaters may perform 50–100 jumps per day, 6–7 days a week, and the force generated from a typical skating jump amounts to eight to ten times the skater's body weight [3]. Because the design of figure skates allows for very little flexion at the ankle, skaters land on their heels, and since the hardness of the ice surface offers almost no shock absorption, most of the force is transferred to the knees, hips, and spine. Most figure skating injuries involve the lower extremity, and many are directly related to the skating boot [4].

Figure skating is the only jumping sport that confines the movement of the ankle joint and calf muscles by the use of rigid boot support [5]. The skate boot is designed with a high heel and inflexible ankle portion that limits ankle plantar flexion, which decreases effectiveness in jump take-off and restricts the ability of the ankle to cushion the landing [5]. The force absorbed by the knee extensor apparatus contributes to occurrence of patellofemoral pain and various overuse injuries. In a study by Dubravic-Simunjak et al., 42.8% of female and 45.5% of male single skaters reported overuse syndromes, the most frequent injuries in females being stress fractures and jumper's knee in males.

Not only does the design of figure skate boots cause injuries, but poor fit can also lead to deformities of the foot. In an article for the US Figure Skating website, Linda Tremain reports that up to 57% of skaters have bunions, while 31% have enlarged navicular bones, likely related to uncorrected pronation problems of the boot and blade or the foot itself [6]. She also found that excess heel slippage has led to the development of Haglund's deformities in 49% of skaters, and hammertoes in

18%. Current research and trials are underway to design an articulated boot that may decrease the magnitude of landing forces by allowing more sagittal plane mobility while still providing the stability required to execute difficult jumps and spins [7].

Speed Skates

In contrast to the unchanged design of figure skates, speed skates have undergone radical changes in the past decade, which have brought about tremendous improvements in both world record and personal best times.

Conventional speed skates featured a low boot with a long, thin blade that was fixed to the boot. A skater would push off until the leg was fully extended, at which point the ankle would naturally want to plantar flex and continue the push. However, this would cause the toe of a conventional skate to dig into the ice, called "toeing-off", which hinders the gliding motion [8]. To prevent the tip of the blade from scratching the ice, speed skaters had to use a technique where plantar flexion was largely suppressed during push off. This limits the efficiency of the stroke because the ankle plantar flexors are prevented from contributing to the push, which also restricts the work done by the calf muscles and knee extensors and causes the skater to lose contact with the ice before the knee is completely extended [9]. Speed skaters often suffered from pain in the tibialis anterior due to this forced suppression on plantar flexion [8].

The klap skate was introduced in 1997 which features a hinge under the ball of the foot that allows the ankle to plantar flex at the end of push off while the blade continues to make contact with the ice. Skating velocity increased by 5% and mean power output improved by 10% due to an increase in both stroke frequency and work per stroke [10]. Surprisingly, this improvement is not simply due to the ability of the ankle to extend at push off, but rather the difference in the center of rotation between the foot and the ice surface [11]. With conventional speed skates, the foot is turned into a long lever because it must rotate around the tip of the skate blade, which is located approximately 10 cm in front of the toes [11]. This extreme frontal location of the center of rotation creates in ineffective push off and makes it difficult to set the foot into motion. The hinge of a klap skate allows the foot to rotate around the ball of the foot, which greatly enhances the effectiveness of plantar flexion in the final phase of push off, leading to increased gross efficiency and mechanical power output [10].

The hinge must be located under the ball of the foot to achieve optimal performance; however, the exact position varies from skater to skater depending upon his or her build and skating technique [11]. Determining the most advantageous location for the hinge is still a question of feel.

Understanding basic skate boot construction along with an understanding of the biomechanics of the sport can assist in making functional interventions in both performance and comfort.

Biomechanics

All the various forms of skating along with the associated footwear are somewhat different. However, the basics of motion, push, and glide are similar as is the performance surface. So for discussion purposes regarding biomechanics we will discuss the biomechanics of power skating.

Power skating in hockey involves skating forward, backward, and with multiple directional changes as the game evolves. It is this ever-changing movement pattern that makes this activity difficult to study from a biomechanical standpoint. It is forward acceleration and striding, however, that are the most consistent and studied aspects of power skating and a commonality that is seen with other forms of skating. The understanding of foot and lower extremity balance on top of a narrow balance point, the skate blade, will allow a practitioner to assist in both improved performance and overuse injury patterns.

In order to better understand the biomechanics of power skating and the clinical injury perspectives that may arise, it is first helpful to compare power skating with the more commonly understood biomechanics of walking. Both walking and skating are biphasic movement patterns that consist of periods of single- and double-limb support. By comparison, it is the support phase of walking that becomes the skating glide. One aspect of skating that makes it unique in the support phase is that the friction on the performance surface is much less than that seen in most walking activities. As a result there are decreased posterior linear shear forces with touchdown due to decreased friction and decreased anterior linear shear forces in the late midstance to propulsion stage. This low-friction surface will necessarily impart a need to abduct the foot by external hip rotation at propulsion [12]. The center of gravity therefore does not progress in a linear sinusoidal path over the foot as seen in walking, but rather the skater and his/her center of gravity move in an opposite direction to the weight-bearing skate.

The acceleration in power skating is divided into two unique stride patterns, the first three strides and the fourth stride, known as the typical skate cut [13]. The first stride pattern usually involves the first three strides. It lasts approximately 1.75 s, involves continual positive acceleration, and has a negligible or non-existent glide phase [14]. It is during this stride pattern that the skater often appears to be "running" on his/her skates.

The second stride pattern often begins on the fourth stride and is considered the typical skate cut [13]. This stride pattern consists of periods of positive and negative acceleration and involves three phases. It starts with a glide during single-limb support which imparts negative acceleration [15]. It continues with propulsion during single-limb support which is accomplished by external rotation of the thigh and the initial extension movements of the hip and knee [16]. This stride pattern concludes with propulsion during double-limb support. During this phase the second limb acts as a balance point to complete propulsion through full knee extension, hyperextension of hip, and plantar flexion of the ankle.

Clinical Injury Perspective

From a footwear and biomechanical perspective there is first the intrinsic foot-to-boot injuries that can be precipitated from the nature of the unique footwear, and second, there are the specific biomechanically produced clinical injury patterns that may arise from overuse.

Biomechanically produced overuse foot and ankle clinical injury patterns can clearly be identified in ice skating. The narrow blade or balance point creates a need for strenuous eccentric muscle control and proprioceptive skills to assist in balance over this small balance point. As a result, general foot fatigue from strain of the small intrinsic muscles of the foot is common. As well as the intrinsic muscle strains, there are the extrinsic tendonopathies that can occur in the posterior tibial tendon and the peroneal tendons and muscles as a reaction to the need for balance.

In comparison to other sporting activities, power skating shows a decrease in the number of contact phase injuries due to he low friction of the ice surface. The overuse injuries in the lower extremity usually show up more proximally in the groin or low back due to the inherent need for skate and skater to be moving in opposite directions as propulsion occurs. Groin injuries in the adductor muscle group (adductor magnus, longus, and brevis) occur when the thigh is externally rotated and the hip is abducted, thus putting this muscle group under maximal strain. Dr. Eric Babins from the University of Calgary has reported a reduction in pain of the lumbar spine and lower extremity along with improved performance with proper fitting of skates, blade alignment, and adjustment for leg length discrepancies as required due to the improved biomechanical balance above the skate blade.

Clinical Biomechanical Balance

There are two steps in the process to assist a skater from a biomechanical perspective. The first is the positioning of the foot within the boot using standard podiatric biomechanical principles. The second is the balance of the blade onto the boot itself.

Step 1: Foot Balance Within Boot-Custom Foot Orthosis

A general podiatric clinician can be confident when dealing with the first step of biomechanical control, which is positioning the foot properly within the boot. A complete lower extremity and foot examination needs to be done as would be done for any athletic population, and a decision on foot orthoses can be made using sound Root biomechanical techniques [17]. These techniques of forefoot to rearfoot and rearfoot to leg control will help to compensate for biomechanical faults, help stabilize the subtalar and midtarsal joints, and help maintain sound structural alignment of the lower extremity from the midtarsal joint to the hip, providing a solid lever for propulsion. This orthosis can then be improved upon by using a general understanding of skating mechanics and applying the newer techniques of foot orthosis control as discussed by Kirby and Blake [18, 19].

As a skater is in single-limb support in the early stages of propulsion, the foot is abducted and the hip externally rotated. The skate and skater are moving in opposite directions at this time while trying to balance on the narrow skate blade. As such, the center of gravity is much more medial with respect to the weight-bearing extremity, and even subtle biomechanical faults, causing excessive foot pronation, will cause a skater to spend too much time on the medial skate edge. Power and efficiency are created by staying on the outside edge as long as possible early in the typical skate cut. Therefore, maximally controlling the medial column of the foot with respect to the subtalar joint axis location can greatly assist a skater with this task. Using both the newer positive cast modifications of medial heel skive and inversion techniques along with traditional biomechanical controlling techniques improves skating power and balance during propulsion.

A typical custom foot orthosis design for skating would include the following features (Fig. 22.5):

1. Neutral suspension casts of feet [17].
2. Trace or send skate insoles with casts to improve boot fit.
3. Intrinsic forefoot posting unless custom extra-depth skate boots are used.
4. Standardly, invert casts 10° using Blake technique to increase medial arch contact and to increase time spent on lateral blade edge. Increase as clinically justified.
5. Standardly, use a 3–4-mm medial heel skive cast modification to help with lateral edge control. Increase as clinically justified.
6. Polypropylene shells are preferable as they be more easily modified as needed to the medial shank of the skate boot.
7. Extrinsic rearfoot posts work if well skived to fit in the heel counter of the boot and when used with a thin cap to decrease heel lift. There should be no motion allowed within the rearfoot posting.

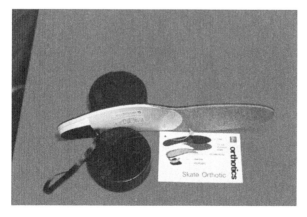

Fig. 22.5 Skate orthosis. (From Humble RN. Podiatric management in ice skating. Podiatry Management November/December 2003, pp. 49–63, with permission.)

8. Use full-length extensions with thin top cover materials of good friction next to the foot for grip and "feel." A thin layer of firm Korex under the extension will protect the forefoot from irritation from the blade housing mounting rivets in the boot.
9. Some skaters like buttress or toe crest pads built into the extension for their toes to grip onto.

Step 2: Blade Balance

The second step in mechanically helping skaters involves blade balance. Blade balance is accomplished using three different techniques: sagittal plane rocker, medial–lateral position of blade, and varus/valgus wedging of blade, which can incorporate limb lifts. These interventions are usually best performed by a professional skate mechanic after medical advice is given.

The sagittal plane rocker of the blade allows for easy response to the center of gravity changes in the sagittal plane. Standardly, the rocker is in the center of the blade with only one inch of the blade in contact with the ice. Some skaters will increase their rocker (decrease contact with ice) in order to improve their maneuverability. Others will decrease their rocker to allow more blades to contact the ice, and this will increase speed but decrease turning capabilities. Adjustments of rockers are more a matter of individual preference for performance and should only be done in the hands of a skilled skate technician.

The medial–lateral position of the blade on the boot has a significant effect on a skater's posture and balance. The standard blade placement is longitudinally from heel center to the second metatarsal head, and second digit. This blade position should provide an inherently stable platform for the foot to sit with only pure sagittal plane rocking (Figs. 22.6 and 22.7).

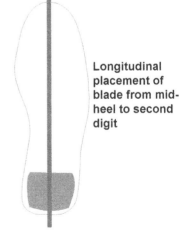

Longitudinal placement of blade from mid-heel to second digit

Fig. 22.6 Standard blade placement. (From Humble RN. Podiatric management in ice skating. Podiatry Management November/December 2003, pp. 49–63, with permission.)

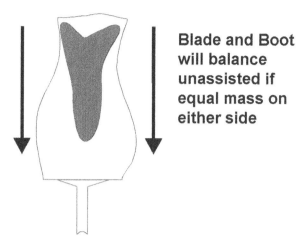

Blade and Boot will balance unassisted if equal mass on either side

Fig. 22.7 Standard blade placement, posterior view. (From Humble RN. Podiatric management in ice skating. Podiatry Management November/December 2003, pp. 49–63, with permission.)

A medially deviated subtalar joint axis will influence the default contact portion of the standardly placed blade. Shifting the blade medially in this circumstance will place the default contact portion of the blade in a more functional position with respect to the medially deviated axis in those patients (Fig. 22.8 and 22.9). In

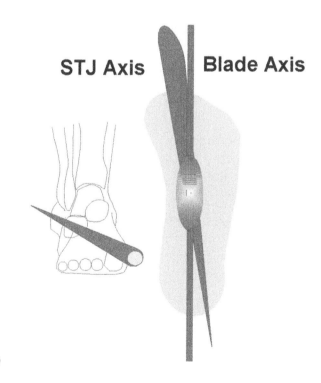

STJ Axis   **Blade Axis**

Fig. 22.8 Standard blade placement compared to subtalar joint axis. (From Humble RN. Podiatric management in ice skating. Podiatry Management November/December 2003, pp. 49–63, with permission.)

Fig. 22.9 Shifting blade medial may put it in a more functional position. (From Humble RN. Podiatric management in ice skating. Podiatry Management November/December 2003, pp. 49–63, with permission.)

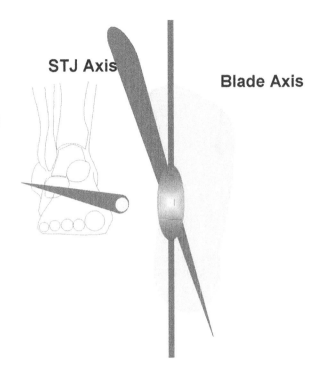

extremely rigid inverted feet, moving the blade laterally on the boot will help to improve balance.

Balancing the blade with wedging is the final blade adjustment technique. After an appropriate orthosis has been made, the rocker has been checked, the blade has been moved medially or laterally as needed, and a decision on using a wedge can be

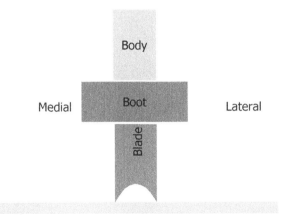

Fig. 22.10 Neutral foot (From Humble RN. Podiatric management in ice skating. Podiatry Management November/December 2003, pp. 49–63, with permission.)

made by looking at the position of the blade edges with respect to the weight-bearing surface. A wedge can assist in balancing the blade to the boot and upper body so that in static stance each edge of the blade balances on the ice surface equally. As odd as it may seem, a supinated or varus foot can require a medial wedge to bring the medial blade edge evenly to the ground. A pronated or valgus foot can require a lateral wedge to bring the lateral blade edge to the ground (Figs. 22.10, 22.11, and 22.12).

Supinated Foot (varus) - Medial wedge

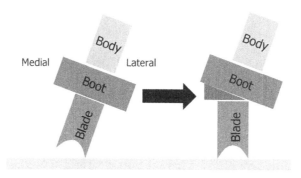

Fig. 22.11 Supinated foot, or lower extremity varum – medial wedge. (From Humble RN. Podiatric management in ice skating. Podiatry Management November/December 2003, pp. 49–63, with permission.)

Pronated Foot (valgus) - Lateral wedge

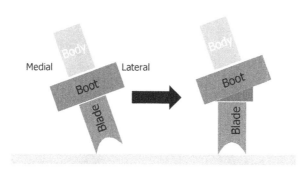

Fig. 22.12 Pronated foot, or lower extremity valgum – lateral wedge. (From Humble RN. Podiatric management in ice skating. Podiatry Management November/December 2003, pp. 49–63, with permission.)

The podiatric management of the skater can be best shown through a series of case examples. Each of these scenarios depicts the management of increasingly complex cases involving both foot-to-boot balance and blade-to-boot balancing techniques.

Case 1: Moderate Pronation

A 10-year-old while boy suffers from medial arch and heel pain predominantly in his day-to-day activities, which carries over into his recreational hockey (Fig. 22.13). He is otherwise fit and healthy and has been diagnosed with plantar fasciitis. A complete podiatric biomechanical examination was performed and the pertinent results were a 2° forefoot varus and a 4° forefoot supinatus bilaterally (Fig. 22.14).

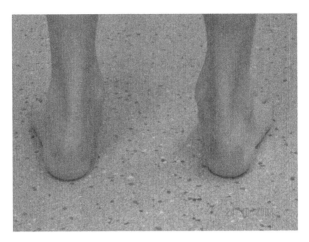

Fig. 22.13 Case number 1: moderate pronation. (From Humble RN. Podiatric management in ice skating. Podiatry Management November/December 2003, pp. 49–63, with permission.)

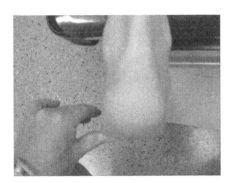
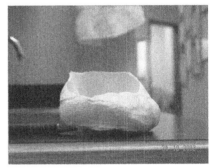

Neutral Position

Neutral Suspension Cast
(no supinatus)

Fig. 22.14 Case number 1: moderate pronation. (From Humble RN. Podiatric management in ice skating. Podiatry Management November/December 2003, pp. 49–63, with permission.)

The first goal in treatment was a daily orthosis to relieve his symptoms and the secondary goal was a skating-specific orthosis to improve his skating performance and his enjoyment of his recreation. The polypropylene skating orthosis was made from a neutral suspension cast with reduction of the supinatus. The forefoot was first posted intrinsically 2° varus and then the casts were modified with 10° of inversion and a 3-mm medial heel skive. A rearfoot post was added to balance the orthosis. A functional skate orthosis with maximal control was used to assist this patient, along with a good-quality and well-fitted skate boot (Fig. 22.15). No blade adjustments were needed, and the blade was left in its standard default position.

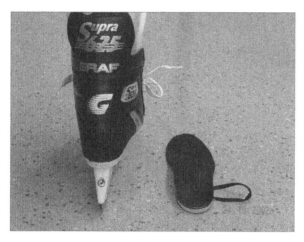

Fig. 22.15 Case number 1: moderate pronation, quality skate, and custom foot orthosis. (From Humble RN. Podiatric management in ice skating. Podiatry Management November/December 2003, pp. 49–63, with permission.)

Case 2: Moderate–Severe Pronation

A 12-year-old boy suffers from medial ankle and knee pain while playing hockey. He is otherwise fit and healthy. After a complete history and physical examination, a diagnosis of posterior tibial tendon strain and patellofemoral pain syndrome was made. The primary etiology of his problems was deemed to be biomechanically produced strain from excessive foot pronation (Fig. 22.16). He functions maximally pronated due to a fully compensated forefoot and rearfoot varus deformity bilaterally of approximately 4° for both.

A custom foot orthosis was manufactured from casts corrected to 25° of inversion using the Blake inversion technique and a 4-mm medial heel skive was added. The forefoot to rearfoot was posted a further 4° of varus and a balancing post was placed on the rearfoot also in 4° of varus (Fig. 22.17). A further mechanical intervention was needed to improve balance, and the blades were moved medially on the skates (Fig. 22.18). The final solution for this patient was a good-quality skate boot appropriately fitted, an aggressive custom foot orthosis, and a blade balancing adjustment (Fig. 22.19).

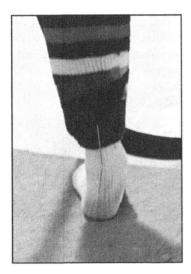
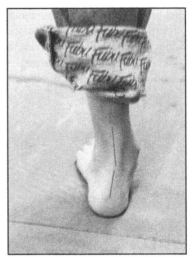

Fig. 22.16 Case number 2: moderate–severe pronation. (From Humble RN. Podiatric management in ice skating. Podiatry Management November/December 2003, pp. 49–63, with permission.)

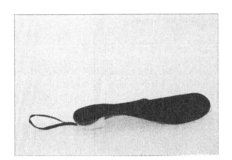
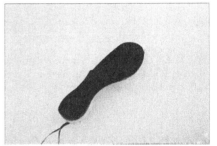

Fig. 22.17 Case number 2: skate orthosis. (From Humble RN. Podiatric management in ice skating. Podiatry Management November/December 2003, pp. 49–63, with permission.)

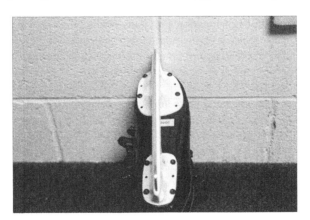

Fig. 22.18 Case number 2: blade adjustment

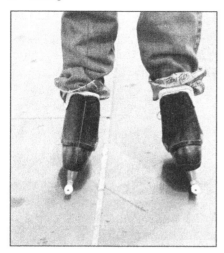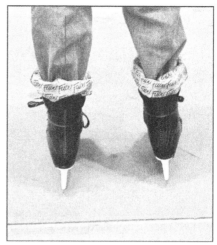

Fig. 22.19 Case number 2: end result. (From Humble RN. Podiatric management in ice skating. Podiatry Management November/December 2003, pp. 49–63, with permission.)

Case 3: Supinated Pes Cavus Foot Type

An 18-year-old Western Canadian Hockey League player suffers from lateral leg and ankle pain, as well as skate balance problems. History and physical examination finds him otherwise fit and healthy. A diagnosis of peroneal tendonitis was made secondary to a rigid forefoot valgus and a limb-length discrepancy (Figs. 22.20 and 22.21).

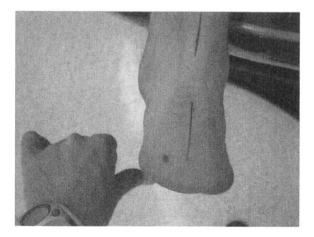

Fig. 22.20 Case number 3: pes cavus with forefoot valgus. (From Humble RN. Podiatric management in ice skating. Podiatry Management November/December 2003, pp. 49–63, with permission.)

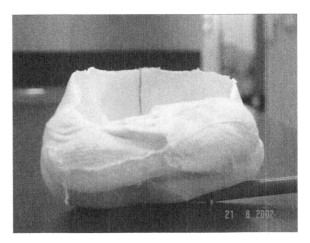

Fig. 22.21 Case number 3: neutral cast. (From Humble RN. Podiatric management in ice skating. Podiatry Management November/December 2003, pp. 49–63, with permission.)

The mechanical solution to this patient's problem was a custom-made, extra-depth skate boot to accommodate an orthosis with an extrinsic forefoot valgus post to the sulcus. Standard Root biomechanical principles were used to make this orthosis and no newer inversion techniques were utilized (Fig. 22.22).

Fig. 22.22 Case number 3: skate orthosis. (From Humble RN. Podiatric management in ice skating. Podiatry Management November/December 2003, pp. 49–63, with permission.)

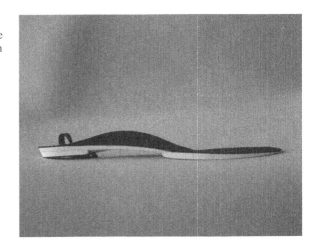

Many blade adjustments were needed to assist in this patient's performance. A limb lift was added full length, the blades were moved laterally on the boots, and a medial wedge was inserted to assist further in bringing the medial edge of the skate blade down to the ground.

Conclusion

Skating in all its various forms is showing increased popularity throughout North America. All footcare practitioners can expect to see ice skaters in their offices. A sound understanding of the footwear used in these sports along with the use of proven podiatric biomechanical management techniques as used in other athletic populations can assist the practitioner in assisting with the pleasure and performance of this unique activity.

References

1. Bradley MA: Prevention and treatment of foot and ankle injuries in figure skaters. Curr Sports Med Rep, 5(5): 258–261, 2006.
2. Bruening DA, Richards JG: The Effects of articulated figure skates on jump landing forces. J Appl Biomech. 22(4): 285–295, 2006.
3. Arnold AS, King DL, Smith, SL: Figure skating and sports biomechanics: The Basic Physics of Jumping and Rotating. Skating. Sept. 2004.
4. Smith AD, Ludington R: Injuries in Elite pairs skaters and ice dancers. Am J Sports Med, 17(4): 482–488, 1989.
5. Dubravic-Simunjak S, Pecina M, Kuipers H, Moran J, Haspl M: Incidence of injuries in Elite junior figure skaters. Am J Sports Med,. 31(6): 511–515, 2003.
6. Tremain L: http://www.usfigureskating.org/content/Boot%20Problems%20and%20Boot%20 Solutions.pdf
7. Bruening DA, Richards JG: Optimal Ankle axis position for articulated boots. Sports Biomech,. 4(2): 215–225, 2005.
8. van Ingen Schenau GJ, de Koning J, Houdijk H: Backgrounds of the slapskate. Faculty of Human Movement Sciences: Dept. of Kinesiology, Vrije Universiteit of Amsterdam. Amsterdam, Netherlands, 1997.
9. van Ingen Schenau GJ, de Groot G, Scheurs AW, Meester H, de Koning JJ: A New Skate Allowing Powerful Plantar Flexions Improves Performance. Med Sci Sports Exerc, 28(4): 531–535, 1996.
10. Houdijk H, de Koning JJ, de Groot G, Bobbert MF, van Ingen Schenau GJ: Push-off Mechanics in Speed Skating with Conventional Skates and Klapskates. Med Sci Sports Exerc. 32(3): 635–641, 2000.
11. Houdijk H: Scientific Explanation for Success of the Klapskate. Netherlands Organization for Scientific Research. May 2001.
12. Roy B: Biomechanical features of different staring positions and skating strides in ice hockey. in, Asmussen E, Jorgenson K (eds.), Biomechanics V1-B, p. 137. Baltimore, MD University Park Press, 1978.
13. Hoshizaki TB, Kirchner GJ: A comparison of the kinematic patterns between supported and non-supported ankles during the acceleration phase of forward skating. Proceedings of the International Symposium of Biomechanics in Sport, 1987.
14. Marino GW: Acceleration time relationships in an ice skating start. Res Q 50:55, 1979.
15. Mueller M: Kinematics of speed skating. Master's thesis, University of Wisconsin, 1972.
16. Marino GW, Weese RG: A kinematic analysis of the ice skating stride. in Terauds J, Gros HJ (eds.), Science in Skiing, Skating and Hockey, pp. 65, 73. Del Mar, CA: Academic Publishers, 1979.

17. Root ML, Orien WP, Weed JH, Hughes RJ: Biomechanical Examination of the Foot, Vol 1. Clinical Biomechanics Corporation. Los Angeles, CA.
18. Kirby KA: Subtalar Joint Axis Location and Rotational Equilibrium Theory of Foot Function. J Am Podiatr Med Assoc 91(9): 465–487, 2001.
19. Blake RL: Inverted functional orthoses. JAPMA 76: 275, 1986.

Chapter 23
Skiing and Snowboarding

Jeffrey A. Ross

Downhill Skiing

Alpine or downhill skiing is a complex skill that requires a series of integrated movements that requires controlled pronation, setting the foot, ankle, and lower extremity on the inside ski edge. Pronation sets the inside edge of the downhill (control) ski and allows for the skier to lean inward against the ski which holds a skidless arc throughout the turn. Even today with wider parabolic skis, the skier drives the shin forward against the stiff wraparound type, or hybrid type boot cuff and swings the hips to the opposite direction. The ski rolls onto its sharp steel edge and bites the snow, creating an arc across the hill [1]. Skiing in the freestyle is like ballet dance on snow, yet at the same time, the skier encounters many centrifugal and G-forces, as turns are created, while simultaneously attempting to keep the center of gravity in line over the center of the ski. Any deviation of normal lower extremity biomechanical balance can alter the skier's ability to carve a controlled turn, thus placing the skier at risk for injury if the biomechanical abnormality is great enough. Before a skier should consider taking part in this demanding sport, three important factors are important in a skier's conditioning and performance, namely flexibility, strength, and adequate range of motion of lower extremity joints. A number of variable factors such as structural deformities, functional deformity, or dynamic imbalance of muscle groups can influence the performance of the skier and also help to predict potential injury. When skiers have pre-existing injuries, i.e., knee instability, quadriceps muscle weakness, posterior tibial dysfunction, chronic peroneal tenosynovitis, etc. this will contribute to muscle weakness, decreased flexibility, and limited range of motion of involved lower leg joints. This will limit the skier's ability to ski efficiently and safely, and as a result, increase the muscular effort required, resulting in greater skier fatigue. Fatigue has been shown to be one of the main factors in the

J.A. Ross (✉)
Department of Medicine, Baylor College of Medicine, 6624 Fannin Suite 2450, Houston, TX 77030, USA

M.B. Werd, E.L. Knight (eds.), *Athletic Footwear and Orthoses in Sports Medicine*, DOI 10.1007/978-0-387-76416-0_23, © Springer Science+Business Media, LLC 2010

incidence of downhill skiing injuries [1], and the same effect occurs in snowboarders as well.

Skiers will typically compensate for structural biomechanical abnormalities through hip and knee pronatory forces in order to hold the skier's edge and to ski in proper control. Ross incorporated the electro-dynogram (EDG) to show that forces are transmitted from both the forefoot and the rearfoot, which is essential in up-and-down weighting, as well as in the completion of proper turns [2]. There were many abnormalities observed with this technology, namely excessive foot pronation, shortened heel contact and excessive propulsive phase on the toes, extreme forward lean of the boot, limb length discrepancy, including asymmetry between the two feet. All of these findings contribute significantly to the skier's efficiency and performance.

The use of custom footbeds and custom foot orthoses in ski boots has been shown to be effective in improving skiing style, edge control, reducing excessive pronation, and other foot imbalances. It has also been shown that custom insoles (made at the ski shop) can help control milder degrees of pronation and other lower leg imbalances (tibial varum, genu valgum). For the more severe rearfoot and forefoot abnormalities, a custom foot orthoses is valuable to provide proper footbed balance and improve ski performance and efficiency [3]. The use of easy-to-customize liners and removable full-length soft support systems has also become a integral part of the comfort and support system. Custom foot orthoses may be substituted for the pre-existing insole.

In order to work effectively with the skier, the foot specialist or sports medicine specialist must have a basic understanding of both boot design and the biomechanics of ski performance in addition to a close working relationship with the ski shop and the boot fitter/ski tech. The foot specialist can assist in the proper selection of the "right" boot, by first determining the skier's foot type, and targeting existing areas of biomechanical imbalances, protruding bony areas of the foot that lead to friction and irritation, circulatory compromise, nerve entrapments, and metabolic disorders (diabetes).

After taking these factors into consideration, the boot fitter can assist the skier in selecting a boot designed for a wide foot, a flat or high-arched foot, a foot that requires large volume, a pure forward entry boot or hybrid (with both overlap and rear-entry design), a narrow heel pocket, or with a thin, thick, or adaptable liner. Early research noted that a majority of National Ski Patrollers, ski racers, and ski instructors wear a custom footbed, insole, or custom foot orthosis in order to achieve biomechanical neutrality while improving skiing efficiency.

Once the unbalanced foot is situated in the ski boot, the bucking down of the boot can result in a significant loss in volume and can also accentuate or aggravate already existing biomechanical imbalances within the foot or lower extremity, which can lead to improper fit of the boot, overuse injury, or a resulting traumatic injury [1]. Ski boot designs change rapidly, with new designs, variations in the inner boots and shells, internal canting and buckle systems, as well as variability of forward lean (Fig. 23.1a,b).

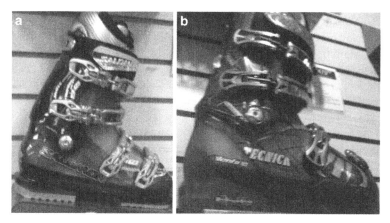

Fig. 23.1 (**a** and **b**) Ski boot designs

Tibial Varum

Tibial varum is a biomechanical abnormality that can have a great deal of negative effect upon the skier's ability to ski normally [4]. Tibial varum is a result of an uncompensated varus deformity of the tibia which transmits instantaneously to the ski–snow interface and causes the skier to ride excessively on the outside edge of the ski. When a skier has more than 8–10° of tibial varum deformity, he or she will have a great deal of difficulty initiating the parallel turn without "catching" the outside edge of the ski. Skiers who chronically ski on the outside edges of their skis when attempted to "set-up" the next turn will have difficulty getting on to their inside edges, and when they do will often cross tips, which can eventually lead to sudden falls and possible injury [1]. High-performance boots of this day and age provide a boot cuff adjustment to accommodate varying degrees of tibial varum in order to create a flat ski surface. One of the simplest and most reliable means of treating tibial varum is to use a full-length, canted, in-boot foot orthosis. The advantage of this method is that the orthosis provides for total foot contact within the boot, affording the skier greater correction of lower extremity imbalances within the foot and leg. Another typical problem that can be eliminated with a balanced footbed or orthosis is the reduction of friction on bony areas of the foot against the boot, while simultaneously affording a comfortable, dependable, balanced footbed that helps to provide effectual edge control [4].

Tibial Valgum

Skiers who have tibial valgum or genu valgum of the knees will be constantly on the inside edges of their skis. The inward position of the knee sets the skier up for potential crossing the ski tips, as well as decreased control of the uphill ski. These skiers will relate that they "caught an edge" even on the flat terrain as a result of this lower leg position. In addition the skier will also complain of medial collateral ligament strain from excessive internal femoral rotation, leading to patellar tracking and patellofemoral joint syndrome pain. Tibial valgum is associated with coxa vara–genu valgum as well excessive pronation of the feet. Orthosis control will typically correct the improper knee position and allow for a more neutral position of the foot on the ski. However, when this is not sufficient the use of a cant may be necessary to provide for lower extremity alignment. The knee position can be visualized to be more frontal when the skier stands on a bench with both the orthosis and the cant in place.

Forefoot Varus

Forefoot varus imbalance can also lead to a forefoot that "rides" on the outside edge of ski, similar to a subtalar varus. When the skier stands on a platform and a vertical plumb line is dropped from the midpoint of the patella, it should drop directly down to the vicinity of the second metatarsal. However, if the line drops more laterally, forefoot varus imbalance may continue to be present. Additional forefoot posting on a full-length orthosis may be required to correct this imbalance. The skier will be able to feel the difference and relate much more stability in the forefoot. It is important not to overcorrect the rearfoot with extrinsic posting which can elevate the heel causing a potential rearfoot boot fit problem, and/or irritation at the posterior aspect of the heel. Skiers have often complained about boot fit and comfort. They often state that their feet hurt, and that they are cold, tight and irritating. Compared to years when first skiing with laced leather boots, technological advances in design and performance have made boot comfort a standard in the industry. Designs have changed over the years, having gone from the traditional overlap design, then through a rear-entry revolution and now having come full circle back to a forward entry and hybrid designed performance boot. From a biomechanical standpoint ski boots have become extremely sophisticated biomechanically. There are a number of adjustable features now on boots which include internal versus external canting systems, adjustable spoilers or shaft-angle adjustments, boot flex, forward lean, internal/external heaters, as well as custom heat-moldable liners made of ethyl vinyl acetate (EVA). To facilitate the use of custom foot orthoses, most ski boots have footbeds that easily can be removed. Most ski shops offer custom insoles that can be made readily by using computer technology or with an apparatus which places the foot in a semi-weight-bearing neutral position, with knee stabilizer apparatus built into the platform to accurately align the knee over the foot, for complete lower leg correction. The traditional prescription can either be made with computer technology and plaster casting in neutral position outside the boot or from an in-boot cast while the skier assumes a neutral ski stance position, quite often functioning which much greater control than the custom insole, due to increased correction and stability in the rearfoot, subtalar joint, midtarsal joint, and forefoot. By locking the midtarsal joint, and controlling excessive pronation/supination, we can achieve greater stability and balance which will afford the skier greater edge control and better performance. When looking at the ski boot, there are five areas of concern:

- Zone 1, the footbed
- Zone 2, the tongue
- Zone 3, the hindfoot
- Zone 4, the shaft
- Zone 5, the forefoot

Alpine skiing has become much more technical but with the advent of parabolic skis, initiating turns with advanced ski boots have made initiating turns much simpler, with much less energy exerted through the hips, knees, and lower extremities. The foot specialist must be cognizant of the various challenges which skiers have to confront. It is imperative that the specialist have a clear-cut understanding of lower extremity biomechanics related to the sport of skiing.

Snowboarding

The sport now almost 20 years old has become mainstream with youngsters and adults alike. Many adults who for years were alpine skiers and/or runners have found snowboarding to be much gentler on the knees. First began as a winter version of skateboard surfing, it has its own inherent risks as does alpine skiing. The snowboarder may find falling a common event due to an exaggerated uphill edge that is required for carving turns. Most injuries from snowboarding occur due to falls, as well as striking obstacles as in tree boarding, or from colliding with other boarders/skiers on the mountain.

Unlike alpine skiing the initiation of a turn from a snowboard takes longer and the carve of the turn takes a longer period of time. This necessitates a wider area for the turn to be accomplished. According to Ganong et al. [5] snowboarders sustain a wide variety of injuries: 44% involve the upper extremity, while 43% are from the lower extremity; 12% head, spine, or torso; and 4% miscellaneous. The most common site of injury is the wrist (trauma and fracture), followed by the knee (sprains) and the ankle (fractures). The abundance of upper extremity injuries is due to the fact that the boarder lacks the freedom of individual leg movement, which unlike alpine skiing does not allow for as quick a recovery. In snowboarding a sudden "hop" is required in order to make that instantaneous correction. Due to a sideway position of the board and the feet and torso facing forwards, when the fall occurs, the snowboarder will usually fall forward on the hands, wrists, and upper extremity. The twisting fall involved in a turn will typically involve the lower leg. Unlike downhill skiing, which uses the integration of foot, knee, and hip motion, snowboarding concentrates its energy on the hips and knees owing to the nature of the short pivoting turns [4]. Biomechanical balancing on the snowboard is equally important as it is on the alpine ski. It is essential that when the snowboarder is riding the board edge the foot be as neutral on the midsection of the board as possible.

Snowboard boots have evolved over the years beginning with a soft design, followed in recent years with a full hard shell and half-shell design. Compared to the harder designs, the softer version snowboard boot allows for greater movement within, which gives the boarder the advantage of tactile sensation and proprioception on the board. However, this boot design may increase the risk of injury compared to the harder designs. Soft boot injuries will typically be seen in the ankles, whereas the more rigid full-shell boots protect the ankles, while allowing for greater forces to be transmitted to the knees. This results in an increased number of knee injuries. The binding systems for the boots have also improved (Fig. 23.2), making snowboarding safer and a higher performance winter sport.

Cross-Country Skiing

Cross-country skiing has increased in popularity over recent years as a cross-training alternative to alpine skiing, and as another exercise activity for all ages that provides an excellent cardiovascular workout. Elson reported that 1 h of cross-country skiing is equivalent to 2 h of downhill skiing, or 2–12 h of tennis, or 4 h of cycling at 5.5 miles per hour [6]. Cross-country skiing, another endurance sport, provides an excellent means of upper body as well as lower body development. Only swimming can achieve as even development of muscular groups with aerobic effects. For runners searching for a safe cross-training winter activity, cross-country skiing is excellent in cases where underdeveloped anterior muscle groups and overdeveloped posterior groups can be equalized.

As opposed to alpine skiing, cross-country skiing has a different technique, as well as application. In downhill skiing, the heel and lower leg are locked in a rigid boot, applying control to the foot's subtalar joint and rearfoot complex. In addition, the skis will typically rest directly beneath the body's center of mass, with a constant parallel location. Whereas in cross-country skiing the heel is repeatedly lifted

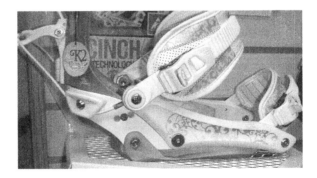

Fig. 23.2 An example of a binding system for snowboarding

from the ski surface and lowered again, allowing for a certain degree of skier imbalance. The classical technique for cross-country skiing is commonly referred to as a swing kick and glide. The poles assist in creating upper body stability and propulsion, while the heel is kicked upward to maintain forward motion, which allows forefoot propulsion on the ski. A smooth alternating gliding motion is attained with a technique referred to as the diagonal stride. By alternating the opposite arm and leg forward, a ski gait is created similar to walking and jogging [7]. Similar to running, as the skier's pace is increased, the forward lean of the body over the skis will increase. This will produce a swing-phase ski that as it touches the snow, will slide forward in a motion better known as the "glide." The opposite-sided ski, known as the stance phase ski, will press down on to the snow surface under full pressure, creating a stable platform which allows for a plant and push-off action to occur.

The velocity of the diagonal stride is affected by three factors: stride length, stride rate, and horizontal skier velocity. The distance that the skier can kick and glide is referred to as the stride length. Duoos-Asche claims that the stride length is one of the most important factors in increased skier velocity [8]. The number of kicks and glides performed in a certain time frame, known as the stride rate, will also have an influence but to a lesser degree than the stride length. The horizontal skier velocity is a total forward velocity achieved from stride length and stride rate. Among racers and those cross-country skiers who want to achieve maximum energy efficiency, achieving the greatest stride length and stride rate is the key [1].

Cross-country boots are quite different than the alpine version. They are an intermediary between back-country and racing boots in both design and support. The cross-country touring boot has a greater freedom of movement, yet sacrificing support. Because the touring skier moves predominantly in sagittal plane motion, this unidirectional sport with only moderate curves involved does not necessitate as great a stability boot. Due to the flexibility of the boot, and a lack of stability, a skier's biomechanical imbalances will be accentuated, thus creating malalignment over the skis.

Biomechanical considerations for the cross-country skier are essential. The patella should be properly aligned over the skis in a bent-knee skiing position. A lighter, more flexible orthosis, rather than the bulkier more rigid device is preferred. The device should be fabricated as thin as possible, in order to provide greater volume for the foot and toes to function [1, 4].

References

1. Ross, JA, Subotnick SI: Alpine Skiing. in, Subotnick SI (ed.), Sports Medicine of the Lower Extremity, 2nd ed., pp. 671–686. New York, Edinburgh, San Francisco: Churchill Livingstone, 1999.
2. Ross JA: Computerized gait analysis in skiing: the electrodynogram and its use in the ski industry. Ski Mag,3:147, 1985.
3. Ross JA, Cohen S: If the boot fits you probably have a custom insole; Ski Mag,10, 82, Oct 1984.
4. Ross JA: Skiing (Sport Medicine and Injuries) Lorimer DL (ed.), Neale's Disorders of the Foot, 7th ed., pp. 351–352. Edinburgh, London, New York, 2006.

5. Ganong RB, Heneveld EH, Beranek SR, Fry P: Snowboarding injuries: a report on 415 patients. Phys Sports Med 20:114, 1992.
6. Elson PR: Ski bound? Ski Canada's 1978 Guide to Cross Country skiing, 2nd ed. Ontario, Canada: Ski Counsel of Canada.
7. Parks RM: Podiatric sports medicine care for the cross country skier; Presentation of American academy of podiatric sports medicine. Phoenix, AZ, May 1989.
8. Duoos-Asche BA: Fatigue and the diagonal stride in cross-country skiing. ISBS – Conference Proceedings Archive, 2 International Symposium on Biomechanics in Sports 1984, http://w4.ub.uni-konstanz.de/cpa/article/view/1414.

Chapter 24
Basketball and Volleyball

James M. Losito

Basketball and volleyball are clearly similar sports with regard to their ballistic nature and the need for lateral (side-to-side) movement. The primary difference is that there is no consistent running in volleyball and basketball does not generally involve lunging or diving on a regular basis. Current design strategies in court shoes are aimed at lateral stability, torsional flexibility, cushioning, and traction control to decrease the risk of injury [1].

The shoes worn in basketball reflect the physical requirements of the sport: the shoe must allow for running, jumping, and lateral movement and while providing primarily lateral stability to the subtalar and ankle joints (Fig. 24.1). Good forefoot cushioning is also desirable because the majority of the impact occurs on the forefoot. Most basketball shoes are composed of a blown or gum rubber outer sole. As with some running shoes, the manufacturer may interpose gel, "air" or other materials placed in the midsole which are often visible on the outer sole. The goal is optimal traction and stability on a wooden or concrete surface. The midsole is generally composed of ethyl vinyl acetate or a polyurethane foam material. Some manufacturers will augment the midsole with pockets of gel, "air" or other systems designed to increase stability and shock absorption. The most recent of these midsoles is a mechanized system by Adidas which can be used to adjust the desired amount of stability or cushion. The battery is included. The fine balance between cushioning and stability is critical and the inverse relationship understood. McKay and associates found that players wearing shoes with cushioning air cells were at greater risk for a lateral ankle injury [2]. Another requirement of the outersole and midsole in a basketball shoe is that the minimum required material is utilized. This allows for the shoe to be kept as low to the ground as possible. The Wade line of shoes by Converse exemplifies the desire for the shoe to maintain a low profile.

The combination of outersole and midsole determines the properties of the shank. It is essential that a basketball shoe has solid shank stability. The shoe should never have sagittal plane flexibility in the shank region. Some manufactures have

J.M. Losito (✉)
School of Podiatric Medicine, Barry University, Miami Shores; Division of Podiatry, Mercy Hospital, 3659 S. Miami Ave., Miami, FL 33133, USA

M.B. Werd, E.L. Knight (eds.), *Athletic Footwear and Orthoses in Sports Medicine*, DOI 10.1007/978-0-387-76416-0_24, © Springer Science+Business Media, LLC 2010

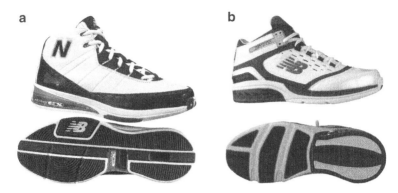

Fig. 24.1 (**a** and **b**) Basketball shoes must allow for running, jumping, and lateral movement, while providing lateral stability to the subtalar and ankle joints. (Courtesy of New Balance, Boston, MA.)

reinforced the shank with fiberglass, plastic, or graphite material in an attempt to reduce bulk but maintain stability. Failure to maintain shank stability may contribute to a variety of problems including plantar fasciitis.

Perhaps the most well-known feature of the basketball shoe is the high-top construction which has characterized the sport (Fig. 24.2a,b). Prior to 1980, the vast majority of basketball shoes were constructed above the malleoli in an effort to provide lateral stability and reduce the incidence of lateral ankle inversion injuries. However, more recently basketball shoes have been increasingly constructed at or below the malleoli (three-quarter or low-cut). The reason for this is probably fashion driven, but the lower cut construction does allow for increased mobility of the ankle and subtalar joints which is certainly beneficial. There is evidence that high-top construction may actually increase shock transmission and reduce both running and jumping performance [3]. Most importantly, research has shown that even the highest top basketball shoe does very little in preventing lateral ankle injuries [4, 5].

Volleyball shoes similarly are designed with the needs of the sport in mind. Gum rubber is the most commonly used outsole material. As with basketball shoes, the midsole is composed of ethyl vinyl acetate or polyurethane foam with occasional augmentation by gels and "air" cells. Volleyball shoes are all low-cut below the

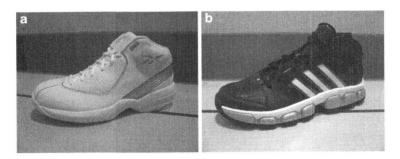

Fig. 24.2 (**a**) High-top Reebok basketball shoe. (**b**) High-top Adidas basketball shoe

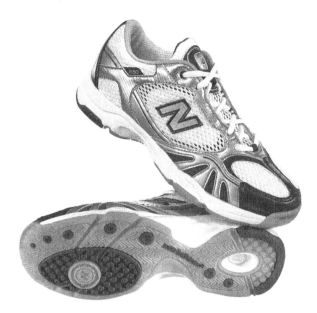

Fig. 24.3 Volleyball shoes are low-cut below the malleoli (Courtesy of New Balance, Boston, MA.)

malleoli to allow for the frequent lunging and diving which occurs (Fig. 24.3). As with many basketball shoes, the desire to keep the shoe low to the ground for improved lateral stability is seen. As with basketball shoes, a stable shank is essential.

Custom Foot Orthoses

Custom foot orthoses usage in basketball and volleyball is common among recreational, collegiate, and professional athletes. Experience estimates that over 50% of basketball players and 30% of volleyball players utilize some type of pre-fabricated or custom foot orthotic device. These orthotic devices are prescribed by podiatric physicians, orthopedic surgeons, athletic trainers, physical therapists, prosthetists, and chiropractors. The variety of devices range from a leather insole with a heel lift and scaphoid pad to a custom functional orthotic device composed of thermoplastic and foam materials. The majority of orthotic devices utilized today are composed of light, resilient thermoplastic materials [6, 7].

In my experience, the most common orthosis requirements in basketball and volleyball are cushioning and stability. There is no true heel to toe progression for any significant amount of time during either of these sports and therefore the concept of the orthosis "functioning" is not possible. The orthosis usually fabricated is a hybrid with features of both a functional and an accommodative device, utilizing a semi-weightbearing casting method, often with foam. Maintain subtalar joint neutral position during casting and capture any forefoot deformity. Non-weightbearing neutral suspension casting technique may be utilized if desired; however, the laboratory should be instructed to use generous amounts of arch fill and lateral heel expansion because these athletes generally do not tolerate orthosis which are biomechanically correct. It is essential to balance any forefoot deformity as this prevents rearfoot compensation and increases subtalar and ankle stability. Malalignment such as forefoot valgus and rearfoot varus may predispose to lateral ankle injury [8]. It is best to apply any forefoot balancing extrinsically as only forefoot contact may occur during activity. In addition, orthoses have been shown to improve postural control which may also improve lateral ankle stability [9]. The typical device is composed of a polypropylene or polyurethane shell with some degree of arch fill composed of soft or medium-density ethyl vinyl acetate. Include a heel cup of at least 16 mm and any other modifications depending on the pathology being treated, and it is common to use a top cover of perforated ethyl vinyl acetate or microcellular rubber (Spenco). If additional cushioning is desired, add 1/16 in. Poron below the top cover. If shoe fitting is a problem, then arch fill can be reduced or eliminated. Forefoot thickness should be at least 1/8 in.

Sport-Specific Pathology

Lateral Ankle Sprain

As with most sports, the lateral ankle sprain is the most commonly encountered injury in basketball and volleyball. In fact, the lateral ankle sprain occurs more commonly in basketball than in any other sport [10]. The best preventive measure and management involves physical therapy and rehabilitative exercise, especially proprioceptive training [11, 12]. Ankle braces have been shown to improve ankle stability and reduce the incidence of inversion ankle sprains without adversely affecting athletic performance [4, 12]. Experience shows that basketball players favor lace-up braces and volleyball players generally prefer a more rigid device. As mentioned previously, custom orthotic devices have also shown some efficacy in the prevention and management of lateral ankle instability. The typical orthosis modifications include forefoot balancing, a lateral heel cup of 18 mm, and a lateral flare to the rearfoot post. In some cases a valgus forefoot post can be used to further stabilize the midfoot.

In cases of severe or chronic ankle sprains such as syndesmotic injuries, a Richie brace ankle foot orthosis is an excellent option for balancing the foot and obtaining maximal subtalar joint and ankle stability. Although this device is frequently used for tibialis posterior tendon dysfunction, it has excellent indications in cases of chronic ankle pain or instability.

Plantar Fasciitis

The second most common pathology encountered in both volleyball and basketball is plantar fasciitis. Both distal and proximal ("heel spur syndrome"). This ubiquitous overuse injury can be instigated by an unstable (flexible) shank and ankle equinus, which is considered to be the primary etiology [13]. With this being said, the most efficacious form of management is Achilles stretching, either manually or with a plantar fascial splint [14, 15]. Physical therapy, non-steroidal anti-inflammatory medications, injectable corticosteroids, orthotic devices, and extracorporeal shock wave therapy have all proven to be effective to some degree [16–18]. Regarding orthotic devices, there is evidence to suggest that pre-fabricated insoles compare favorably to custom orthotic devices [19]. However, in resistant cases, the use of a custom device, derived from a non-weightbearing neutral position cast with emphasis on plantarflexion of the first ray during casting is recommended. Balance the forefoot in slight valgus with a reverse Morton's extension to further promote first ray plantarflexion. This will reduce the tension on the plantar fascia [20]. Varus posting should be avoided as this will increase tension on the fascia [21].

Other Injuries

A variety of other injuries are frequently encountered in both basketball and volleyball. These include sesamoiditis, metatarsalgia, metatarsal phalangeal joint capsulitis, first metatarsal phalangeal joint sprains ("turf toe"), Achilles tendonitis, tibial fasciitis ("Shin splints"), Jones fractures, and digital nail problems. Tibial fasciitis or "shin splints" is the most common overuse leg pain encountered in basketball and volleyball [22, 23]. The etiology is generally overuse in combination with ankle equinus, anterior leg muscular weakness, and biomechanical flaws [22–24] Excessive subtalar joint pronation is a frequent contributor to this injury as well. Orthotic devices can control excessive subtalar or midtarsal joint motion and may be useful in the prevention and management of shin splints [22].

Jones Fracture

The Jones fracture is a type of stress fracture located at the metaphyseal–diaphyseal junction of the proximal fifth metatarsal. This injury seems to be more common in basketball than in volleyball. The Jones fracture has a poor prognosis for healing with conservative care, with the non-union rate as high as 50% in some studies [25, 26]. Therefore, surgical intervention is therefore the treatment of choice for many athletes. Following surgery and immobilization, a custom orthosis may be useful in the prevention of recurrence, using a custom orthotic device with a modification designed by William Olson, DPM (2000, personal communication). The Jones fracture modification involves expanding the lateral aspect of the positive cast to produce an accommodation for the fifth metatarsal in the orthosis shell. A high lateral flange is then created which is directed over the metatarsal and the device is flat-posted (0 degrees of motion). As with most custom sports orthoses, polypropylene is the material of choice. As previously noted, the shoe must provide a stable shank and lateral (side-to-side) stability.

Summary

Clearly, there exist many available orthosis modifications in the prevention or management of basketball and volleyball injuries. An orthotic device with a metatarsal bar or raise along with forefoot accommodation is useful incases of metatarsalgia or metatarsal phalangeal joint capsulitis. A reverse Morton's extension with accommodation plantar to the first metatarsal phalangeal joint may be useful in the management of sesamoiditis. A thin, rigid extension plantar to the first metatarsal phalangeal joint may be useful in cases of structural hallux limitus, but may increase the likelihood of gastrocnemius strain or shin splints.

References

1. Reinschmidt C, Nigg BM: Current issues in the design of running and court shoes. Sportverletz Sportschaden, 14(3): 71–81, Sept. 2000
2. McKay GD, Goldie PA, Payne WR, Oakes BW: Ankle injuries in basketball: Injury rate and risk factors. Br J Sports Med, 35(2): 103–108, April 2001
3. Brizuela G, Liana S, Ferrandis R et al.: The influence of basketball shoes with increased ankle support on shock attenuation and performance in running and jumping. J Sports Sci, 15(5): 505–515, Oct. 1997
4. Handoll HH, Rowe BH, Quinn KM: Interventions for preventing ankle ligament injuries. Cochrane Database Syst Rev, (3): CD000018, 2001
5. Barrett JR, Tanji JL, Drake C, et al.: High – versus low-top shoes for the prevention of ankle sprains in basketball players. A prospective randomized study. Am J Sports Med, 21(4): 582–585, Jul-Aug 1993
6. Olson W: Orthoses: An analysis of their component materials. JAPMA, 78: 203, 1988
7. Hunter S, Dolan MG, Davis JM: Foot orthotics in therapy and sport, pp. 8–9. Human Kinetics, Champaign, IL, 1995.
8. Weil L, Moore J, Kratzer CD, Turner DL: A biomechanical study of lateral ankle sprains in basketball. JAPA, 69(11): 687–690, Nov. 1979
9. Richie DH: Effects of foot orthosis on patients with chronic ankle instability. J Am Podiatr Med Assoc, 97(1): 19–30, Jan-Feb 2007
10. Garrick J: Ankle injuries: Frequency and mechanism of injury. J Natl Athletic Trainers Assoc, 10: 109, 1975
11. Mohammadi F: Comparison of 3 preventative methods to reduce the recurrence of ankle inversion sprains in male soccer players. Am J Sports Med 35(6): 922–926, 2007
12. Thacker SB, Stroup DF, Branche CM, et al.: The prevention of ankle sprains in sports: A systematic review of the literature. Am J Sports Med, 27(6): 753–758, 1999
13. Wolgin M, Cook C, Grahm C, Mauldin D: Conservative treatment of plantar heel pain: Long term follow-up. Foot Ankle, 15: 97–102, 1994
14. Gill L, Kiebzak GM: Outcome of non-surgical treatment for plantar fasciitis. Foot Ankle Int, 17: 527–531, 1996
15. Martin RL, Irrgang J, Conti S: Outcome study of subjects with insertional plantar fasciitis. Foot Ankle Int, 19: 803–810, 1998
16. Thomson CE, Crawford F, Murray GD: The effectiveness of extra corporeal shock wave therapy for plantar heel pain: a systematic review and meta-analysis. BMC Musc Disord, 22 (5): 19, April 2005
17. Ogden JA, Alvarez RG, Levitt RL, et al.: Electrohydraulic high-energy shock-wave treatment for chronic plantar fasciitis. JBJS, 86-A(10), 2216–2228, Oct. 2004

18. Kudo P, Dainty K, Clarfield M, et al.: Randomized, placebo-controlled, double-blind clinical trial evaluating the treatment of plantar fasciitis with an extracorporeal shock wave therapy (ESWT) device: a North American confirmatory study. J Orthop Res, 24(2): 115–123, Feb. 2006

19. Pfeffer G, Bacchetti P, Deland J et al.: Comparison of custom and prefabricated orthoses in the initial treatment of proximal plantar fasciitis. Foot Ankle Int, 20 (4): 214–221, 1999

20. Kelso SF, Richie DH, Cohen IR et al.: Direction and range of motion of the first ray. J Am Podiatr Med Assoc, 72:600, 1982

21. Kogler GF, Veer FB, Solomonidis SE, Paul JP: The influence of medial and lateral placement of orthotic wedges on loading of the plantar aponeurosis. JBJS 81–A: 1403, 1999

22. Thacker SB, Gilchrist J, Stroup DF, Kimsey DC: The prevention of shin splints in sports: a systematic review of the literature. Med Sci Sports Exerc 34(1): Jan. 2002

23. Edwards PH, Wright ML, Hartman JF: A practical approach to the differential diagnosis of chronic leg pain in the athlete. AM J Sports Med, 33(8) 1241–1249, 2005

24. Rauh, MJ, Macera CA, Trone DW, Shaffer RA, & Brodine SK: Epidemiology of stress fracture and lower-extremity overuse injury in female recruits. Med Sci Sports Exerc, 38(9): 1571–1577, 2006

25. Larson CM, Almedkinders LC, Taft TN et al. Intramedullary screw fixation of Jones fractures; Analysis of failures. Am J Sports Med, 30(1), 55–60, 2002

26. Sammarco GJ: Be alert for Jones fractures. Phys Sports Med, 20(6), 101–110, June 1992

Chapter 25
Aerobic Dance and Cheerleading

Jeffrey A. Ross

Aerobic Dance

For over 30 years, aerobic dance has been one of the most popular forms of cardiovascular exercise in America. Step/bench aerobics has evolved from a high-impact aerobic "exercise dance" form with a high degree of lower extremity injuries to a safer form of low-impact dance. The reduction of impact shock to the lower extremities has aided in the reduction of the number of lower leg and foot injuries seen by the sports medicine specialist. Initially, aerobic dancers would participate in their workouts on a floor consisting of a thin carpet and padding overlying an unrelenting concrete floor. Both exercise physiologists and sports medicine specialists saw the need for change in the surface and promoted the high-tech air-suspended wooden floor surfaces. The reduction in these injuries has been multi-factorial. For instance, the aerobic dance instructors and the participants are better trained and much more informed than they were years ago. Cross-training and new facets to the exercise routine with the addition of "kickboxing" and "urban rebounding" have helped to break up the routine and help to reduce injuries. Health magazines, instructor certification, improved aerobic and cross-training shoe design, better supervised instructors, and a better educated medical community have all led to the improvement and prevention of injuries [1].

Approximately 20 years ago aerobic dance evolved into a new form utilizing a "bench" platform and created an aerobic exercise equal if not better in its cardiovascular benefits, while reducing the impact forces to the lower extremity. The exercise routine is performed on a "step" that is 43 in. long by 16 in. wide by a minimum of 4 in. high (109 cm × 40 cm × 10 cm). At the onset it was thought that the higher the bench, a harder and more vigorous workout could be accomplished. However, over the years, and with research on the sport, it was determined that with elevations of one, two, and three block increments, the risk of overuse injury increased [2].

J.A. Ross (✉)
Department of Medicine, Baylor College of Medicine, Houston, TX 77030, USA

M.B. Werd, E.L. Knight (eds.), *Athletic Footwear and Orthoses in Sports Medicine*,
DOI 10.1007/978-0-387-76416-0_25, © Springer Science+Business Media, LLC 2010

In addition to the new equipment used in the dance studio, a new vocabulary aimed at directing the participants to specific dance steps had to be developed (Table 25.1). For the beginner aerobicizer, learning this new language was imperative, otherwise participating in the early stages of the routine could become very frustrating [1].

The foundation to any sport is the shoes the participant wears. As in running or other sports technological advances in design have led to a much more stable, high-performance shoe (Fig. 25.1). Additional changes in design have led to the newer breed of shoe known as the *cross-trainers*. These shoes permit the participant to perform aerobic dance while engaged in minimal short-distance jogging. With increased running incorporated into the routines, combined with lateral and back-peddling dance movements, the cross-trainer is a vital part of the aerobicizer's standard foot wear.

One of the most important factors in injury prevention in step/bench aerobics is the keen observation of the instructor. Most aerobic instructors agree that technique is very important in the avoidance of dance injuries and that repetition is dangerous.

Table 25.1 Terminology for aerobic dance

Helicopter move (half-hop turn)
Inner thigh
Diagonal lunge
Power knees
Leg extensions
Over the top
Straddle the bench
Double-knee with jog
Jack and jump
Karate and squat

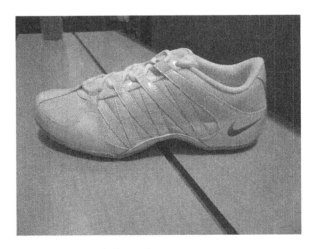

Fig. 25.1 Nike Musique IV women's dance shoe

A study conducted of aerobic dancers has shown that an aerobic dance routine performed at a cadence that was extremely fast (over 128 beats per minute) did not allow for the participant to secure his/her entire foot on the bench. This can cause the foot to hang over the edge of the bench, causing strain or an enthesis of the Achilles tendon, as well as the posterior tibial tendon or the peroneal tendons. This can also lead to a strain of the medial or central bands of the plantar fascia, or the intrinsic musculature of the plantar aspect of the foot [1, 2]. Additionally, an over the top step off the bench can lead to a number of overuse impact injuries. These can include stress fractures of the lesser metatarsals, navicular as well as the tibia or fibula, sesamoiditis, tarsal tunnel syndrome, or the interdigital neuroma formation. Biomechanical considerations, and the use of prefabricated insoles or custom foot orthoses, may be needed for these foot conditions. If the participant extends the foot too far backward off the bench, hyperextension of the ankle with concomitant traction of the Achilles tendon can occur. If left undetected, and with repetitive loading, a chronic Achilles tenosynovitis, paratendinitis, or insertional calcinosis can develop. Knee alignment is also crucial in relation to the lower leg, as well as the placement of the foot on the bench. It has also been reported that striking the floor from the bench with repetitive impact can cause chondromalacia patella, patellofemoral joint syndrome, or chronic posterior shin splints [2]. It is imperative that the aerobics instructor surveys the participants before initiating activity to determine if any have pre-existing overuse injuries, or if there is a high risk for developing an injury. A pre-dance evaluation by the sports medicine foot specialist can determine – using visual or computerized gait analysis – if the participant is at risk for developing an overuse injury. Recommendations on flexibility stretching, proper shoe gear selection, and improved range of motion to foot, ankle, and knee can be made.

Older instructors who have been teaching for over 10 years, and have taken the proper certifying courses, seem to teach safer classes and know how to prevent the pitfalls of overuse injury. On the other hand, inexperienced younger instructors who have not yet developed those supervisory skills may be more likely to induce injury to participants.

There are a number of factors that can help lower the incidence of these overuse injuries: certifying instructors, carefully selected music (pacer per minute), smooth choreography, cueing to the beat of the music, as well as the participants taking the class. The predicament for the instructor is to choose between a safe and an efficient workout, while providing for an aggressive and challenging one that could lead to an overuse injury [2].

Prevention of injuries for the aerobic dancer athlete should be a concern for the sports medicine specialist. These aerobicizers train at high levels and often ignore the potential for injury. Many may actually dance through an injury similar to runners who run through an injury in order to continue to participate and avoid downtime. Many of these participants may have physical or psychological disorders (i.e., amenorrhea, anorexia nervosa, osteoporosis – the "female triad") which can have serious repercussions when they first begin an aerobics class. The sports medicine specialist should be on the alert when interviewing the patient during the history taking, since any one of these diagnoses can render clues as to the underlying injury. Extreme weight loss, and/or stress fractures (particularly in the young female athlete), should raise suspicion for the sports medicine practitioner to look beyond the easily definable diagnosis and consider referral to the appropriate specialist [1, 3].

In a preliminary investigation by Ross of 329 participants surveyed, 153 claimed that they had suffered some discomfort or pain due to step/bench aerobics, whereas 163 claimed that they were symptom-free [1, 2]. Of those injured, 43 claimed that they had sought treatment by a foot specialist. Shoes seem to be another consideration, with 105 responding that they had some problem with their shoes (i.e., blisters, improper fit, not enough support, cutting off circulation, irritation), while 197 denied any problems with their shoes. The most common sites for the incidence of injury were the (1) knee, (2) calf, (3) Achilles tendon, (4) foot, and (5) shin.

Instructors interviewed during the study made the following recommendations:

1. Keep the knees slightly bent, never locking the knee.
2. Bring the foot all the way up to the bench, so that the heel is not hanging off.
3. Keep the knee over the ankle (creates less strain on the knee).
4. Push off with the heel (not with the knee) with either squats or lunges.
5. Keep the head up and the chest tall (to prevent lower back strain).
6. Avoid stepping too far away from the bench.
7. Avoid stepping overenthusiastically or ballistically off the step.
8. Maintain the same pace and avoid stepping too quickly.
9. Do not be afraid to lower the bench to a level more suitable to your abilities to avoid injury.

It was important to note that the instructors felt (1) the class size was important in order to observe properly, (2) keeping the pace of the step at 128 beats per minute, whereas exceeding the pace would not allow the entire foot to rest on the bench, (3) technique was extremely important to avoid injury, (4) excessive repetition of the steps can lead to injury, (5) keeping the height of the benches under three platforms: hyperextension of the knee can occur with more, and (6) stretching and warm-up prior to activity is essential to avoid injuries.

Step and bench aerobics have become a very popular form of exercise workout for the enthusiast. Careful monitoring of the participants has been shown to be helpful in avoiding injuries. For the sports medicine practitioner, understanding the mechanics of the sport, the terminology, as well as the biomechanics of the individual participant can help predict what injuries may occur and how to properly diagnose and treat when the occasion arises.

Urban Rebounding

Other forms of aerobic dance have surfaced over those few years, with one exciting form of aerobic workout entitled *urban rebounding*. The urban rebounding system was created by J. B. Berns, a practicing martial artist. The workout has its roots in the martial arts and core body postures, resulting in a non-stop abdominal workout, which strengthens the core and improves balance and coordination. The workout begins with the use of a small trampoline referred to as the urban rebounder.

The warm-up consists of a series of jumps and toe taps. The exercise consists of about 30 min of a combination which progressively adds moves to include "straddle hops," "knee-ups," and jumping jacks. The next part of the workout includes interval training in which a series of jogs is followed by sprints, picking the knees up as high as possible. The spring in the rebounder allows for recoil without the impact of a floor aerobics program or jogging. Certain movements are able to be performed on the rebounder such as a basic bounce, straddle, lateral knee raise, jumping jacks, twists/double twists, 180 degree turns, military press, forward jump, upright row, and forward knee abdominal crunch. There are also sports-specific moves including the four jog sprints, vertical jumps, 180 degree spins, and power jump/knee tucks [4].

Biomechanical considerations for this whole workout is as important as with step/bench aerobics. Foot position on the rebounder is essential. Proprioception of the foot and ankle on the rebounder is also critical. A rebounder participant should not participate if previous ankle injury or ankle instability is present. Since there are so many deep knee lunges (similar to alpine skiing – great preparation), a participant with chondromalacia patella should avoid this workout as well. Quadriceps strengthening for this workout would also be recommended. Shoe consideration is also important, with worn out or distorted shoe counters a reason for elimination. Balanced, stable motion control shoes are essential for this workout program. Biomechanical balancing with orthoses may also be necessary. This core body and lower extremity workout has many advantages over the high-impact or bench-type aerobics program; however, lower extremity considerations are very apparent and need to be focused prior to initiating this workout.

Kickboxing

This aerobic exercise routine combines martial arts and aerobics together. With upper body arm movement and leg extensions and kicks, this intense workout can help to build upper body as well as lower body strength. Proper lower extremity flexibility is essential before knee flexion and extensions are attempted. Balancing on one foot and attempting to extend the opposite foot can place increased strain upon the support limb. Rotation of the hip and extending the lower limb again places stress upon the support limb. Kickboxing has been shown to be an excellent form of aerobic training which increases cardiovascular endurance. Foot balance and lower extremity strength is essential in order to perform the movements properly. As in step/bench proper instructor supervision of the participants' movement can help to avoid overuse injury.

Cheerleading

Cheerleading's roots can be traced back to a cold day in the 1880s on the Princeton campus when the "locomotive cheer" first came upon the scene. In 1884, Thomas Peebler, a graduate of Princeton University, took the locomotive cheer and shared with his students at the University of Minnesota the first cheer. On a crisp fall day, November 2, 1898, on the Minnesota campus, Johnny Campbell began the first official cheerleader "yell." The father of modern cheerleading was Lawrence "Herkie" Herkimer from Southern Methodist University, who eventually formed the National Cheerleading Association.

In cheerleading various movements are important. Jumps, stunts, basket tosses, and tricks, and lunges are just to name a few. Beginning with the motions and cheers that cheerleaders engage, leg positions are a vital part of the cheer. Three leg positions are involved, namely the lunge, back lunge, and the wide. The lunge is performed by keeping the front leg bent and the back leg straight. The straight leg classifies the lunge as either "right" or left. The back lunge is accomplished with the front leg bent. The hips should face forward and the other leg should extend back. Weight is on the back leg. The wide position is created by keeping the leg stance open, slightly wider than the shoulder width apart [5].

The second important category is jumps. The most popular jump is the toe touch, followed by other jumps such as the front or side hurdler, double nines, and around the world. In the toe touch the position creates the appearance of a hyper-extended jump. It requires a strong hip flexor together with a powerful jump off the ground. In the front hurdler the cheerleader snaps his/her front leg up to the chest, keeping the back leg bent behind the body. On the jump, the arms are extended directly in front of the athlete. The side hurdler is accomplished in the same fashion but with the torso facing the side direction, rather the forward. The around the world jump is performed by creating a front pike that opens up into a toe touch. The double nine is not as common and is performed by making the shape of the figure nine. There are a number of jump drills that the cheerleader can perform in order to perfect their jumps. The straight jumps, the tuck jump, frog jump, snap-ups, standing one-leg snap-ups, seated leg raises, and repetitive jumps are just a few. These jump drills are a part of the practice and help to improve jumping skills.

Stunting is probably the most colorful part of the cheerleading experience and can be one of the most dangerous in terms of injury (Fig. 25.2.). Each cheerleader has a specific role and position in stunting and should rotate in their participation just to understand what their teammates' roles are like. The various roles are the following: the flyer, who will be tossed and flies through the air; the base (or bases) who perform the toss, holds, and supports the weight of the flier; the third, responsible for the back portion of the stunt and assists the bases with tossing, holding, and supporting the flier. The third is regarded as another base member. The spot (or fourth) is there to "spot" and ensures the safety of the stunt and to assist with the stunt as necessary [5].

Spotting drills are very important and help to ensure the success and safety of the stunt. They also help to build trust with each member of the "team." The various

Fig. 25.2 Each cheerleader has a specific role and position in stunting. (Courtesy of All-Girl Cheerleading Club on NC State University, Raleigh, NC)

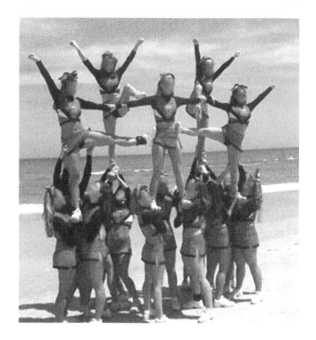

drills used are the step off where the athlete practices both stepping off (flyer) and catching (base) roles. The platform will gradually be raised to increase the level of difficulty. The lower down is the next progression from the step off drill. The athletes load the flyer up into a stunt and then slowly lower her to the ground level. The fall-back cradle is where the athlete familiarizes themselves with being caught in a cradle. The cheerleaders should familiarize themselves with holding the flyer in the cradle catch before attempting to catch a flyer from a backward fall [5]. These drills are intended to help prevent injury to the flyer. Each member of the team has a specific role and is vital to the success of the stunt and to the safety of the flyer. The dismount of the flyer is the way in which they are brought back to the ground. The most common dismounts are the "pop down" and the "cradle." Multiple bases and multiple pyramids are developed to enhance the various stunts and to optimize the trajectory of the flyer. Many of these designs can be quite complex and take a significant amount of coordination, particularly with the toss and catch of the flyer.

Pre-conditioning, flexibility, strengthening, and coordination are essential for success in the cheerleader's routines. Injury prevention is essential; however, injuries do occur. Ankle strains are probably one of the most common injuries encountered in this sport: stress fractures of the foot, knee injuries, and overuse muscular injuries, just to name a few. The sports medicine specialist is an important part of the cheerleader program and should regard these athletes as important as the football or basketball players whom they cheer for. When injuries do occur to the cheerleader, "downtime" can be just as devastating as to the athlete on the field or court. Psychological as well as physical support is just as important.

Cheerleading has become a very popular sport with serious competitions between teams as seen on the nationally televised scene. Cheerleading clubs in addition to scholastic cheerleading squads have become just as popular for the young athlete. Dance routines, acrobatics, and gymnastic skills have become integrated in the cheerleading routines, which have added to their complexity. Again, the sports medicine specialist should be familiar with many of the terms, and movements of the sport, to understand how injuries may occur.

References

1. Ross JA, Subotnick SI: Step/Bench Aerobic dance and its potential for injuries of the lower extremity, pp. 657–660. in Subotnick SI (ed.), Sports Medicine of the Lower Extremity, 2nd edn. Churchill Livingstone, New York, Edinburgh, San Francisco, 1999.
2. Ross JA: A study of step/bench Aerobic injuries, Presented at the American College of Sports Medicine Scientific Meeting, May 1998, Orlando, Florida.
3. Ross JA: Step/Bench Aerobics; Sports medicine and injuries, pp. 346–347. in Lorimer DL (ed.), Neale's Disorders of the Foot, 7th edn, Churchill Livingstone, London, Edinburgh, New York, 2006.
4. JB Berns: Urban Rebounding, 2008, Web Site   www.urbanrebounding.com
5. Wilson L: The Ultimate Guide to Cheerleading, pp. 69–75. Three Rivers Press, New York, 2003.

Chapter 26
Dance

Lisa M. Schoene

Lower Extremity Biomechanics and Considerations in the Evaluation of the Dancer

Today the dancer's body appears in many shapes and sizes, due to an increasing interest in dance forms other than ballet, i.e., tap, modern, jazz, hip hop, and Irish dance. Dance for many years has only been seen as an "art form," now we must realize the rigors and athleticism that is necessary to perform. The differing styles of dance all place high demands on the body which parallels or supersedes that of any other demanding sport. "Only the astronaut in our society is a more selected individual than the professional ballet dancer," according to Dr. William Hamilton [1].

There are variances within each of the dance forms, so the stresses on the lower extremity may be different. The traditional starting point for a dancer is the five universal ballet positions which are taught during ballet classes. These positions are carried throughout the dancer's career as ballet is the staple to which most forms of dance training work from. Traditional female ballet dancers dancing on pointe will have different stresses on the lower extremity and body than a modern female barefoot dancer who may be lifting another female dancer or performing on the floor using acrobatic movements. Understanding the universal but different nuances within each style of dance can help the evaluation and treatment process. Dancers have lower extremity injury rates well over 50% and it is noted that dancers have been shown to sustain more lower extremity injuries than that of collegiate athletes [2, 3].

A biomechanical evaluation of the lower extremity should include the foot, knee, and hip. Flexibility and strength tests should be performed as well as evaluating functional dance movements. The dancer should have on shorts or a leotard in order to accurately see alignment.

L.M. Schoene (✉)
Gurnee Podiatry & Sports Medicine, Park City, IL 60085, USA

M.B. Werd, E.L. Knight (eds.), *Athletic Footwear and Orthoses in Sports Medicine*,
DOI 10.1007/978-0-387-76416-0_26, © Springer Science+Business Media, LLC 2010

The Foot

A non-weight-bearing and weight-bearing examination should be performed to access the range of motion of the joints and the strength of the muscles. The weight-bearing examination should include measurements of resting and neutral calcaneal stance position (Fig. 26.1), forefoot position as it relates to the rearfoot, assessment of arch height, and a "releve" (up on toes) check (Fig. 26.2). Evaluation of the first ray and first MPJ is very important to help assess the ability of the dancer to be able to properly rise up onto demi-pointe. Normal range of motion (ROM) for the first metatarsal phalangeal joint (MPJ) in an adult is 65 degrees. For the dancer, approximately 90 degrees of dorsiflexion of the first MPJ is necessary for proper demi-point

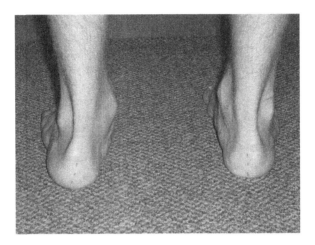

Fig. 26.1 Resting and neutral calcaneal stance position

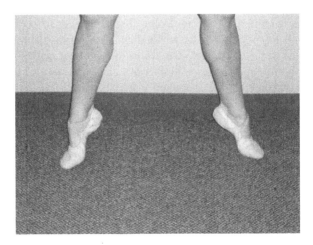

Fig. 26.2 Releve of the foot

stance. The peroneus longus is continually activated when up onto demi-pointe and it is the primary plantarflexor of the first ray. The peroneus longus EMG studies peak at the time of jumping and toe-off [4]. In the abnormally pronating foot, the peroneus longus loses the effective pull, thus allowing for dysfunction of the first ray and first MPJ. Testing the first ray should be done by loading the foot off weight bearing and checking it standing. When the arch is corrected by aligning the subtalar and midtarsal joints out of a pronated position the first MPJ ROM should improve (Fig. 26.3).

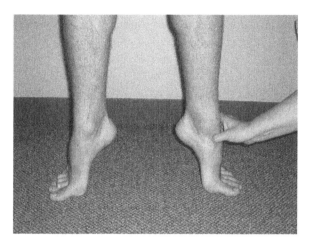

Fig. 26.3 Releve with proper alignment

The Functional Examination

The functional examination should include having the dancer perform all five dance positions on releve and with demi-plies in each position, simple jumps can be used for the evaluation process as well. The foot while on the floor should have a three-point balancing system, the first and fifth MT and the heel. This triangle forms a base, so the foot can work in a strong and supported system [5]. As the dancer rises onto demi-point, plies, or jumps the alignment should remain consistently aligned through the ankle, subtalar, midtarsal, and MPJ joints (Fig. 26.4a, b).

Weight-bearing foot x-ray evaluation is always helpful to assess the biomechanics of the foot. Growth plate evaluation should be considered for the adolescent dancer. Functional x-rays while up on pointe or demi-pointe can be taken to see if abnormal toe or metatarsal positions are present. It is not uncommon to see increased cortical bone along the metatarsals in experienced dancers due to increased loading of the foot. Early recognition of foot deformities, i.e., bunions and hammertoes, can be halted by early intervention with dance and street shoe gear changes and orthotic devices to prevent abnormal pronatory forces.

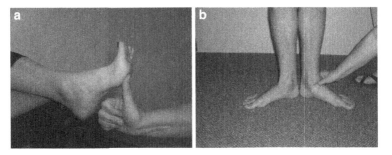

Fig. 26.4 (**a**) First ray testing non-weight bearing. (**b**) First ray testing weight bearing

The Knee

The knee should be evaluated non-weight bearing and weight bearing. Traditional ligament and patellar testing should be performed. The alignment of the patellofemoral joint is very important; evaluating the Q angle helps to assess for increased risk of patellofemoral syndrome or dislocation. If there is an increased Q angle of over 15 degrees, abnormal lateral pulling on the patella may occur. Rotational and jumping movements require excessive lateral pull of the patella upon takeoff, so an increased Q angle may predispose the dancer to injury. Other overuse injuries like patellar tendonitis can also occur from continual plies and releves during class and rehearsal [6]. Medial knee strain can occur due to limited external hip rotation and increased turnout from the knee, overpronated feet causing internal tibial rotation, or weak hip musculature. When evaluating the adolescent, keep in mind that the knee goes through the genu varum and genu valgum stages prior to straightening out at approximately 8 years of age. It is not uncommon for dancers with ligament laxity to have slight genu recurvatum as well. When treating the dancer it is important to address the abnormal biomechanics creating these alignment issues when possible.

The Hip

Proper ROM of the hip is critical for the dancer to attain the correct alignment for esthetic purposes and to safely perform the necessary movements. Normal adult external rotation is approximately 45–50 degrees. Ninety degrees of external rotation is desired in the classical ballet dancer. As young dancers are working on the turnout *en dehors*, teachers should allow it to develop safely and under supervision as it can take many years of training. If the dancer does not attain at least 60–70 degrees of turnout before advancing onto pointe work, it may be advised to hold on this advanced work. When evaluating for proper ROM and strength, the examination should include hip extended and flexed to check for soft tissue or bony limitations. The weight-bearing examination should test the functional movements of dance; this can be evaluated using the rotation disk (Fig. 26.5). External hip values are

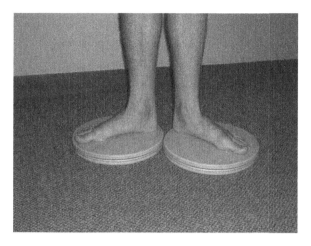

Fig. 26.5 Rotational disk

attained through femoral neck bony adaptations by exercises and stretching up to approximately 12 years of age; after this age, bony architecture shows less plasticity. It is thought that soft tissue stretching can help turnout position primarily through stretching the iliofemoral ligament. Evaluating the hip functionally with lunges, squats, and jumps can alert the evaluator to hip weakness. Improper hip turnout will potentially lead to soft tissue stresses and injury similar to that seen at the knee.

General Flexibility and Strength

The question is always do these athletes choose dance or does dance choose them? Inherent ligament laxity is quite typical of the adolescent and professional dancer, as extreme flexibility and joint position demands are high. These extreme ranges are not typically required by other sports. Age appropriate, safe flexibility and strength exercises should always be administered to the dancer. Simple foot and lower extremity exercises can be done regularly using rubber tubing, which can be stored in dance bags for easy use (Figs. 26.6a–d and 26.7a–d). Pointe work should require good strength, good balance, and proper alignment of the foot, knee, and hip. The standard requirement of the ankle is for the dancer to be able to perform 25 heel raises [7]. Proper abdominal strength can be tested with a plank test, a double-leg lowering test, or the above-mentioned lunges or squats and or jumps. General balance and coordination may differ among dancers, especially adolescents. Just as the dancer is improving and preparing to go on pointe, the balance and proprioception abilities may regress. When the dancer finishes up the last growth spurt, the balance and proprioception will typically be secured once again. The last growth spurt can be completed up to 17 years of age. Teacher and parent guidance and discussion will help to soothe away worry.

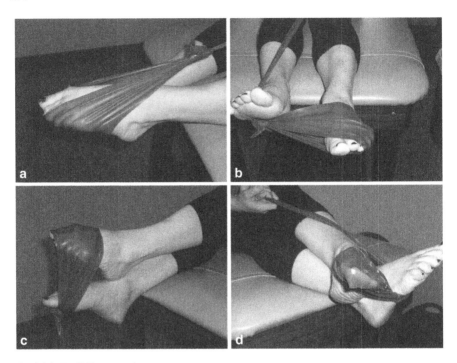

Fig. 26.6 (**a–d**) Foot exercises

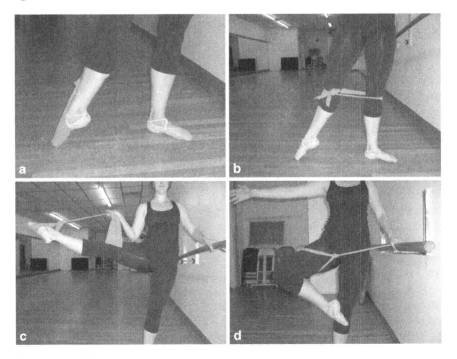

Fig. 26.7 (**a–d**) Hip exercises

What to Look for at the Foot and Ankle

Due to the nature of the various forms of dance the foot and how it functions is an extremely valuable asset. For the ballet dancer, a foot examination is common by teachers at an early age. The desired shape, function, and esthetic will get the dancer far as it relates to injury and possibly job security. A dancer may put upward of four times body weight on each foot per jump with only a ballet slipper on the foot, as opposed to that of a runner wearing a thick cushioned shoe [8]. The best shape for the dancer's foot is having all the toes or at least the first three toes the same length. Reports of varying toe lengths may predispose the dancer to stress fractures and other soft tissue injury [9]. A nicely formed longitudinal arch is ideal; many dancers will work the arch by stretching it to help produce the proper degree and esthetic of the pointed position. Dangerous practices of extreme stretching still exists, so stressing the importance of safe and progressive strengthening and stretching is paramount.

The Ankle Joint

Normal adult plantarflexion is approximately 50 degrees; in a dancer approximately 90 degrees is needed for proper pointing positions and movements. A quick check for enough plantarflexion of the ankle can be done using a pencil on the talus; when the foot is fully pointed, the pencil should line up parallel with the tibia [10] (Fig. 26.8).

The Midtarsal Joint

The midtarsal joint is also called the *coup de pied*. This joint should have ability to rotate plantarly like the ankle. There are five secondary plantarflexors of the

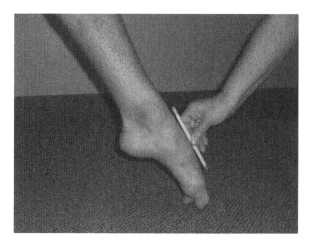

Fig. 26.8 Pencil test

foot (peroneus longus, peroneus brevis, tibialis posterior, flexor digitorum longus, and flexor hallucis longus); they all assist to produce that strong pointed foot. Contraction only of the two primary plantarflexors (gastrocnemius and soleus) without the aid of the secondary muscles due to weakness will contract and pull the calcaneus into equinus, allowing the talus to slide down and forward creating a "locked"-like affect, not allowing the midtarsal joint to plantarflex properly. This ultimately leads to the dancer forcing the foot to point distal to the midtarsal joint. In order for this to happen, the pointed appearance is really coming from the tarsometatarsal joints, i.e., Lisfranc's joint. Although this foot may look properly pointed this foot is not stable, due to the fact that the talus is not gliding properly. The dancer may complain of a "jammed"-like feeling and the inability to point the foot properly (Fig. 26.9).

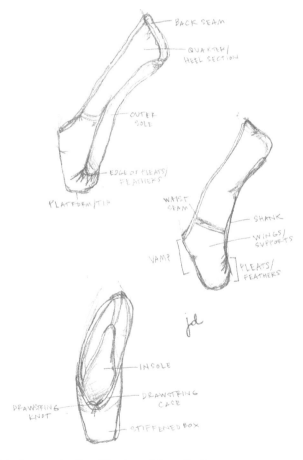

Fig. 26.9 Pointe shoe construction. (Courtesy of the author)

Footwear Recommendations and Modifications

Footwear is limited or non-existent in ballet, modern, and Irish dance. Most often the dancer will take class in socks or a ballet slipper. For the modern dancer they will take class barefoot or use a thin jazz shoe. Even when shoe use is limited it is important that proper fit be considered. The ballet slipper or jazz shoe comes in canvas cloth or leather. As the shoe stretches, the fit will change. The toe area should be snug but not too tight as pressures on the metatarsal joints, soft tissue, and/or nerves may be compromised. Often adding one size to a shoe can reduce foot pain. Some thin plastazote or poron padding can be added in the ball of the foot to add cushioning for the metatarsals. The pointe (toe) shoe comes in a satin material over layered paper or fabric which is dipped with glue. The fitting process can be challenging even for the professional dancer, as there are many shoe makers many being out of the United States. Depending on the skill level, the shoe can be made with varying shank stability, vamp shape, wing stiffness, and platform shapes.

The standard for the new pointe dancer is a harder shoe at first then as she becomes stronger, she can progress into the softer shoe: Some dance schools suggest a de-shanked pointe shoe for the dancers preparing to go up onto pointe, as it makes the dancer work harder to point the foot, and adds some weight at the toe area to prepare the dancer for regular pointe work[11]. The typical age for going up onto pointe is approximately 11. Pointe shoe fitting is critical and should be done by a professional fitter. With proper fitting, the formation of blisters and calluses should be minimal. Lamb's wool is the preferred choice of material to fill inside the toe box, as silicone or rubber padding may restrict movement of the toes. Very thin padding (poron or plastazote) can be added inside the ballet slipper or Irish dance slipper as well or point shoe to help with metatarsal pains or loss of fat padding. Some point shoes will accommodate a very thin digital corn pad to prevent soft corns that may start if a shoe is too snug in the toe box. Traditional podiatric longitudinal metatarsal pads can usually fit into a soft slipper, or slightly loosened pointe shoe if a foot injury exists or to prevent abnormal pronatory forces. The Braver ballet orthosis has the ability to help re-align the foot and can be used in ballet shoes as well. Tap shoes have a larger internal volume and can usually accommodate a small pad or thin orthosis. Lacing of the shoe can be changed to snug the heel fit or give more arch support. The hard Irish dance shoe is like a combination of a pointe shoe and a tap shoe harder in the toe box, and heel counter, but very flexible through the arch. This shoe is snug and only small amounts of padding can be added. Athletic tape is the best option for these tight-fitting dance shoes.

Foot Hygiene

Proper callus, blister, and toenail care are very important and can prevent infections. Barefoot dancers may sustain floor burns, or splinters, and may contract potential skin infections if the skin is repeatedly cracked or callused. Tapes or light bandages that are skin colored can be used under most dance shoes and stockings or for barefoot dancers without much notice. These various tapes can be used to support an injured tendon or ligament or to cover a blister or painful callus. Proper first aid treatments should be initiated immediately if there is a problem. It is important to keep ballet and jazz shoes dry in order to extend the life and prevent trapped moisture. The use of powders and shoe trees for the more structured shoes will help to keep the shape. Street shoes are an important consideration for the dancer. When rehabbing a lower extremity injury, avoid wearing unsupportive shoes, flip flops, or going barefoot. While rehabbing an injury, proper foot and arch support will aid in the speed of recovery.

Proper and thorough examination of the dancer will alert the examiner to instabilities, weaknesses, and biomechanical abnormalities. With this knowledge the dancer can improve his or her technique and possibly prevent unnecessary injuries.

References

1. Hamilton W: Ballet: The ideal body type, Cleveland clinic organization paper, November 2004
2. Garrick J, Requa R: Ballet Injuries: An analysis of epidemiology and financial outcomes. Am J Sports Med, 21:586–590, 1993.
3. Mayers L, Judelson D, Bronner S: The prevalence of injury among tap dancers. J Dance Med Sci, 7:121–125, 2003.
4. Travel J, Simons D: Myofascial pain and dysfunction, The trigger point manual, pp. 370–396. Butler J (ed.), Peroneal Muscles. Williams and Wilkins, Philadelphia, PA, 1992
5. Spilken T: The dancer's foot book, Barrett R (ed.), Princeton Book Company,7–14, 1990.
6. Brown T, Micheli, L: Where artistry meets injury. Biomechanics,: 13–22, 1998.
7. Lunsford BRP: The standing heel rise test for ankle plantarflexion: criterion for normal. Physical Therapy, 75:694–698, 1995.
8. Spilken T. The Dancers Foot Book, Barrett R (ed.), Princeton Book Company, 1–6, 1990.
9. Kahn K, Brown J, Way S et al.: Overuse injuries in classical ballet. Sports Med, 5:341–357, 1995.
10. Novella T: An easy way to quantify plantarflexion in the ankle. J Back Musculoskelet Rehabil, 8, 1995.
11. Barringer J, Schlesinger S: The Pointe Book, pp. 19–31. Princeton Book Company, Princeton, NJ, 1998.

Suggested Readings

1. Braver R: Insights on orthotic treatment of ballet injuries. Podiatry Today, 13:21–26, 2000.
2. Leanderson J, Eriksson E, Nilsson C et al.: Proprioception in classical Ballet dancers. A prospective study of the influence of an ankle sprain on proprioception in the ankle joint. Am J Sports Med, 24:370–374, 1996.
3. Macintyre J, Joy E: Foot and ankle injuries. Clin Sports Med, 10:351–367, 2000.
4. Kravitz S, Murgia C: Common dance injuries: Why they occur. Podiatry Today, 10:38–44, 1997.
5. Lasser M: The dance: DPM's keep performers in step. Podiatry Today, 10:22–36, 1997.
6. Theresa H: Beyond the satin: How to judge a shoe. Pointe, 3:61–63, 2002.

 7. Cunningham B, DiStefano A, Kirjanov N et al.: A comparative Mechanical analysis of the pointe shoe. Am J Sports Med, 26:555–561, 1998.
 8. Van Dijk CN, Poortman A, Strubbe EH et al.: Degenerative joint disease in female ballet dancers. Am J Sports Med, 23:295–300, 1995.
 9. Bronner S, Ojofeitimi S, Rose D: Injuries in a modern dance company. Am J Sports Med, 31:365–373, 2003
10. McGuinness D, Doody C: The injuries of competitive irish dancers. J Dance Med Sci, 10: 35–44, 2006.

Chapter 27
Baseball and Softball

Tim Dutra

Baseball and softball are very popular sports at all levels of play and are considered limited contact sports. Recreational players typically have a poor level of conditioning, and many softball players will play well into their adult years. The evolution of baseball and softball cleats has basically followed the same pattern as football and soccer shoes. Surfaces are natural or artificial turf in the field and dirt or clay on the infield base paths. Metal cleats are primarily for high school, college, and professional players; however, metal cleats are allowed in some junior and senior divisions in Little League Baseball. In recent years there has been an explosion of female participation in softball leagues from youth through professional teams.

Lower Extremity Biomechanics and Considerations of Baseball and Softball

There are unique motions in baseball as compared to other sports in regards to throwing and hitting, which are complex motions. Throwing and hitting require transferring weight to achieve the maximum force and balance. Baseball and softball involve straight ahead sprinting, rounding bases, sliding, batting, throwing, and pitching. Sprinting involves running the bases and fielding the balls. Side-to-side movements include taking leads, running bases, and fielding balls. The feet remain neutral to give the body an increase in stability for the lower extremity to compensate for the upper body force exerted. There is also more demand on the right foot and shoe due to running on the base paths, where the shoe contacts the inside corner of the base. Pitchers also have the increased demand of pushing off during their pitching motion, so the more rigid the sole of the shoe the better support during push off. The catcher requires more flexion in the ball of the foot as the position

T. Dutra (✉)
Student Health Services, California State University, East Bay, Hayward, CA, USA

M.B. Werd, E.L. Knight (eds.), *Athletic Footwear and Orthoses in Sports Medicine*,
DOI 10.1007/978-0-387-76416-0_27, © Springer Science+Business Media, LLC 2010

requires that most of the time they are in the squatting position, with weight equally distributed on both feet. There is no predilection of foot types with rectus, planus, and cavus foot types equally applicable for baseball or softball.

General Footwear Recommendations

As a rule when fitting shoes for athletes, the shoes should feel comfortable from the start and they should not require a break in period. Shoes offer protection, support, and cushioning for the athlete, but ill fitting shoes will cause blisters and nail problems. Shoe characteristics and features for baseball and softball cleats should address the following [1–3]: (1) firm heel counter, (2) torsional rigidity, (3) shoe flexion in the forefoot, (4) stable upper material with hard leather preferable, (5) single density midsole, (6) external last – straight last increases control, (7) internal last – board lasted, (8) outsole with cleats usually square made of molded rubber, polyurethane-like material, or metal (Figs. 27.1 and 27.2). Some models have detachable replacement cleats. Turf cleats have shorter and more numerous rubber studded cleats, and (9) cushioning-EVA-wedged midsole increases cushioning. Lacing techniques include conventional techniques – diagonal or chevron, and parallel. Socks include cotton sanitary hose; a player may use synthetic sock underneath sanitary hose made from acrylic, polyester, polypropylene, or nylon.

Fig. 27.1 Men's molded cleat baseball shoe. (Courtesy of New Balance, Boston, MA)

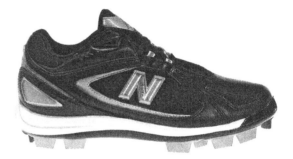

Footwear Modifications

Pathology Specific (Acute and Chronic)

Shoe and lacing considerations are the same as for general recommendations. Prefabricated insoles can provide some cushioning and support for acute or mild problems. As a general rule, the slower athletic movements require more medial support, which is best provided by straight lasted shoe. A curve lasted shoe is better adapted for faster movements which increase stress on the outer aspect of the foot. Variable width lacing is very helpful for wide or narrow foot types. Uppers are usually leather with a padded tongue and collar for comfort. A rigid heel counter

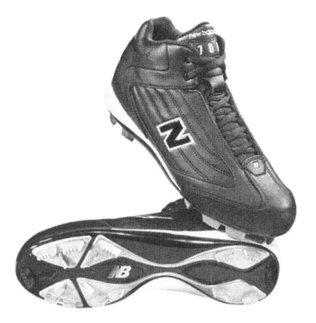

Fig. 27.2 Men's high-top baseball cleats with non-metal spikes. (Courtesy of New Balance, Boston, MA)

is needed for support and to prevent heel slippage, as well as a soft and flexible Achilles tendon heel pad. Metal cleats usually have the split cleat with three cleats in front and two in the heel. Some models come with removable versions. Softball cleats are usually lightweight and have multi-studded cleats. Pitchers often require a toe cap for toe drag to help prevent excessive wear to the front of the shoe. Most of the baseball and softball shoes are patterned after running shoe technology, with a wider, deeper toe box, more rigid heel with Achilles pad, lacing pattern, and a sock liner/insole with more cushioning and support. Many brands and models are available to choose from – including team colors. Popular brand names include Adidas, Easton, Mizuno, New Balance, Nike, Puma, Reebok, and Under Armour, and most baseball shoes will allow adequate room for a low-profile custom foot orthosis.

Special features of baseball and softball cleats include the following:

- Ankle strap for increased lock down
- Flex grooves in forefoot of shoe
- Full-length midsole to increase cleat pressure dispersion
- Multidirectional pattern outsole for maximum traction
- Nylon pull tab in heels
- Molded EVA sock liner
- Lightweight synthetic and mesh upper combination
- Molded heel for lateral support
- Different number of spikes for traction

References

1. Cheskin MP: The Complete Handbook of Athletic Footwear. Fairchild Publications, New York, 1987.
2. Denton J: Athletic shoes. in Valmassey RL (ed.), Clinical Biomechanics of Lower Extremities. St. Louis, Mosby, 451–462, 1996.
3. Segesser B, Pforringer W: The Shoe in Sport. Year Book Medical Publishers, London, 1989.

Chapter 28
Special Olympics

Patrick Nunan and Shawn Walls

Mentally and physically handicapped individuals, such as those afflicted with Down syndrome and cerebral palsy, have gait problems that progress with age. These gait abnormalities frequently lead to the eventual development of foot pain if not corrected. No matter what the etiology, foot pain can lead to a decrease in activity and mobility and, for the mentally handicapped, the eventual removal of community participation [1]. Studies have found that early identification and correction with conservative care of lower extremity foot deformities commonly seen with the mentally and physically challenged can lead to improved development of the individual both physically and socially [2, 3]. This chapter covers orthoses, shoe gear, and shoe modifications to help with the most common pedal problems associated with active mentally and physically challenged individuals, with the hope of improving physical activity and wellness.

In 1948, Sir Ludwig Guttman held the first organized sporting event for the physically handicapped. The Paralympic games, founded by Guttman, included athletes with visual and physical impairments, such as those with amputations and those requiring wheelchairs [4, 5]. Other programs have since been created that allow for the participation of a wide variety of athletes, including those with mental and physical disabilities, in national and international competitions. One of the most noted organizations today is the Special Olympics. The Special Olympics is dedicated to providing training for 2.25 million mentally challenged athletes in 160 countries, promoting improvement in both physical and mental fitness [6]. In the United States, there are an estimated 2–3 million active athletes with mental and physical disabilities [5].

There is a vast volume of literature covering the physical improvements that exercise and physical activity can have on the human body. This literature mainly covers normal developing adults. Little research has been generated for the physically and mentally handicapped active population [4]. The small amount of research that has

P. Nunan (✉)
Fit Feet/Healthy Athletes/Special Olympics, Inc.; Podiatry Section, The Jewish Hospital of Cincinnati, 7797 Joan Dr., West Chester, OH 45069, USA

M.B. Werd, E.L. Knight (eds.), *Athletic Footwear and Orthoses in Sports Medicine*,
DOI 10.1007/978-0-387-76416-0_28, © Springer Science+Business Media, LLC 2010

been conducted is dedicated to showing that with an increase in activity and inter-active events such as sports, mentally and physically handicapped persons show improvements in daily activity, health, and social interactions [3–5, 7].

Before a handicapped individual participates in athletic events a thorough physical should be performed to assess physical limitations. Athletes with mental and physical challenges can have physical limitations and health risks that are non-conducive to certain athletic events. Physical limitations that should be considered before participation in individual sporting activity include endurance, strength, and mobility. Severe health risks, including those that can cause loss of body control or even death, need to be identified. For instance, in individuals with Down syndrome up to 25 percent have atlantoaxial instability from ligament laxity. Increased ligamentous laxity can allow subluxation of the C1 vertebrae on the C2 vertebrae. Vertebral subluxation will cause compression on the spinal cord by the dens. Spinal cord compression can present as abnormal neurological manifestations, quadriplegia, and death [1, 8]. In individuals with cerebral palsy, 40 percent of all children have an associated seizure disorder [3]. Seizure disorders need to be identified, addressed, and monitored by a medical professional before athletic clearance can be given.

A brief discussion on normal gait and the development of the lower extremity is warranted. During a normal child's growth the lower extremity rotates inward and outward around a central axis at three key osseous locations: the hip, knee, and ankle. The rotation is caused by a balance of soft tissue development and the growth of long bones. There are three key periods of growth that occur at approximately ages 1, 6, and 15. At each age the bones of the hip, knee, and ankle are rotating either inward or outward, ultimately causing the foot to retain an inward or outward position. Key rotating bones are the femur, fibula, and tibia at the tibial condyles and malleoli. Differences in femoral and tibial bone rotation result in bringing the knee into a progressively decreased varum position, rotating the knee inward, and bringing the knees closer together throughout skeletal maturity. At the ankle, the external malleolar position increases with age.

The result of the combined bone rotation at all levels of the lower extremity causes out-toeing or an externally rotated flatfoot from 0 to 2 years old. Flat foot and out-toeing can be considered normal from birth to 2 years old as a child will be unable to form a foot arch due to lack of maturity of the neurological system until after age 2. Intoeing, or "pigeon toe," will be present from 4 to 6 years old and again at 13–15 years old. At the age of skeletal maturity, 15–18 years old, the malleoli should be rotated 18–23° of external rotation forming the normal mildly everted foot position of about 18° from the body's sagittal cardinal plane [9].

Common foot problems affecting normal gait can be classified into three general categories: pes planus, pes cavus, and equinus. These pathologies are the result of one or a mixture of three main biomechanical mechanisms: pronation, supination, and ankle equinus. Other problems commonly associated with mentally challenged athletes include hyperhidrosis syndromes.

Ankle equinus is the inability of the foot, at the ankle joint, to dorsiflex 10° past perpendicular to the leg. It is a common deforming force in the foot, typically causing the foot to pronate. Pronation is a frequent biomechanical compensation in normal gait. Primary manifestations of ankle equinus without biomechanical compensation, such as tiptoe walking, are not commonly seen except in certain neuromuscular diseases such as muscular dystrophy and cerebral palsy. Conservative treatment for ankle equinus consists of intrinsic and extrinsic heel lifts and will be discussed with the conservative treatments of pes cavus and pes planus.

Pes planus, or flat foot, is one of the most common foot conditions globally [10]. Flexible flat foot has been shown to occur in 44 percent of children aged 3–6 years old [11]. Some experts consider flat foot a normal developmental stage in children up to 6 years old [12]. The most common cause of flat foot is excessive pronation at the subtalar joint.

Pronation of the foot inhibits mechanical dampening mechanisms by the bone and soft tissues, preventing internal rotation of the leg during heel contact and leading to foot and joint pain. Pronation is considered to be the foot at the subtalar joint functioning at maximum eversion. Quantitatively pronation can be described as a measurement equal to or greater than $10°$ eversion at the subtalar joint, leaving the calcaneus in a valgus position [8, 13].

Pronation can be visually identified in several ways: (1) an everted heel; (2) flat medial arch on or off weightbearing; (3) prominent talar head or midtarsal bones; (4) the inability of the heel to supinate with performance of the Jack's test or Hubscher maneuver, activating the windlass mechanism to form the medial foot arch; (5) forefoot abduction causing "too many toes sign" on weightbearing evaluation; and (6) the lateral border of the foot appearing shorter than the medial border [13, 14]. Appearance of a midtarsal bony collapse with a pronated foot is usually an indicator of more severe pes planus problems [13]. The degree of abnormal pronation leading to pes planus depends on a variety of factors.

Flat foot disorders can be classified as either pathological or physiological. Pathological disorders are commonly seen at birth and cause rigid abnormalities. Examples of pathological disorders include vertical talus syndrome, trauma, and spastic conditions. Physiological disorders result from developmental abnormalities that cause a foot to gradually lose an arch throughout the first decade of life [11, 14].

Pes planus etiologies can be further classified as either genetic or acquired. Acquired pes planus is seen with (1) osseous fractures, (2) ligamentous tears, (3) muscular imbalances, (4) degenerative joint diseases, and (5) postural problems, resulting, for example, from obesity or pregnancy [10]. Genetic etiologies include (1) tarsal coalition, (2) obliquity of the ankle joint, where the medially located tibia grows faster than the fibula, (3) failure of tibial torsion, (4) Achilles tendon shortening, (5) ligamentous laxity (which is seen in Down syndrome, Ehlers–Danlos syndrome, and Marfan's syndrome) [10, 15], and (6) increase or decrease in muscle tone, which can cause more complex forms of pes planus. Low muscle tone is seen in neurologically delayed subjects with or without anterior horn loss, in primary muscle damage, and in collagen pathology. There is debate on whether latent cognitive and neurological system development of the cerebellum has an impact on abnormal physiological development causing ligamentous laxity, such as that found in Down syndrome. It is general consensus that a delay in cerebellar development does delay the age at which ambulation begins [1, 16].

High muscle tone pathology causing flat foot is seen with spastic peroneal muscles, the primary cause of a progressively rigid flat foot [8, 10, 13, 17]. Flat foot caused by peroneal spasticity can be corrected with a scaphoid pad, varus heel wedge, and orthosis [8].

Osseous developmental problems resulting in pes planus include acetabular dysplasia, hip dislocation syndromes, metabolic syndromes such as Blount's disease, and physiological tibial varum [3, 7, 13]. These pathologies should be treated by surgical means. In the foot pathologies include metatarsus adductus, hallux valgus, metatarsus primus varus, ligamentous laxity, joint hypermobility, foot and ankle equinus commonly caused by a tight Achilles tendon, pes cavus, forefoot supination, rigid forefoot varus, tarsal coalition, and foot rigidity [2, 16]. Most foot pathologies resulting in pes planus can be treated with appropriate shoe gear as long as the pes planus has not progressed to a symptomatic rigid state [7, 14].

Of the genetic disorders with associated flat foot, Down syndrome is the most common. It occurs in 1 in 660 live births [1, 2]. Down syndrome individuals are active and commonly participate in athletic events. Half of all people afflicted with Down syndrome have gait abnormalities appearing as gait imbalance and abnormal walking posture [1, 2]. Problems with ambulation are attributed to a delay in neurological development, ligamentous laxity, and muscular hypotonia, all of which are found in 88 percent of individuals with Down syndrome [1]. Ligamentous laxity and muscular hypotonia also allow for joint hypermobility causing increased foot width and potentially disabling osteoarthritis leading to rigid foot deformities if left untreated [1, 2, 16]. Flexibility, ligamentous laxity, and muscle hypotonia associated with Down syndrome decrease greatly with age but never fully resolve [1, 16].

Down syndrome individuals are also affected by osseous variations in bone torsion in the lower extremity. Developmental deformities include hip retroversion causing severe external rotation in hip flexion and extension and resulting in an out-toe gait. Hip dysplasia and dislocation can also be found; these are treated surgically. Knee problems are generally secondary to foot abnormalities. Knee pathology, which is relatively uncommon, includes patellofemoral instability, patellofemoral dislocation, knee flexion contracture, external tibial rotation, genu valgum, and rotary tibiofemoral subluxation. Knee pathologies are generally not inhibitory to activity or gait and tend to be well tolerated. Treatment consists of wearing a patellar sleeve during ambulation. At the ankle, the tibia is externally rotated causing an externally rotated foot [1, 7]. Although these examples of lower extremity problems are seen with Down syndrome, they are not limited to it and can be found in other congential pathologies [18].

Any deviation from normal development of the lower extremity will decrease the efficiency of gait in an active individual. Gait alteration with conservative measures that provide biomechanical and postural correction can dramatically improve activity and structural development in the lower extremity [2, 18].

Biomechanically, flat foot is a complex deformity. Pes planus can be caused from biomechanical imbalances in one body plane or a combination of all three: sagittal, transverse, and frontal. For pes planus treatment to be successful it must be addressed on the deformity's main cardial plane [13, 17].

Structurally the foot is designed to bear weight on the rearfoot, lateral column, and the first and fifth metatarsal heads [10]. In pes planus, as the medial foot arch collapses the foot shifts laterally along the lateral column shortening it and lengthening the medial column. The forefoot is hypermobile, allowing the first metatarsal to shift dorsally and medially, transferring weight further up the medial column which is not designed for weightbearing. The first metatarsal and sesamoid bones normally support 33 percent of the body's weight during the normal stance phase. This percentage of weightbearing decreases with abnormal pronation, resulting in increased weightbearing in other areas of the foot [10].

In pes planus the rearfoot does not supinate on the forefoot, preventing locking of the midtarsal joints. If the forefoot joint complex is unlocked it is unstable. An unstable foot platform decreases the effectiveness of gait and allows joint subluxation to occur. Repetitive subluxation will result in eventual degenerative joint disease, foot pain, and possibly rigid foot deformities. Flat foot deformities that become painful and symptomatic are referred to as pes planovalgus deformities.

There are two modes of thought about correction of flat foot deformities during early limb development. Some practitioners theorize that flexible flatfoot should be left alone. The rationales are that only 20 percent of infants with flexible flat foot will not outgrow the deformity within the first decade of life, tight Achilles tendons can be stretched, and most flatfoot individuals do not become symptomatic [14, 18].

Other practitioners theorize that flexible flatfoot should be treated aggressively by using casting techniques and orthoses. These authors point out that there is no way to determine which individuals will outgrow their flat foot deformity; therefore, prophylactic treatment should be performed before the occurrence of possible latent pathological symptoms that require difficult conservative or surgical treatment [1, 8].

With genetic etiologies like Down syndrome and others involving low muscle tone and ligamentous laxity, these factors do not resolve with age. The individual will not outgrow their pes planus deformity and will eventually develop a painful, rigid symptomatic flat foot.

Regardless of the etiology of flatfoot, methods of conservative care remain the same. Conservative treatment options used for active individuals include shoes with or without intrinsic and extrinsic modifications, bracing, and orthoses. Treatment should also include consideration of the appearance of the prescribed device. People with mental handicaps have a sense of style; thus shoes and shoe modifications have to be cosmetically acceptable [1].

Casting therapy should be employed before the child can ambulate or during crawling age and will not be discussed.

The foot and associated pathologies need to be evaluated before appropriate conservative treatment is selected. Rigid foot types need shoes that will provide smooth ambulation such as a rocker bottom sole. Flexible foot types need shoes with a mixture of rigidity and flexibility along with a sturdy shoe upper. If there is an associated drop foot or muscle hypotonia due to neuromuscular conditions, bracing needs to be considered. Width and depth of the shoe must be evaluated to accommodate a wider foot type and for use of orthoses [8]. Special shoe modifications and orthoses should be employed after independent walking starts.

Shoes in general should have a strong heel counter, inflexible rearfoot and midfoot, and a forefoot which should be flexible at the metatarsal heads. The shoe upper should have sufficient strength to hold the foot in alignment [8]. For mild flat foot with younger children, a rigid shoe should not be used. The flexible foot will not conform to the shoe shape; instead it will bend around the shoe's rigid construction, eliminating the supportive effect. For mild pes planus, a standard last, leather shoe without a rigid shank but with a firm heel counter should be used. This combination will allow for foot flexibility needs while still maintaining biomechanical control [8]. For rigid deformities the sole should have a rocker bottom to allow a smooth transition from rearfoot to forefoot, forefoot clearance at toe off, and better propulsion.

Trying to alter the shape of a developing foot with alternative shoe lasts should be performed at an early age, well before bony maturity. The theory behind early conservative care is that if the foot is held in an anatomically correct position before epiphysis closure, the soft tissue supporting the bone will alter accordingly [8]. For patients with hypotonia and ligamentous laxity, a straight last, open-toed shoe with a rigid heel counter and a rigid, wide, flat sole should be used. The straight last shoe can be further enhanced using an orthosis [1].

Further biomechanical stability can be accomplished by using high-top shoes for ankle instability. Shoe sizing should be done at the end of the day when ligaments are at their most lax. If orthoses or bracing are to be used, it is important that the shoes have removable insoles and are able to accommodate the orthoses or bracing. Shoe insoles should be replaced with the orthosis to allow for proper shoe fit. To maintain the best limb alignment in pes planus, the choice of wide flat soled shoes increases the available weightbearing surface, allowing for better propulsion for individuals with a potentially unsteady gait such as is found in Down syndrome [1].

Shoe modifications can be classified into intrinsic and extrinsic modifications. For young children with a mild to moderate flat foot that displays prominent midtarsal bones, notably the talar head, a scaphoid pad can be used. Thickness of the pad depends on the talar head prominence and ranges from 3/8″ to 5/8″. The pad elevates that talar head back into bony alignment. If the foot is in severe pes planus a longitudinal felt or foam pad can be placed along the medial arch [8]. Extrinsic modifications include a Kirby heel skive, a special triplanar wedge, which acts as a medial rearfoot varus wedge when placed in the rearfoot of a shoe. The Kirby heel skive causes the calcaneus to maintain an inverted position and helps prevent eversion of the calcaneus through the contact and stance phase of gait. A neoprene medial buttress can also be placed on the outsole of a shoe to allow for an increase in weightbearing surface and shoe stability [1].

Heel cups and heel lifts can be added to shoes or orthoses, providing more STJ motion stability and bringing the ground to the heel to correct ankle equinus or limb length discrepancy. A heel lift can be intrinsically or extrinsically incorporated into an orthosis or shoe. If the limb length discrepancy is at or over 2 cm, the heel lift should be made as an extrinsic orthosis modification or incorporated into shoe modification. Other extrinsic shoe modifications include insole varus heel posts and rocker bottoms [1]. Shoes with layered midsole construction are better for creating intrinsic shoe modifications.

Orthoses are classified as either functional or accommodative. Accommodative orthoses are designed for pressure offloading in stance phase only and for minimally active individuals. Functional orthoses are designed for biomechanical correction during activity. They have a rigid heel counter, limiting calcaneal movement, and thus subtalar joint motion. Modifications that can be performed for increased biomechanical efficacy include flares, deeper heel cups, and intrinsic and extrinsic corrective posting.

Functional orthoses can be prefabricated or custom molded. Prefabricated insoles, such as Spenco and Powerstep, provide a low-cost alternative for biomechanical correction of pes planus. Prefabricated insoles do not provide the level of support that custom orthoses can provide but they will provide an improvement in the support of a properly fitting shoe [1]. Prefabricated insoles also offer a low-cost alternative for individuals who do not perform athletic activities on a routine basis.

Custom foot orthoses should be created from a cast of an individual's foot, not from Styrofoam foot impressions. Styrofoam impressions or similar materials can create an improperly fitting orthosis due to lack of control of the subtalar joint while obtaining the foot impression [1]. A foot cast should try to precisely capture the foot in subtalar joint neutral with possibly a mild to moderate pronatory exaggeration of the heel in the biomechanically corrected position. The success of orthosis treatment is inversely proportional to the rigidity of the foot deformity. For more rigid deformities, bracing should be used to hold the deformity in place rather than altering biomechanics [13].

Three types of custom foot orthoses are generally recommended for pes planus in individuals affected with Down syndrome: leather, rigid polyolefin, and polypropylene orthoses from the University of California Berkley Laboratory (UCBL).

Leather orthoses tend to be the most accommodative fit for a variety of athletic shoes. Leather orthoses are pliable and adjustable and will expand and compress to accommodate a variety of shoe widths. Leather orthosis expansion provides comfort in tighter shoes and orthosis compression offers more support. To improve biomechanical function, leather orthoses should be four ply, have a deep heel cup, and have high medial and lateral flanges [1].

Rigid polyolefin offers the best biomechanical support by providing exceptional pronation control. It tends to be the least forgiving biomechanically if casting and manufacturing are performed incorrectly. Rigid polyolefin orthoses that are too wide will subtract from shoe support due to their inability to offer lateral compression. Those that are too narrow will irritate the foot from the creation of abnormal pressure points [1].

UCBL orthoses are best suited for individuals with severe flexible flat foot deformities such as those seen with Down syndrome. UCBL orthoses are rigid and thin, provide the ability to create a very deep heel cup along with high medial and lateral flanges, and allow for some lateral compression [1]. For severe pes planus cases, an addition of a plastic heel cup with medial arch extension can be used for biomechanical correction to a UCBL orthosis. These orthosis modifications may not be effective for individuals 12 years or older [8].

Patients with pes planus deformities from hypotonicity and ligamentous laxity may not be biomechanically controllable until skeletal maturity when hypotonicity and laxity decreases. During this time, supramalleolar ankle–foot orthosis (SMO) or ankle–foot orthosis (AFO) should be considered. AFO and SMO can promote foot control in all three body planes [13].

Some practitioners feel that supramalleolar ankle–foot orthoses offer little advantage over properly fitting shoes and orthoses. Furthermore, supramalleolar ankle–foot orthoses may need modified shoes for a correct fit [1]. Due to the limited advantages that a supramalleolar ankle–foot orthosis may provide, an ankle–foot orthosis should be considered for severe flexible or rigid pes planus. Ankle–foot orthoses can be non-articulated or articulated, generally at the ankle joint, to allow for sagittal plane motion. Ankle–foot orthoses can provide excellent control in all three body planes. Modifications include a proximal extension for sagittal plane control, anterior extension to limit transverse plane malposition, and high medial and lateral flanges with extensions from the plantar aspect of the device to the digits to help control subtalar joint pronation. AFOs are designed to hold a lower extremity deformity in a static position rather than altering biomechanical motion [13].

Pes cavus is another common foot abnormality associated with active individuals and athletes. It is biomechanically defined as the rearfoot being dorsiflexed on the forefoot, the forefoot being plantarflexed on the rearfoot, or a combination of both occurring in the midfoot. The overall result is a plantarflexed forefoot on the rearfoot.

Pes cavus deformities occur predominantly in the sagittal plane, with a majority occurring in the forefoot. Forefoot deformities are frequently referred to as forefoot equinus or pseudoequinus. Ankle equinus is another common associated deformity found with pes cavus. Of individuals affected with pes cavus, 66–75 percent has an associated neuromuscular disease [17, 19].

Pes cavus appears visually as a high medial arch which may reduce with weightbearing. If a high arch remains during weightbearing, the deformity is typically more rigid in nature. Pes cavus can be associated with either pronation or supination depending on foot flexibility and involvement of ankle equinus. Typically the rigidity of a frontal plane deformity and the severity of ankle equinus affect whether the heel maintains neutral, inverted, or everted position on weightbearing [17]. It is not uncommon for the cavus foot to be supinated off weightbearing and pronated upon weightbearing.

Forefoot pes cavus with normal foot pathomechanics, and without progressive muscle disease, has six typical forms: flexible forefoot varus or valgus, rigid forefoot varus or valgus, and plantarflexed first ray that is flexible or rigid. Each form will cause a high arch either on or off weightbearing. Flexible deformities will usually cause pronation on weightbearing.

Supination is defined as an inward roll of the foot during gait [19]. Biomechanically a supinated foot maintains a plantarflexed, adducted varus position. If the subtalar joint remains in a varus position during the contact and stance phases of gait, biomechanical dampening mechanisms are prevented. Without biomechanical dampening, increased joint subluxation will occur, causing osteoarthritis and spasticity of the muscles trying to maintain biomechanical stability.

While supination can cause biomechanical faults, the mixture of pes cavus, ankle equinus, and self-perpetuating myostatic contracture can cause excessive pronation in physically handicapped individuals such as those afflicted with cerebral palsy. The excessive pronation results in an equinovalgus foot orientation during ambulation, resulting in joint destruction throughout the foot. The additive effects of abnormal biomechanics plus the progressive nature of muscle contracture and increase in foot rigidity further found in neuromuscular disease aid abnormal physiological positions, making orthosis management eventually inadequate as a treatment. Individuals with progressive neurological physical handicaps ultimately require management through bracing techniques that attempt to hold the extremity in a stable, static position [13].

Pes cavus is often the first sign of neuromuscular conditions. Conditions associated with pes cavus can be acquired or genetic. Acquired diseases include spinal cord tumors, spinal cord lesions, and syphilis. Genetic diseases that cause pes cavus are typically neuromuscular in origin and include Charcot–Marie–Tooth disease, Friedreich's ataxia, poliomyelitis, progressive muscular dystrophy, and cerebral palsy [9, 17].

The most noted neurological condition associated with pes cavus is cerebral palsy. Cerebral palsy is the result of malformations in the central nervous system during gestation or immediately after birth [9, 20]. The ratio of children born with cerebral palsy is 1–5 per 1000 live births [3, 20]. There are six types of cerebral palsy, each described on the basis of associated pathological movement relating to muscle spasticity, balance, motor control, and weakness [5, 9]. Cerebral palsy types include spastic, athetoid, ataxic, rigid, tremor, atonic, and mixed [9, 17]. Cerebral palsy is further grouped by associated anatomical patterns which include quadriplegia, diplegia, hemiplegia, and other [5].

The most common form of cerebral palsy is spastic cerebral palsy, encompassing 70 percent of all cases [9]. Spastic cerebral palsy individuals have abnormal and primitive reflex patterns and atypical increase in muscle tone, which affects ambulatory gait as well as balance, posture, and movement [3, 19]. Cerebral palsy is a non-progressive neuromuscular disease, but due to muscle spasticity and a tendency toward inactivity, progressive rigidity often occurs as an individual becomes older [3, 9, 17, 20]. Sports activity, routine physical therapy, and stretching can reduce the progression of muscle weakness, muscle spasticity, and rigid deformities [3].

Gait patterns vary depending on the cerebral palsy type. In spastic diplegia cerebral palsy the lower extremity has exaggerated knee flexion, increased hip adduction and internal rotation, and associated ankle equinus. With spastic hemiplegia cerebral palsy the hip and knee are either fully flexed or extended and the foot remains in ankle equinus on the affected side [19]. Other associated deformities affecting the lower extremity include hip instability, patellofemoral chondromalacia, metatarsalgia, bunions, and hammertoe deformities resulting from extensor tendon substitution compensating for ankle equinus [5].

Spastic cerebral palsy individuals are able to walk and run, though gait techniques are modified. Individuals with cerebral palsy increase their gait velocity through increasing cadence rather than stride length. This is attributed to spasticity, contractures, and muscle weakness throughout the lower extremity. Running cadence is conducive with the normal anatomical posture of spastic cerebral palsy patients with their natural tendency for hip extension, knee flexion, and ankle equinus giving the appearance that they can run better than they walk. Nonetheless, the running style used by cerebral palsy patients has been found to be biomechanically inefficient [21].

Injuries to athletes with spastic cerebral palsy are generally caused from stress-induced disorders created by trying to overcome the limitations of contractures, spasticity, and muscle weakness [5].

Conservative treatment revolves around preventing progression of contractures and loss of muscular strength. Minimal loss of strength can result in large deficits in activity, impacting mobility, and independence [5]. Standards in conservative care include stretching, strength training, physical therapy, shoes, orthoses, and bracing.

Shoes are generally used in conjunction with orthoses and brace management and are not a primary treatment for moderate to severe pes cavus and rigid foot deformities. For mild flexible pes cavus, a running shoe with a higher arch support and a strong heel counter should be considered. Shoe design must be wide and deep enough to accommodate orthoses. The midsole should be layered to allow for intrinsic varus or valgus modifications and for incorporation of heel lifts to treat ankle equinus. The entire sole of the shoe can also be elevated in the case of limb length discrepancy. For the individual with a dyskinetic, spastic, or equinus gait, modifications such as rocker bottom soles may be incorporated to allow for ground clearance at toe off.

Orthosis management is good for both flexible and mild, rigid pes cavus. A weightbearing evaluation should be performed to identify pronation or supination compensatory factors and orthoses should be designed accordingly. Orthosis design is intended to bring the ground up to the foot, keep the foot in biomechanical correction, and, with neuromuscular disease, try to prevent the progression of contractures [13]. With progressive muscle spasticity, as seen with cerebral palsy, orthosis therapy will eventually become inadequate. Orthosis therapy used in neuromuscular disease is designed to improve ambulation and function, but also to delay inevitable surgical intervention [22]. In active individuals with neuromuscular disease the functional status of the foot is already impaired limiting the benefits of functional orthosis. Orthoses tend to be designed as a soft accommodative device to offload areas of abnormal pressure.

Orthoses can be modified similar to that of pes planus, with intrinsic or extrinsic varus or valgus wedges, medial or lateral flares, and heel cups with or without heel lifts to compensate for ankle equinus. As with pes planus, the heel lift should be incorporated into the orthosis intrinsically if under 2 cm and extrinsically if over 2 cm.

For individuals with moderate and inflexible pes cavus deformities, supramalleolar foot–ankle orthosis may be employed. Some practitioners argue that supramalleolar foot–ankle orthoses do not offer enough biomechanical support for individuals with neuromuscular disease; they instead promote the use of ankle–foot bracing [13].

Most individuals afflicted with neuromuscular disease will eventually need bracing orthoses. Orthosis bracing's primary function is to keep a lower extremity deformity in a static state. When utilizing bracing for individuals with neuromuscular disease such as cerebral palsy, movement should be incorporated to prevent muscle group weakness and progression of muscle spasticity. Common bracing includes ankle–foot orthosis and dynamic ankle–foot orthosis (DAFO). The DAFO is a thinner and more flexible brace than a regular AFO and allows for ankle joint plantar flexion. AFOs are commonly used as conservative treatment in individuals affected with diplegic and hemiplegic spastic cerebral palsy [19, 22]. Studies have shown that AFOs can improve stride length, increase velocity, and allow single-limb support in young adolescents, but the improvements degrade with age becoming non-beneficial in one study after age 7 [19, 22]. After adolescent years AFO and DAFO are used to hold static deformities stable, reduce muscle tone during weight-bearing situations, offload pressure points, and to allow for greater freedom of movement by reducing the effort required for movement [20].

Hyperhidrosis is the final subject matter to be covered. Mentally handicapped athletes and children in general have excessive foot perspiration, called plantar hyperhidrosis. The cause of hyperhidrosis is unknown [23]. Up to 5 percent of the general population is affected by primary focal hyperhidrosis or excessive sweating [23, 24]. Plantar hyperhidrosis tends to cause moist socks and shoes along with foot odor which can socially impact a patient [23].

There is no conservative treatment for plantar hyperhidrosis that is completely effective. Various conservative treatments for plantar hyperhidrosis can be added to one another for increased results. Frequent changing of socks and shoes is a common and effective treatment. Using alternative sock material such as rayon and nylon which do not retain moisture but allow easy passing of moisture through the material is a viable option. Using non-absorptive material along with absorptive power, such as talc, and/or anti-perspirants, such as Drysol, or roll-on deodorants with anti-perspirants, can help prevent sweating and absorb excess moisture.

Individuals with mental and physical disabilities involved with sports can benefit from conservative care. Whether or not these individuals are international athletes or active amateurs, the benefits of exercise and daily social interaction can be immeasurable. Without treatment, many of these individuals will eventually develop pedal pathology, limiting or eliminating participation in physical activities. Any removal of activity can greatly impact the physical and social health of mentally and physically handicapped individuals. The use of conservative management can effectively delay, reduce, or prevent the progression of lower extremity pathology.

References

1. Caselli M, Cohen-Sobel E, Thompson J, Adler J, Gonzalez L: Biomechanical management of children and adolescents with down syndrome. J Am Podiatr Med Assoc, 81(3): 119–127, 1991.
2. Concolino D, Pasquzzi A, Capalbo G, Sinopoli S, Strisciuglio P: Early detection of podiatric anomalies in children with down syndrome. Acta Paediatrica, 95: 17–20, 2006.
3. Carroll K, Leiser J, Paisley T: Cerebral Palsy: Physical Activity and Sport. Curr Sports Med Rep, 5: 319–322, 2006.
4. Banta J: Athletics for people with disabilities. Dev Med Child Neurol, 43: 147, 2001.
5. Wind W, Schwend R, Larson J: Sports for the physically challenged child. J Am Acad Orthop Surg, 12:126–137, 2004.
6. The Special Olympics Website. http://www.specialolympics.org/Special+Olympics+Public+Website/English/About_Us/default.htm. 2007
7. Winell J, Burke S: Sports participation of children with down syndrome. Orthop clin North Am, 34(3): 439–443, 2003.
8. Trott A: Children's foot problems. Orthop Clin North Am, 13(3):641–654, 1982.
9. Watkins L: Pocket Podiatrics 3rd ed., 203–207, 490–491, 505, 2003.
10. Lawrence D: Pes planus: A review of etiology, diagnosis, and chiropractic management. J Manipulative Physiol Ther, 6(4):185–188, 1983.
11. Pfeiffer M, Kotz R, Ledl T, Hauser G, Sluga M: Prevalence of flat foot in Preschool-aged children. Pediatrics, 118(2):634–639, 2006.
12. Chambers H: Ankle and foot disorders in skeletally immature athletes. Orthop Clin North Am, 34:445–459, 2003.
13. Genaze R: Pronation: The orthotist's view. Clin Podiatr Med Surg, 17(3):481–503, 2000.
14. Cappello T, Song K: Determining Treatment of flatfeet in children. Curr Opin Pediatr, 10:77–81, 1998.
15. Disease Database. http://diseaseesdatabase.com/result.asp?glngUserChoice=22o53&bytRel=2&blnBW=False&strBB=RL&blnClassSort=True. 2007
16. Angelopoulou N, Tsimaras V: Measurement of range of motion in individuals with mental retardation and with or without down syndrome. Percept Mot Skill, 89:550–556, 1999.
17. Banks A, Downey M, Martin D, Miller S: McGlamry's Comprehensive Textbook of Foot and Ankle Surgery 3rd Ed. New York: Lippincott Williams and Wilkins, 2001.
18. Finidorf G, Rigault P, de Grouchy J, Rodriguez A, Pouliquen J, Guyonvarch G, Fingerhut A: Osteoarticular abnormalities and orthopedic complications in children with chromosomal aberrations. Ann Genet, 26(3):150–157, 1983.
19. The Way You Walk. http://walking.about.com/od/shoechoice/a/wayyouwalk.htm 2007.
20. Bill M, McIntosh R, Myers P: A series of case studies on the effect of a midfoot control ankle foot orthosis in the prevention of unresolved pressure areas in children with cerebral palsy. Prosthet Orthot Int, 25:246–250, 2001.
21. Davids J, Bagley A, Bryan M: Kinematic and kinetic analysis of running in children with cerebral palsy. Dev Med Child Neurol, 40:528–535, 1998.
22. Bjornson K, Schmale G, Adamczyk-Foster A, McLaughlin J: The effect of dynamic ankle foot orthoses on function in children with cerebral palsy. J Pediat Orthop, 26(6):773–776, 2006.
23. Nuanhainm K: Hyperhydorsis. http://www.sts.org/doc/4097
24. Zhou, Y: No Sweat! A New Way To Control Excessive Sweat. http://www.sweating.ca/articles/art_4.html

Part III
Coding and Billing

Chapter 29
Durable Medical Equipment and Coding in Sports Medicine

Anthony Poggio

The use of durable medical equipment (DME) is a common part of a sports medicine practice. Proper documentation and billing protocols must be followed to insure proper payment and to attest to medical necessity and reasonableness of the item(s) dispensed. Medicare covers certain durable medical equipment, prosthetics, orthoses, and supplies (DMEPOS) items. Items are covered for both chronic and acute conditions (i.e., postoperatively) as long as the coverage criteria are met. Other insurance carriers have their own specific policies regarding coverage of DME items.

In this chapter, we discuss common DME items used in a sports medicine practice and insurance company coverage and billing protocols of these items. To begin with you must determine if you even want to dispense DME from your office. As a DME provider, you are classified as a supplier not a physician. There are insurance company, state, and federal rules and regulations you need to be aware of and comply with. Space may also be an issue to adequately stock the various products, sizes, etc. Staff needs to be trained to explain, fit, and ultimately bill properly for the various products. For any DME item, you need to be aware of coverage issues, deductibles, co-pay/co-insurance, and any restrictions. Some items may have a specific exclusion when prescribed for the foot (as is common for foot orthotics), or only allowed for certain diagnosis, i.e., covered for tendonitis but not neuroma, covered only for the diabetic patient, etc.

Definition

Each carrier defines DME per their contract provisions. Furthermore the carriers define what they will cover and under what circumstances. This is where clear and thorough documentation in your chart is critical to ensure that the carrier

A. Poggio (✉)
Private practice, 2059 Clinton Ave., Alameda, CA 94501, USA

M.B. Werd, E.L. Knight (eds.), *Athletic Footwear and Orthoses in Sports Medicine*,
DOI 10.1007/978-0-387-76416-0_29, © Springer Science+Business Media, LLC 2010

understands what you are requesting and why so that it can make an accurate coverage determination according to its policy.

Centers for Medicare and Medicaid Services (CMS) defines DME as any equipment that provides therapeutic benefits or enables the member to perform certain tasks that he or she is unable to undertake otherwise due to certain medical conditions or illnesses and

- can withstand repeated use; and
- is primarily and customarily used to serve a medical purpose; and
- generally is not useful to a person in the absence of an illness or injury; and
- is appropriate for use in the home but may be transported to other locations to allow members to complete instrumental activities of daily living, which are more complex tasks required for independent living.

All requirements of the definition must be met before an item can be considered to be durable medical equipment.

Durability

An item is considered durable if it can withstand repeated use, i.e., the type of item, which could normally be rented. Medical supplies of an expendable nature such as lamb's wool, pads, ace bandages, and elastic stockings are therefore not considered "durable" within the meaning of the definition. There are other items that, although durable in nature, may fall into other coverage categories such as braces, prosthetic devices, artificial arms, and legs.

Medical Equipment

Medical equipment is that which is primarily and customarily used for medical purposes and is not generally useful in the absence of illness or injury. Dispensement of such equipment may require documentation to determine medical necessity. This is based upon the standard of care and carrier policy guidelines. If the equipment is new on the market, obtaining prior authorization is recommended to obtain information from the supplier or manufacturer explaining the design, purpose, effectiveness, and method of using the equipment in the home as well as the results of any tests or clinical studies that have been conducted.

Medically Necessary

Durable medical equipment is considered *medically necessary* when *all* of the following criteria are met:

- The requested item has not otherwise been identified as not medically necessary or investigational/not medically necessary by a specific policy guideline/restriction.
- There is adequate documentation in the medical records or in the claim submission of *all* of the following:

  - The documentation substantiates that the physician exercised prudent clinical judgment to provide for a patient for the purpose of preventing, evaluating, diagnosing, or treating an illness, injury, disease, or its symptoms and that are in accordance with generally accepted standards of medical practice.
  - There is a clinical assessment and associated rationale by the doctor for the requested DME in the home setting.
  - There is documentation substantiating that the DME is clinically appropriate for the patient's diagnosis in terms of type, quantity, frequency, and accepted by community standards as being effective for that patient's condition.
  - The documentation supports that the requested DME will assist, restore, or facilitate improvement in the patient's ability to function better in normal day-to-day activities.
  - The requested DME is not primarily for the convenience of the patient.
  - The DME is not more costly than other options/items which may be equivalent as far as effectiveness and therapeutic outcome.

Not Medically Necessary

Any item that does not meet the above criteria would not be considered medically necessary and reasonable. Carriers may impose other restrictions affecting what is medically necessary and

- the DME item is intended to be used for athletic, exercise, or recreational activities as opposed to assisting the patient in day-to-day activities; or
- the DME includes additional features that are added primarily for the comfort and convenience of the member (e.g., multiple pairs of orthoses, customized options on wheelchairs, crutches); or
- the DME item represents a product upgrade to a current piece of equipment that is either fully functional or replacement of a device when the DME can be cost-effectively repaired.

Licensure

For Medicare you must have a separate durable medical equipment regional carrier (DMERC) license to dispense DME from your office. If you do not have a valid DME license, you cannot dispense and bill the patient for a covered item, *even if the patient agrees to pay you for it.*

In the DMERC system, a physician is referred to as a "supplier." You may choose to be a "participating supplier" or a "non-participating supplier" under DMERC. This decision is linked to your current participation status under Medicare Part B. You cannot be a "participating" physician under Medicare Part B and a "non-participating" supplier under DMERC or vice versa.

You may need to re-apply for a DMERC number if you have not submitted claims for four consecutive quarters. You must call and ask for a re-application form. If you do not have a DMERC number, call the National Supplier Clearing House at 866-238-9652 to obtain an application. No surety bond is required at this time when filling out your application. Part of your application process will be an *unannounced* on-site inspection.

Other requirements include that you must have your hours of operation posted on your door, and you also need to have a complaint form available and a complaint resolution protocol established.

For other insurance carriers/HMOs/IPAs, make sure that you are designated as a DME supplier (beyond being a physician provider) and that their insured may be able to obtain these items from you. If you are not a designated supplier and if you dispense that DME item, you may not be reimbursed. Trying to collect for this item from the patient may be difficult and create ill will toward your practice if they could have gotten this item covered at an outside/designated facility. If you are allowed to dispense DME items, make sure you understand all of the carrier's rules, restrictions, and billing protocols.

Assignment

Participating Supplier

Participating supplier accepts assignment on *all* cases. There is no "limiting charge" for any DME supplies. The supplier bills Medicare. Medicare will pay 80% of the allowable charge or the reasonable and customary fee (after deductible has been met). The supplier may collect the remaining 20% and any amount that went toward the deductible from the patient at the time of service (if the amount is known) or after payment is received from Medicare. It is advisable, however, to delay billing the patient until receipt of their payment determination to ensure that the allowed charges or remaining balance is accurately shown. A violation of the assignment agreement occurs if the physician collects (or attempts to collect) from the patient any amount that, which when added to the benefit check, exceeds the Medicare allowance. For non-covered services a "participating supplier" may collect at the time of service.

Non-participating Supplier

Non-participating supplier under DMERC can elect on a case-by-case basis to accept assignment or not. If the supplier agrees to accept assignment, the above scenario applies. If the supplier does not accept assignment on a covered item, the payment may be collected from the patient when the item is actually dispensed and not when initially ordered. A claim is submitted to Medicare and the insurance check would then be sent directly to the patient. For non-assigned claims you may bill your usual and customary fee. Medicare will still pay 80% of the allowable fee for that item (after deductible has been met) or 80% of billed charges, which ever is lower. *However, the patient is responsible for the balance in full, not just the 20% of the allowable charges.*

There is no need to inform patients when services exceed $500 whether you participate or not under DMERC as there is with Medicare Part B.

As a designated supplier for Medicare, you may accept orders/prescriptions to dispense DME items from other physicians. In this capacity your relationship to the patient is only that of a supplier not a physician. You would bill the insurance company or the patient only for the item prescribed. You would not bill this as a professional consultation in addition to supplying the item unless the prescribing physician specifically requests a consult, *and* if all of the medical necessity and documentation requirements for a consultation (per CPT criteria) are met. Yet if you feel that the item requested is incorrect, it would be appropriate in the spirit of offering top quality care to the patient to contact the prescribing physician and voice your concerns.

There is a question if a podiatrist/DME supplier could dispense other DME supplies such as splints and orthotics for other body parts, glucose strips, etc. This may depend on state requirements as well as individual plan provisions. This is a bit of a gray area and you should consult with an attorney who specializes in health care as well as your malpractice carrier before proceeding with dispensing "non-podiatric" DME items.

FEE Schedule

When an insurance company covers an item, you are held to their fee schedule and any policy/protocols listed in your contract with the insurance company. For example, certain services pertaining to the DME item such as casting, dispensement, or adjustments, patient training/education in the use of the item may be included in the fee allowance for the device, similar to the global fee concept with surgery. For non-covered devices, you are not bound to any fee schedule, and hence you may charge your usual and customary fee. It is recommended to have a single fee schedule for all of your services, provided including DME whether they are covered or not.

You should also check with current and any new insurance carriers regarding their fee schedule. This is especially true for HMOs and capitated programs. You may find that their fee allowance is not acceptable to you. You should try to renegotiate your contract to a more acceptable allowance. Or, you may elect not to provide DME to that insurance company's insured. Make sure this does not violate terms of your contract. You cannot bill the patient a "surcharge" to make the fee more acceptable.

If you are in a capitated program, you may consider "carving out" the DME portion out of your capitation fee if the DME fee reimbursement schedule is unacceptable. This way you can charge your usual and customary fee schedule for those "carve out" items.

Communication

Whenever you speak with an insurance carrier, always record the date, time, and name of the person you spoke with. Be specific as possible and record what you were told. This information may be vital when formulating an appeal for denial of payment. Make sure you ask the telephone representatives to check on any specific foot exclusions. An inexperienced telephone person may state that DME is a covered benefit as a general policy but they may not look deeper into the fine print and find that there may be certain exclusions. If they state there are no exclusions, document this.

Office Forms/Policies

You should have a clear policy in your office with regard to DME items, especially orthoses. It is recommended to utilize preprinted forms describing the device, coverage issues or possible non-coverage, and other charges associated with the devices (i.e., casting fee, orthosis fees). That way there are no surprises and the patent is fully aware of any out-of-pocket costs.

You should also have a policy dealing with complaints that patients may have with the device and a protocol for resolution of complaints. Be prepared to address issues beyond the device itself. Patients may have concerns regarding the appearance of the device, fit in various shoes, etc. Specifically with dispensement of shoes, patients may have issues with the appearance, color, laces vs. Velcro, etc.

Billing Protocols

When billing for a DME item submit a CMS-1500 claim form using the appropriate Healthcare Common Procedure Coding System (HCPCS) code. If you are unsure of the proper code to submit, SADMERC (Statistical Analysis DMERC) at 877-735-1326 or write: Palmetto Government Benefit Administrator, P. O. Box 100143 Columbia, SC 29202-3143. Describe the item, model number (if any), manufacturer, and any other information you may have and they will see if there is an appropriate HCPCS "A" or "L" code.

Check with the involved carrier regarding billing for DME. Many carriers including Medicare will want you to bill for DME when the item is dispensed not when ordered or molds obtained. This is important if the insurance company gave you an authorization with a fixed time frame. If so, make sure the item is molded, fabricated, and dispensed within that time frame. When billing multiple separate items there is no need to add a −51 modifier to subsequent items. Each item is fully reimbursable at its allowable fee.

For orthoses or other bilateral devices some carriers may prefer you to use RT/LT modifiers. In this case bill each item line by line. Other carriers may prefer to bill single line items but use the appropriate "units" when billing in box 24G of the CMS-1500 claim form.

NPI Number

If you do not have a National Provider Identifier (NPI) number, you should obtain one immediately. CMS had mandated that NPI numbers be utilized on the CMS claim form in May 2007. The deadline has been extended, but it is unclear at the time of this printing when the new deadline may be. List the NPI number of the referring physician and yours in boxes 17b and 33a, respectively, on the new CMS-1500 form. If the NPI number of the referring physician is not known or if you do not have an NPI number, list the existing legacy number in boxes 17a and 33a but add a 1C and a space before the legacy number (i.e., 1C XXXXXXX).

Place of Service

The place of service should be shown on your claim form as the place where the item, equipment, or supply would be used. Since the item would be used at home, the proper place of service would be "home" or place of service "12" even if it was dispensed in your office. Medicare only pays for place of service "12" (home), "33" (custodial care facility – NOT SNF/NH), "54" (ICF/mental retardation), "55" (residential substance abuse treatment facility), and "56" (psychiatric residential treatment center). Medicare will also pay for DMEPOS in place of service code "34" (hospice) as long as the item being billed is not for the primary diagnosis they are on hospice. DMERC does not cover DME to the supplier in place of service "31" (SNF) or "32" (nursing home). However, they do cover prosthetics, orthotics, and related supplies and surgical dressings as part of the facility's services.

Obtaining a Denial

Specifically for Medicare, orthoses are not covered unless they are part of a shoe which is attached to a brace. Since this service is not covered by statute, no Advance Beneficiary Notice (ABN) is required. For non-Medicare patients you should generate an office form (similar to an ABN) that you have the patient sign, indicating that the item is not covered by their plan and that they agree to pay for the device in full. Again this may help minimize any billing confusion later on.

The primary insurance may not cover a specific DME item but the secondary insurance carrier might. In this case you must bill the primary insurance carrier first to get the denial and then you may bill the secondary carrier. For Medicare, bill your DMERC carrier not the carrier that provides Medicare Part B services for you to get the proper DME denial.

To obtain the proper denial from Medicare for a non-covered DME item, append the HCPCS code with the GY modifier, indicating that this item is not covered by statute. An incorrect denial message may adversely affect coverage by the secondary carrier. If the primary insurance carrier deems an item not medically necessary so may the secondary carrier. But if the denial reads not a covered service, then the secondary carrier would implement its coverage criteria and determine if payment is allowed under its plan.

Medicare does not require claims to be submitted for any *non-covered* item or service that is excluded from coverage by Medicare statute. The exception to this is if the patient requests a claim to be submitted if they believe the item maybe covered or to obtain a formal Medicare determination. It is a patient's/beneficiary's right to such a determination. In this instance, bill the item with a –GA, –GZ modifier, indicating a potentially non-covered item or service was billed for denial or at the patient's request. Other carriers may require that all claims be submitted for adjudication whether the service is covered or not.

Incorrect or Overpayment

If you know that the item was paid for incorrectly, the monies should be returned to the carrier. If the determination is based upon "medical necessity" and hence you cannot know if it may be paid or not, then you may deposit the monies. If the insurance company comes back at a later time and wants a refund, you do have legal rights. If you acted in good faith, called the carrier (and it is documented), and submitted a proper claim for a medical necessary and reasonable item, then you may not have to return such monies. There are state laws protecting providers from such refund demands. Check with an attorney or your state association for state laws in this regard.

Modifiers

- *GA modifier:* Add this modifier when billing for a Medicare item or service that the provider feels (1) may be deemed a not medically necessary service, (2) the patient has been informed of such and given the specific reason why the doctor feels it may be deemed medically not necessary, and (3) that an ABN is on file.
- *GZ modifier:* It is similar to the –GA modifier except that it is used when an ABN is not on file.

- **GY modifier:** This modifier indicates that the supply is not a covered benefit of Medicare and that a denial is required such that a secondary insurance company may be billed.
- **KX modifier:** Some items have specific Medicare policies and requirements for coverage. This indicates that certain specific requirements found in the documentation policy have been met and evidence of this is available in the supplier's record such as documenting diabetes with PVD or ulcer history to validate the necessity for a therapeutic shoe.
- **NU modifier:** Certain items require this modifier (especially for Medicare DMERC) if the item was dispensed as new item.
- **RR modifier:** Certain items require this modifier (especially for Medicare DMERC) if the item was rented.
- **UE modifier:** Certain items require this modifier (especially for Medicare DMERC) if the item was dispensed as used.

Deductibles and Deposits

For covered DME items, you may or may not be allowed to collect a deposit. Make sure that collecting a deposit does not violate your contract with the carrier. For most carriers you are allowed to collect any co-pay or unmet deductible portion at the time the device is dispensed.

For non-covered items you can collect the entire fee upfront at the time of ordering the item or obtaining the mold. It is recommended to at least obtain a deposit, which covers the hard cost of the DME item before proceeding with fabrication of the item. This way if the patient changes their mind or does not return to pick up the device at least you will cover the laboratory fees.

Sales Tax

With any DME item dispensed from your office, check with your state regarding requirements for collecting sales tax. Medicare does not pay for sales tax separately. State laws may vary as to what is considered a "medical device." In some states, shoes (including "diabetic shoes") may have a separate classification when it comes to medical devices and may be subject to sales even though other medical devices are not.

Dispensing Requirements

You should have the patient sign a form indicating that they received the DME item (the item should be itemized as to device and any associated additions/modifications to the device), the device fit well, and patient instructions were reviewed. The HCPCS codes, description of the device, and associated items/additions should be listed as well. For Medicare patients, you should also dispense the 21-point supplier standards. You do not have to indicate the specific costs and charges billed to the carrier.

Patient Education

Dispensing the orthosis and associated patient education is generally including the fee allowance for the orthosis itself. CPT codes 97760–97762 are for orthotists not physicians.

Replacement Interval

The term *durable* medical equipment implies that the item, as the name implies, is durable and should last for some time. This time interval may vary between carriers. This may range from 1–5 years for certain DME items. Items can break, wear out prematurely, or the patient's condition, and therefore their prescription, may change as well. You need to be aware of each carrier's policies on this and potential appeals processes to obtain replacement DME items for your patient. Documentation is very important in this regard. Be very clear how and why the item broke or wore down and what are the changes in the patient's status that warrant a new device earlier than expected.

Especially with orthoses, multiple pairs are often necessary to accommodate various styles of shoes. You should be aware of each carrier's rules regarding multiple DME items. A patient may be involved in different work duties at their job, which requires different shoe gear. Contrast this with a patient wanting several pairs for personal preference. Many athletes may have a locker at a gym and want to leave a pair there or in their gym bag for convenience. Many orthotic laboratories keep molds on file for many years. You should consider developing a formal office policy on obtaining multiple pairs of orthoses when multiple pairs are not covered by the insurance plan.

Inability to Deliver DME

If a custom-made device was fabricated but not dispensed to the patient because the patient died, no longer needed it, etc, payment can be made based upon the supply cost of the item. Use the date the patient died or order canceled as the date of service. Indicate such on the claim form. It is recommended to submit this as a paper claim with an explanation attached.

Specific Items

Orthoses

There are two categories of orthoses: prefabricated insoles or custom foot orthoses. Most insurance companies will not pay for prefabricated insoles even when dispensed in your office. They may sometimes pay (incorrectly?) for them as a supply code 99070. Generally, prefabricated insoles are a CASH item.

Custom Foot Orthoses

Most insurance companies have policies regarding custom foot orthoses. Medicare does not allow coverage for orthoses unless they are dispensed as part of shoe, which has a brace attached. Many insurances follow that guideline as well. There may be separate allowance for diabetic orthoses when dispensed as part of the diabetic shoe program, which will be discussed later.

The fabrication of an orthotic device includes many components. First there is the determination as to whether an orthotic device is an appropriate treatment option or not for the patient's presenting problem. This is an Evaluation and Management service (E/M). As with any E/M service, document your history and examination and decision-making, select the most appropriate E/M code level *based upon your documentation in the chart not the eventual diagnosis*. Insurances will also use this documentation to determine medical necessity as per its guidelines.

Use of or prior history of use of prefabricated insoles or good results with a foot strapping (as a diagnostic or therapeutic tool) may also help validate the medical necessity of formal orthotic devices.

Medicare does not cover foot orthotic devices by statute. The orthotic device and all services directly related to the molding, fabrication prescription writing, dispensement, and adjustments are not payable either. Other insurances may follow this same protocol. Some may allow portions of the orthoses and its related services paid.

If the patient presents in your office and the decisions are made to proceed with custom orthotic devices and the mold is obtained, the E/M service should be payable. The orthoses and related services may or may not be.

If the athlete is rescheduled to return to the office at a later date for casting or biomechanical evaluation, then there is no separately identifiable E/M service, which should be billed on that day. The examination has been performed and the decision has been previously made to proceed with an orthosis.

There is no specific CPT code for casting for orthotic devices. The recommended code to use is CPT 29799, the unlisted casting procedure code. This code is billed once for obtaining molds for a pair of orthoses. This code also includes the plaster, foam block, or other casting materials. Do not use HCPCS codes A4580 and A4590 as this implies the use of an entire roll of plaster material. Insurance companies may recognize CPT 29799 code for separate payment or the casting component may be included in the overall fee allowance for the orthotic device.

The use of CPT 29515 is also not appropriate as this is a code to apply a posterior splint not casting for an orthotic device.

The use of machines that scan the foot and generate a "mold" may or may not be payable separately. Billing a CPT code implies that a professional service was performed. Is there a professional service preformed having the patient stand on a machine? Was the foot held in corrected position, mid tarsal joint locked, first ray plantarflexed, etc. Check with each insurance carrier to determine their policy on foot scanning machines.

Biomechanical Examination

Commonly performed tests as part of an orthosis workup include the manual muscle testing and the range of motion examination. CPT code 95831 is described as muscle, testing manual with report, extremity. Therefore a complete testing of each muscle in that extremity needs to be performed, recorded, and formal interpretation/report must be generated. Simply stating "muscle-testing WNL" is not acceptable. The next component is if such a test is medically necessary and reasonable. Does the patient have a myopathy or muscular dystrophy, which requires a complete extremity examination vs. healthy runner with arch strain? Just performing the test does not mean it should/will be paid.

The next test commonly billed is CPT 95851 range of motion measurements and report each extremity. Again this implies all joints in the extremity are tested, measured, recorded, and an interpretation/report generated. You must also document the medical necessity and reasonableness of doing this examination. Listing WNL is not appropriate. Is checking the hip and knee range of motion medically necessary to create an orthotic for hallux limitus? Document why each test is required.

When medically necessary and reasonable CPT 98531 and 95851 should be billed as 95831-RT and 95831-LT and CPT 98551-RT and 95831-LT

Gait Analysis

Gait analysis should generally be included as part of your E/M workup on the patient. Do not use CPT code ranges 96000–96004. The introduction section of this codes series in the CPT book specifically states that these codes are to be used when the gait analysis is performed in a designated motion analysis laboratory utilizing true 3D analysis, multiple video cameras, etc. Watching the patient walk back and forth in your hallway or videotaping alone does not qualify for this code series. Patients who generally qualify for this type of examination are those with neuromuscular gait abnormalities, muscular dystrophy, etc. When purchasing gait analysis machines make sure that you check with your principle insurance companies to make sure that they will pay on the use of that machine/code or you may spend a lot of money with no revenue source.

Orthoses HCPCS Codes

There are several types of custom orthotic devices.

- Orthosis code L3000s are listed in orthoses and prosthetic manuals as UCBL devices. The description indicates a device molded to a patient model and shows a device with a heel cup and heel support/stabilization with a post. This most closely resembles the classic custom foot orthoses.
- Orthosis code L3020 is also molded to a patient model but does not have a heel cup nor is it posted.
- Orthosis code L3030 is a device molded directly to a patient's foot. Therefore, if a cast is not made of the foot, clearly this is not an appropriate selection.

Orthosis Modifications

There are various HCPCS codes for orthosis repairs in the code range L4205–L4210. Most orthotic companies will offer some type of guarantee for their products for premature breakage or incorrect prescription. As far as repairs, many insurance carriers do not pay for such services. Adjustments to the orthoses such as modifying the post, adding modifying forefoot extensions, and grinding down a rough area may not be payable separately. You could charge the patient directly for these repairs.

Sending orthoses back for minor repairs can be expensive and time consuming, plus the patient does not have the device. As a practice management tool, being able to perform minor repairs may be a great practice builder. Patients like the efficiency of having you repair the device promptly vs. a week or more wait if the orthosis is sent back to the orthotic laboratory. During this time the patient is without the use and benefit of the orthotic device. Plus this allows you an opportunity to review the orthosis and consider additional changes/modifications; see if the patient would benefit from a second pair of orthoses or possibly attempt other non-orthosis-related treatments, i.e., physical therapy for some residual pains.

There are several modifications that can be made to orthoses and shoes listed in HCPCS code range L3300–L3649 and for AFO-type devices HCPS code L1900–L2999. Again, these may or may not be payable. Clearly document why modifications need to be made.

E/M Services with Regard to Orthosis Management

Be clear in your chart note the basis for the office encounter. If the patient came in solely to have the orthosis adjusted because there was a sharp edge or it was a bit too long and irritating the patient, some insurance may not pay for this as it may be deemed included within the orthosis fee allowance. No office visit may be allowed in that regard as there is no E/M service performed. Contrast this with the patient returning for evaluation of their plantar fasciitis, which is improving, but reached a plateau. In the latter case the E/M service would be allowed as you are addressing the plantar fasciitis, possibly changing treatment algorithm and/or adjusted the orthosis or post the device to try to increase the control of the orthosis to make it more effective.

Postoperative/Wooden Shoes/Cast Shoes

Medicare does not cover these under any circumstances. They are therefore billable to the patient directly. An ABN is not required since this item is never covered. There is no limiting charge. The appropriate L-code for this shoe is L3260. The denial will read – not a covered service. This would therefore allow you to bill a secondary carrier. Non-Medicare payers may or may not cover these items as a separate item.

Covered Items

For items/supplies dispensed from the office, some are covered, many are not. Many are included in the surgical fee allowance. The following items are covered:

- Removable ankle brace (stirrup type) – L4350
- "Cam" walkers: non-pneumatic –L4386; pneumatic-type L4360. (Note: for any Cam Walker, they are not payable when used to off-load the foot as part of treating foot ulcers as of 4-1-04. They should be billed with a –GY modifier to designate they are not a covered item.)
- Fixed AFO L1930
- Ritchie Brace L1970
- With drop foot hinge L2210 per hinge
- Arizona (gauntlet) AFO+ L2280
- Take home supplies for wound care such as Duoderm, hydrogels, and Polymem. They are not covered when you use them in the office.
- Night splints: There is no specific code for this item. However for DMERC regions C and D, after June 2, 2004, use L4396 with ICD-9 code 728.71. For other regions and possibly other insurance carriers submit this L-code, a description of the splint, model number, product literature, etc., and medical necessity. Another option is to use HCPCS code L2999 for the night splint. The claims will be manually processed since an unlisted code is used.
- Crutches E0110-E0117
- Walker E0130-E0147
- Canes E0100-E0105

Non-covered Items

- Ace bandage, in-office bandages, gauze, Coban, and roll gauze dispensed to patient not covered above.

- OTC splints, prefabricated insoles, pads, heel cups, tape, and other commercial type products.
- Prescription medicines dispensed in the office such as pain pills, antibiotics, antifungal preparations, and topical steroids.

These are billable to the patient, with no ABN and no limiting charge.

Strapping

This procedure is payable when medically necessary and reasonable. The supplies are included in the allowance for the procedures. For Medicare, strappings are not paid when performed on the same day as an injection.

Casts

Application of a BK or AK casts are payable per medical necessity. The supplies are paid in addition to the cast application CPT code. Bill HCPCS code A4580 for plaster supplies and A4590 for synthetic supplies bill for each roll applied by listing that number of rolls used in box 24 G as units #X.

For Medicare use the appropriate Q code for cast supplies. Bill this as unit 1 not per roll. Other supplies such as stockinet and under padding are not payable separately. Many insurance companies will not pay for cast shoes, so these would be billed as a cash item directly to the patient.

Billing Scenario

Visit 1

A new patient, 25-year-old runner, presents with AM pain in the right heel after increasing his mileage for the past few months. Pain is a 6 on a scale of 1–10. He denies any specific trauma. Pain is described as a dull ache in his heel. It is especially worse in the morning or after he has been off of his foot for >30 minutes. He has tried ice and ibuprofen with out any improvement. He may have had a similar set of symptoms a few years ago but those responded quickly with rest, ibuprofen, and buying better running shoes.

His past medical history is unremarkable. He takes OTC allergy medication PRN seasonal allergies. He denies any drug allergies. There is a history of rheumatoid arthritis in the family.

Vascular: 3+/4 DP and PT pulses B/L. There is no clubbing or cyanosis of the digits. There is no pedal edema.

Neurologic: DTR are 2+/4 B/L; there is no sensory loss noted in the foot, there is no Tinel's sign with percussion of the PT nerve.

Dermatologic: Good skin temperature, texture, and tone. There is mild contusion on the right hallux nail but no infection noted.

Musculoskeletal: Tenderness is along the course of the right plantar fascia. There is no pain on the left side. There is maximum pain at the insertion point of the fascia into the heel. There is no edema, erythema, or ecchymosis. There is no ankle, STJ, or MTJ pain with ROM. There is no crepitus. He has a very flexible mid foot. There is good muscle strength in all four-muscle groups B/L. He has a mild HAV but that is asymptomatic.

The assessment is plantar fasciitis in the right foot.

Reviewed etiology and treatment options for plantar fasciitis. Obtained x-ray (two views), which did not reveal any spur formation. There were no fractures. Bone stock was normal, no degenerative joint disease noted.

Injected plantar fascia at the heel insertion area with 1% xylocaine plain mixed with 0.5% bupivicaine plain and 1 cc triamcinolone acetate 10. Reviewed possible steroid flare. To continue with ice TID for 15 minutes and rest.

Sample Billing

CPT 99203
CPT 73620-RT
CPT 20550

J3301 (steroid only, local anesthetic not payable nor is syringe, needle, etc.).

Notes: 99203 appropriate level of service based upon documentation, no need for contralateral x-rays since symptoms localized to the right heel and evaluation of the left heel would more than likely not affect the treatment plan for the right.

Visit 2

F/U patient doing better. Good initial relief but benefits waned as the week went on. No change in activities. Physical examination unchanged. Pains continue to be at the insertion point of the fascia. Suggest repeat injection with 1% xylocaine plain and 0.5% bupivicaine plain and triamcinolone acetate 10.

Sample Billing

CPT 20550
J3301

No significant or separately identifiable E/M service rendered on this day, as H&P was more of an update with no new findings.

Visit 3

Patient still only 25% better. Pains the same. He mentions that his brother was recently diagnosed with some "different type" of arthritis. He notices that he is limping more on the right. No change in physical examination except he is walking with the right foot held more abducted. Still fascia insertional pain. Some medial foot pain noted as well especially at the navicular bone. Posterior tibial tendon strong and intact. Will apply a strapping to stabilize the arch and order arthritis panel blood tests

Sample Billing

> CPT 99212-25
> CPT 29540

This evaluation required additional workup and change in treatment plan, hence E/M payable in addition to procedure.

Visit 4

Patient still not any better overall and in fact it may be worsening, although the strapping did temporarily seem to make the foot feel more secure. He did spend 3 hours at a local mall last Sunday. Now there is more of a tearing-type sensation in the arch. Blood tests taken at the last visit are normal. Still localized pain at the fascia insertion point into the calcaneus. He is much more sensitive today to direct palpation of the plantar medial tubercle of the calcaneus. There is no sensory loss or Tinel's sign noted. Will order MRI to evaluate fascia for partial tear or even stress fracture in bone. With his flexible mid foot will schedule for bio-evaluation and orthoses fabrication. Orthoses are not covered by his insurance carrier. Patient understands this and wishes to proceed with the orthoses anyway. Orthoses payment form dispensed.

Sample Billing

> CPT 99213

Additional workup required and decision making to alter treatment course, obtain additional testing, etc.

Visit 5

Bio Eval performed including muscle testing, ROM examination. See attached bio-evaluation form. Patient casted for orthoses, plaster molds obtained.

Sample Billing

CASH $400 for orthoses and associated non-covered services [per insurance company guidelines. If this would be covered suggest obtaining prior authorization for orthoses and associated biomechanical testing. Obtain insurance company's preferred CPT code casting for orthoses as there is no specific CPT code for casting. If covered bill L3000-RT and L3000-LT for the orthoses].

Further Follow-Up

Office called patient and informed them that orthoses have arrived, appointment made. Also informed patient that MRI did not indicate any obvious bone pathology and there is only mild thickening of the fascia consistent with plantar fasciitis. Adjacent ankle ligaments and tendons normal.

Document any conversation with patients, not billable to insurance.

Visit 6

Office staff dispensed device and instructed in break in process. No pressure areas noted by patient. They fit well in the shoes.

Sample Billing

Possibly CPT 99211 as there was no encounter with the doctor. Some insurance companies may lump the dispensement and fitting of the orthoses the cost of the device and not payable separately.

Visit 7

Patient came complaining that front edge binds under first met head. There was a ridge in the distal edge of the orthosis and this was reduced. Patient noted good relief.

Sample Billing

Not billable to insurance as no patient evaluation performed per se. Any orthoses-related services may not be reimbursable separately. For those insurance companies that do not cover orthoses, any orthoses-related service would also not be covered. If the carrier covers the device, such minor adjustments would more than likely be considered included in the allowance for the orthoses. Unless otherwise stated in your insurance company contract you could bill the patient directly/cash for the orthosis adjustment.

Visit 8

F/U on plantar heel pain. Patient states he is 40% better. He noticed good initial relief when he started wearing the device but then the improvement has leveled off symptom quality and location unchanged, just decreased pain level. Patient walks with less of a limp. There is less tenderness with palpation of the heel area. Suggest one additional injection of 1% xylocaine plain mixed with 0.5% bupivicaine plain and 1 cc triamcinolone acetate now that he has good biomechanical support. To continue ice, stretching, and 600 mg ibuprofen BID-TID PRN. Will augment his home stretching program with in-office physical therapy. Will perform ultrasound and icing three times per week for 3 weeks.

Sample Billing

> CPT 99212-99225
> CPT 20550
> J3301

E/M payable as there is a more involved evaluation, including additional treatment options.

Visit 9

Patient presents for physical therapy. Ultrasound performed for 10 minutes on the plantar aspect of the right heel and along the entire course of the plantar fascia. Icing applied after ultrasound.

Sample Billing

> CPT 97035

Ultrasound based upon 15 minute increments, ice packs not payable as that is a modality that the patient can do themselves at home. Six total physical therapy visits performed and documented.

Visit 10

At the seventh PT visit patient states he is still at the 40% improvement level, the injection and physical therapy did not offer any additional benefit. He is becoming more frustrated and his boss seems to be getting less sympathetic with him and his lower productivity at work. Physical examination unchanged with continued cal-caneal insertional pain. No neurologic loss. Slight limp still noted in gait. Will stop physical therapy and cast the patient to rest his foot (BK synthetic cast). Even though he has stopped running he still walks and stands at least 5 hours at work.

Sample Billing

> CPT 99212-99225
> CPT 29425
> A4590 X 4 rolls

Visit 11

Three weeks later patient is no better. Reviewed etiology of plantar fasciitis. Reviewed treatment options common for this condition. Reasonable conservative treatment course completed and only remaining option at this point is surgical intervention if symptoms warrant. Reviewed ESWT, EPF, and the open procedure. Reviewed risks, benefits, and complications for each surgical procedure. Reviewed success rates with each option. Reviewed recovery times and anesthetic choices. Total time spent with patients 45 minutes.

Sample Billing

> CPT 99214

This is based upon documented face-to-face time spent with the patient in consultation. At this visit no significant history was obtained and any examination was cursory. The bulk of the encounter was in consultation.

Conclusion

Since DME is a common part of a sports medicine practice, the proper documentation and billing protocols must be followed to insure proper payment. Medicare and other insurance carriers have their own specific policies regarding coverage of DME items. To dispense DME from your office, you are classified as a supplier and not a physician. Insurance company and state and federal rules and regulations must be complied with to be a DME provider, as discussed in this chapter.

Index